PROGRESS IN CLINICAL AND BIOLOGICAL RESEARCH

1983 TITLES

Please see pages following the index for previous titles in this series

13th International Cancer Congress, Part E

CANCER MANAGEMENT

13th International
Cancer Congress, Part E

CANCER MANAGEMENT

**Proceedings of the 13th International Cancer Congress
September 8–15, 1982
Seattle, Washington**

Editors

Edwin A. Mirand
Roswell Park Memorial Institute
Buffalo, New York

William B. Hutchinson
Fred Hutchinson Cancer Research Center
Seattle, Washington

Enrico Mihich
Roswell Park Memorial Institute
Buffalo, New York

ALAN R. LISS, INC. • NEW YORK

Address all Inquiries to the Publisher
Alan R. Liss, Inc., 150 Fifth Avenue, New York, NY 10011

Library of Congress Cataloging in Publication Data

International Cancer Congress (13th : 1982 : Seattle, Wash.)
13th International Cancer Congress.

(Progress in clinical and biological research ; 132)
Includes bibliographies and indexes.
Contents: pt. A. Current perspectives in cancer -- pt. B. Biology of cancer (1) -- pt. C. Biology of cancer (2) -- pt. D. Research and treatment -- pt. E. Cancer management.
1. Cancer--Congresses. I. Mirand, Edwin A., 1926–   . II. Hutchinson, William B. III. Mihich, Enrico. IV. Title. V. Title: Thirteenth International Cancer Congress. VI. Series. [DNLM: 1. Medical oncology--Congresses. W1 PR668E v.132 / QZ 200 I604 1982z]
RC261.A2I56 1982a   616.99'4   83-48399
ISBN 0-8451-0132-3 (set)
ISBN 0-8451-0178-1 (pt. E)

Contents

IX. BIOLOGICAL RESPONSE MODIFIERS

X. THE ENVIRONMENT AND CANCER: RECENT EPIDEMILOGIC DEVELOPMENTS

XI. ECONOMICS OF CANCER CARE

XII. CANCER NURSING: AN INTERNATIONAL PERSPECTIVE

XIII. HOSPICE: CONCEPT AND ROLE

XIV. SCREENING FOR CANCER

Contributors

Catherine Adonis, Oncology Division, University of Paris, Bobigny, France **[423]**

Etienne-Emile Baulieu, INSERM U 33, Lab Hormones, Bicêtre, France **[167]**

J. Bruce Beckwith, Children's Orthopedic Hospital and Medical Center, Seattle, WA **[159]**

Ernest C. Borden, Departments of Human Oncology and Medicine, Wisconsin Clinical Cancer Center, University of Wisconsin, Madison, WI **[287]**

David A. Boyes, Cancer Control Agency of British Columbia; and Department of Obstetrics and Gynecology, University of British Columbia, Vancouver, British Columbia, Canada **[483]**

H. Busch, Department of Pharmacology, Baylor College of Medicine, Houston, TX **[229]**

R.K. Busch, Department of Pharmacology, Baylor College of Medicine, Houston, TX **[229]**

Kenneth C. Calman, Department of Oncology, University of Glasgow, Glasgow, Scotland, **[13]**

A.C. Carter, Department of Medicine, Downstate Medical Center, Brooklyn, NY **[183]**

P.K. Chan, Department of Pharmacology, Baylor College of Medicine, Houston, TX **[229]**

Louis A. Chedid, Department of Experimental Immunotherapy, Institut Pasteur, Paris, France **[261]**

G.M. Clark, Department of Medicine/ Oncology, University of Texas Health Science Center, San Antonio, TX **[183]**

D.C. Dumonde, Department of Immunology, St. Thomas' Hospital, London, United Kingdom **[83]**

Sándor Eckhardt, Department of Chemotherapy, National Institute of Oncology, Budapest, Hungary **[145]**

Richard Edelstein, Department of Medical Oncology, CHU Avicenne, Bobigny, France **[35]**

Abdelmoumen Grefft-Alami, Department of Medical Oncology, CHU Avicenne, Bobigny, France **[35]**

John W. Hadden, Immunopharmacology Program, University of South Florida Medical College, Tampa, FL **[273]**

Zeev T. Handzel, Clinical Immunology Unit, Kaplan Hospital, Rehovot, Israel **[297]**

Lennart Hardell, Department of Oncology, University Hospital, Umeå, Sweden **[357]**

Oscar Hechter, Northwestern Medical School, Chicago, IL **[175]**

Renilda Hilkemeyer, Staff Asst. to President, Prof. Oncology (Nursing), The University of Texas System Cancer Center, Houston, TX **[413]**

The number in brackets is the opening page number of the contributor's article.

Thomas A. Hodgson, National Center for Health Statistics, Department of Health and Human Services, Hyattsville, MD **[373]**

Robert W. Hoffman, Kings County Medical Blue Shield, Seattle, WA **[383]**

Jimmie C. Holland, Psychiatry Service, Memorial Sloan-Kettering Cancer Center, New York, NY **[21]**

F.C. den Hollander, Organon Scientific Development Group, Organon International BV, Oss, The Netherlands **[83]**

Julius S. Horoszewicz, Department of Biological Resources, Roswell Park Memorial Institute, Buffalo, NY **[315, 327]**

C.A. Hubay, Department of Surgery, Case Western Reserve University, School of Medicine and University Hospitals, Cleveland, OH **[183]**

Heizaburo Ichikawa, National Cancer Center Hospital, Tokyo, Japan **[495]**

Toshifumi Iizuka, Department of Surgery, National Cancer Center Hospital, Tokyo, Japan **[495]**

Lucien Israel, Medical Oncology Service, CHU Avicenne, Bobigny, France **[35]**

H. Jan Keizer, Department of Oncology, Free University Hospital, Amsterdam, The Netherlands **[121]**

D. Kelsey, Department of Pharmacology, Baylor College of Medicine, Houston, TX **[229]**

Hiroshi Kobayashi, Laboratory of Pathology, Cancer Institute, Hokkaido University School of Medicine, Sapporo, Japan **[305]**

Robert A. Kyle, Division of Hematology and Internal Medicine, Mayo Clinic and Mayo Foundation, Rochester, MN **[45]**

Brian C. Lentle, Alberta Cancer Board, Edmonton, Alberta, Canada **[395]**

Susan S. Leong, Department of Biological Resources, Roswell Park Memorial Institute, Buffalo, NY **[327]**

Z.R. Li, Institute of Material Medica, Chinese Academy of Medical Science, Peking, China **[107]**

R.J. Lukes, Department of Pathology, University of Southern California School of Medicine, Los Angeles, CA **[203]**

Robert MacLennan, Queensland Institute of Medical Research, Brisbane, Australia **[347]**

Nobuo Maeda, Section of Social Security, The Institute of Public Health, Tokyo, Japan **[403]**

W.L. McGuire, Department of Medicine/Oncology, University of Texas Health Science Center, San Antonio, TX **[183]**

Jun Minowada, Department of Molecular Immunology, Roswell Park Memorial Institute, Buffalo, NY **[215]**

Edwin A. Mirand, Roswell Park Memorial Institute, Buffalo, NY **[315, 327]**

Grace Powers Monaco, Law Firm of White, Fine, and Verville, Washington, D.C. **[387]**

National Wilms' Tumor Study Group, Philadelphia, PA **[153]**

Eberhard Nissen, Central Institute of Cancer Research, Academy of Sciences, Berlin, German Democratic Republic **[129]**

William D. Odell, Department of Medicine, University of Utah School of Medicine, Salt Lake City, Utah **[247]**

Donna Park, Memorial Sloan-Kettering Cancer Center, New York, NY **[441]**

J.W. Parker, Department of Pathology, University of Southern California School of Medicine, Los Angeles, CA **[203]**

O.H. Pearson, Department of Surgery, Case Western Reserve University, School of Medicine and University Hospitals, Cleveland, OH [183]

Herbert M. Pinedo, Division of Biochemical Pharmacology, Netherlands Cancer Institute; and Department of Oncology, Free University Hospital, Amsterdam, The Netherlands [121]

R.L. Prentice, Fred Hutchinson Cancer Research Center; and Department of Biostatistics, University of Washington, Seattle, WA [69]

Melanie S. Pulley, Department of Immunology, St. Thomas' Hospital, London, United Kingdom [83]

Paul Robel, Lab Hormones, Bicêtre, France [175]

Julia Rowland, Psychiatry Service, Memorial Sloan-Kettering Cancer Center, New York, NY [21]

Y.M. Rustum, Department of Experimental Therapeutics, Roswell Park Memorial Institute, Buffalo, NY [107]

Eizo Saito, Department of Medicine, Toho Medical University, Tokyo, Japan [247]

Yoshio Sakurai, Cancer Chemotherapy Center, Japanese Foundation for Cancer Research, Tokyo, Japan [3]

Raymond Samak, Laboratory of Human Tumors Immuno-Biology, UER de Médecine, Bobigny, France [35]

H.K. Slocum, Department of Experimental Therapeutics, Roswell Park Memorial Institute, Buffalo, NY [107]

Barbara M. Southcott, Department of Radiotherapy, Charing Cross Hospital, London, United Kingdom [83]

W.H. Spohn, Department of Pharmacology, Baylor College of Medicine, Houston, TX [229]

Ellen M.K. Strak, Dr. Daniël den Hoed Kliniek, Rotterdamsch Radio-Therapeutisch Institut, Rotterdam, The Netherlands [427]

Philip Strax, Guttman Institute, New York, NY [465]

Stephan Tanneberger, Central Institute of Cancer Research, Academy of Sciences, Berlin, German Democratic Republic [129]

C.R. Taylor, Department of Pathology, University of Southern California School of Medicine, Los Angeles, CA [203]

D.M.P. Thomson, Department of Immunology, Montreal General Hospital Research Institute, Montreal, Quebec, Canada [193]

Robert Tiffany, The Royal Marsden Hospital, London, United Kingdom [435]

Nathan Trainin, Department of Cell Biology, The Weizmann Institute of Science, Rehovot, Israel [297]

Mary L.S. Vachon, Clarke Institute of Psychiatry, Toronto, Ontario, Canada [451]

Joseph Wybran, Department of Immunology and Hematology, Erasme Hospital, Université Libre de Bruxelles, Brussels, Belgium [95]

Ernst L. Wynder, American Health Foundation, New York, NY [339]

Lu-yi Yu, Cancer Hospital, Shanghai First Medical College, Shanghai, China [475]

Rina Zaizov, Department of Pediatric Hematology and Oncology, Beilinson Medical Center, Petah-Tikva, Israel [297]

Marvin Zelen, Harvard School of Public Health and the Dana-Farber Cancer Institute, Boston, MA [57]

Foreword

The papers presented in the Plenary Lectures and the Congress Symposia at the 13th International Cancer Congress, September 8–15, 1982, Seattle, Washington, are included in these volumes. The United States was the official host of the Congress, which was held under the auspices of the International Union Against Cancer (UICC), and the Fred Hutchinson Cancer Research Center, Seattle, Washington was the host institution.

Dr. William B. Hutchinson of the Fred Hutchinson Cancer Research Center was the Congress President and Dr. Edwin A. Mirand of Roswell Park Memorial Institute, Buffalo, New York, was the Secretary-General.

The scientific program of the Congress contained over 4,000 presentations. The National Program Committee, chaired by Dr. Enrico Mihich of Roswell Park Memorial Institute, felt that it would be appropriate to include only the papers from the Plenary Lectures and the Congress Symposia to keep the number of volumes at a reasonable level. These papers are presented in five volumes.

Volume A — Final Report of the Secretary-General that includes the organizational details of the scientific program
         — Plenary Lectures

Volumes B & C — Basic science topics in oncology

Volumes D & E — Clinical oncology topics

Since it would be impossible to cover all the areas of oncology presented at the Congress, by presenting the plenary and symposia sessions, we attempted to select the most rapidly advancing and promising areas of clinical and basic research. A good index of the growth in the field of oncology can be obtained by comparing the publications of this meeting with the last cancer congress publications (12th International Cancer Congress) held in Buenos Aires from October 5–10, 1978.

Looking over the topics covered herein, one can only marvel at the tremendous rate of progress and the increase in interest in oncology in the past four years. This reflects the developments in molecular biology as it relates to cancer viral and chemical carcinogenesis, in the design and evaluation of clinical trials, biological response modifiers, cancer nursing, psychosocial aspects of cancer, etc.

On behalf of the Congress officers, we wish to express our gratitude to the National Program Committee and to all the scientists, physicians, dentists, nurses, and other participants engaged in oncology who attended this Congress and who made it a success. I am sure that both the scientific and social interchange which was experienced at the Seattle meeting will have a positive, lasting effect on our lives. We hope to see you at the 14th International Cancer Congress to be held in Budapest, Hungary in 1986 to further the scientific and social interaction.

The editors are deeply indebted to all the authors for their outstanding contributions to these volumes.

We wish to express thanks and appreciation to Catherine O'Leary, Lisa Barone, Linda Beverage, Kevin Craig, Ann M. Gannon, Ramon Melendez, Amy Mirand and Lucy Mirand, all of whom aided in various ways in the preparation of these volumes.

Finally, we wish to acknowledge the support of the National Cancer Institute, American Cancer Society, Pacific Northwest Regional Commission for their generous support of the 13th International Cancer Congress.

Edwin A. Mirand

Preface to Part E

Surgery, radiation therapy, and chemotherapy are viewed as the major treatment modalities for cancer. Each treatment has spawned the other when the first has reached its limit. However, today the combination of these three treatments has improved cancer patient survival to approximately 50%.

As researchers work to improve the "standard" treatments, other scientific horizons have begun to show promise. Studies on immunopharmacology, hormone receptors, cellular and hormonal markers of cancer cell activity, and biological response modifiers have all given evidence of potential in treating cancer.

In this volume, authors present the status in certain cancers as well as an update on these newer research endeavors.

The volume also deals with cancer screening, cancer economics, hospice care and the environment, all of which have become important issues as cancer detection and treatment methods have improved.

Edwin A. Mirand

CONGRESS SYMPOSIA

ADJUVANT CHEMOTHERAPY Perevodchikova, N., USSR,
Chairman; Hoogstraten, B., USA, Co-Chairman;
Playhouse

Experimental Basis of Adjuvant Chemotherapy.
*Sakurai, Y., Tokyo, Japan.

Adjuvant Chemotherapy of Breast Cancer.
*Senn, H-J., Jungi, W-F. and Holdener, E. E.,
St. Gallen, Switzerland. (By Title Only)

Adjuvant Treatment of Colo-Rectal Cancer.
*Holyoke, E.D., Buffalo, NY USA (By Title Only)

Chemotherapy of Osteosarcoma. *Holland, J. F.,
New York, NY USA. (By Title Only)

The Use of Adjuvant Chemotherapy in Gynecologic
Cancers. *Young, R. C., Bethesda, MD USA.
(By Title Only)

Please note: Papers that are listed as "By Title
Only" were presented at the 13th International
Cancer Congress, but are not included in these
volumes.

1

13th International Cancer Congress, Part E
Cancer Management, pages 3–10
© **1983 Alan R. Liss, Inc., 150 Fifth Avenue, New York, NY 10011**

EXPERIMENTAL BASIS OF ADJUVANT CHEMOTHERAPY

Yoshio Sakurai, Ph.D.

Director, Cancer Chemotherapy Center,
Japanese Foundation for Cancer Research
Toshima-ku, Tokyo 170   JAPAN

A promising aspect of adjuvant chemotherapy has been demonstrated recently both in experimental studies with various model tumors and in clinical trials. It was proved that the mammary tumor in C3H mouse could be cured neither by resection nor by chemotherapy alone, but if these two modalities were combined with an adequate time sequence, cure rates of more than 50% were obtained (Schabel 1977). Recently, a review was published on the results of clinical trials of adjuvant chemotherapy of breast cancer using combination protocol of cyclophosphamide, methotrexate, and 5-fluorouracil, in which it was emphasized that an intensity of chemotherapy seemed to be more critical than treatment duration (Senn 1982).

The aim of adjuvant chemotherapy to surgery is to obliterate invisible, microscopic cancer cells which are left or disseminated in the body after surgial resection of the main tumor. From an experimental point of view, success of adjuvant chemotherapy depends on effective prevention of metastatic formation or metastatic tumor growth after removal of the local tumor mass. The regimen of chemotherapy should be selected so as to be certainly effective to the tumor but not so toxic to the host. It is thought that medication for a too long period is uncecessary to eradicate the minute tumor burden left after surgical resection, and we must avoid side effects of drugs which might run counter to the effects desired. Needless to say, we have to look for more reliable animal models which can suggest the proper protocol of adjuvant chemotherapy to clinical trials. To prevent metastatic recurrence of tumor after so-called curable surgical operation, the following process should be noticed. The one is to hamper the tumor cells, remaining in the blood stream, to form an extravascular tumor. The other is to prevent the growth of this tumor. Inhibition of tumor growth might be attained by chemotherapy, but it might also be possible to suppress the growth by any mechanisms mediated by some host responses.

As for the formation of metastasis, we must recognize that the pattern of metastasis is influenced by certain rules based on properties of individual tumor and inherent host factors, which have not yet been well elucidated. However, implantation and eventual growth in capillary beds seems to be the most influential factors in metastatic formation. By cinemicroscopical technique, it was clarified that the tumor cells implanted in the carotid artery reached the mesenterium within a few seconds and embolized at the entrance of meta-arterioles. The embolized cells passed through the capillary in due time which became attached to the endothelium of venules and then form extravascular tumor. (Sato 1967) In these processes, there have been many findings concerning the role of thrombocytes or thromboplastic activity of the tissues. Thromboplastin-active substances released from the embolized tumor cells help the lodgement of the tumor cells, by initiating the clotting sequence that leads to entrapping of cells in the capillary bed. It is said that a postulated cancer coagulative factor (CCF) plays an important part in the entrapping process, but the substance which provides a fibrin stroma over which tumor cells can migrate, can be released not only from the tumor cells but also the normal tissues at the site of metastasis (Holyoke 1972). A series of findings have been reported that the high thromboplastin activity and formation of fibrin at the site of metastatic formation favored metastatic formation, while thrombocyto-penia or altered platelet function or administration of anti-coagulant like heparin decreased metastasis. A metastasis hampering effect of a series of xylan sulfate was also found, and a good correlation between activities of anticoagulation and suppression of metastasis formation was pointed out (Tsubura 1977). Experimental evidences were also presented with animal models that plasmin inhibitors like tranexamic acid enhanced blood-borne metastasis. A simple adhesiveness of tumor cells to glass or some other material surfaces indi-cates a tendency of frequent lung metastasis. However, it was also stated that the factors favoring the lodgement of tumor cells involve more complicated biological responses. (Nicolson 1975)

It seems an ordinary behavior of each tumor to metasta-
size preferentially to a certain organ, for example, a transplantable reticulum-cell sarcoma of C3H/Pi mouse metastasized
selectively to the spleen, even when it was inoculated in the
kidney (Pilgrim 1969). However, the lung is a very suitable
soil to disseminated cancer cells. The pieces of lung,
kidney, heart, skin, and thyroid tissues were implanted subcutaneously in mice and Cloudman melanoma cells were inoculated
intravenously , which metastasized only in the transplanted
lung tissue (Kinsey 1960). Therefore, hardness or easiness
of metastatic formation depends on each mutually related properties of the tumor and the tissue, to which the tumor metastasizes. Elucidation in the future of these complicated but
very important mechanism of establishment of metastatic tumor
will afford a great profit in progress of adjuvant chemotherapy.

However, thinking of efficacy of adjuvant chemotherapy,
the most essential problem is suppression of growth of metastatic tumor. The characteristic properties of metastatic
tumors are minute but sites of tumor might be plural in some
cases. A careful consideration is therefore necessary to
distribution or route of administration of drugs. The second
point is that the tumor cells in metastatic sites are the
selected cell population through the process of metastasis.
The difference in drug sensitivity among the cell lines of
spontaneous metastases derived from the same parental tumors
were frequently observed (Tsuruo, Fidler 1981). K-1735 melanoma of mice was inoculated into the footpad of C3H/HeN mice
and the cells were isolated from 2 lung metastases, 1 lymph
node metastasis, and 1 brain metastasis. Sensitivity of these
4 cell lines were compared in vitro to adriamycin, AMSA, bleomycin, vincristine, vindesine, and DIC. Most of the cell
lines from the metastatic sites appeared less sensitive to
all drugs tested than the parental line with a few exceptions.
The significant difference in sensitivity suggests a difficulty to choose a proper drug to treat metastasis effectively.
If plural metastatic sites exist in the different tissues, a
rationally prepared regimen of combination chemotherapy will
only proffer a good result. An experimental results showed
the mouse colon tumor C26 increased frequency of lung metastasis by the following procedure. (Tsuruo 1982) The tumor was
inoculated subcutaneously into BALB/c mice and a fragment of
the lung was retransplanted subcutaneously into the normal
BALB/c mice immediately before death of tumor-bearing mice.
No tumor nodule was visible in the lung tissue at this stage,

but after 26 times repetition of this procedure, the transplanted mice became to yield a great number of visible metastatic foci in the lung. Tsuruo then made 50 clones from
this highly metastatic line of C26, each of which were transplanted to mice and frequency of lung metastasis was compared.
The most interesting point was that, among the 50 clones, a
few clones exhibited a very high frequency of metastasis (NL-
17, NL-22, NL-33) but most of them were less metastatic than
the parent population, from which the clones were derived.
A few clones like NL-14 or NL-26 showed no visible metastasis
at the time of tumor death of mice. A clone, NL-17, was a
very high metastatic population when it was inoculated into
the vein, but yielded very small number of metastatic foci in
the lung tissue if it was inoculated subcutaneously. On the
contrary, NL-22 yielded a large number of metastatic foci even
when it was transplanted subcutaneously. These results suggest an extremely complicated mechanism of metastatic formation. Further fundamental research on metastasis will be
necessary to elucidate the problems in clinical metastasis.

The drug sensitivity of tumor at the site of metastasis
mainly depends on property of cells themselves, but it should
be influenced in part either by immunological response of the
host or by the pattern of drug distribution to the tissues.
A very slight difference of histocompatibility antigen between
the hosts could give an influence on metastatic formation of
syngeneic tumor. (Yokoro 1981) A reticulum cell sarcoma,
spontaneously produced in BCF_1 mouse (C57BL/Ka x C3H/He),
metastasized vigorously to the brain, lung, liver, spleen,
kidney, ovary, and lymph nodes when transplanted to the same
host, while, if this tumor was transplanted to $6HF_1$ (C57BL/6 x
C3H/He), the tumor grew well only at the site of transplantation with no metastasis, unless the mouse was given total body
irradiation to suppress immunological reaction.
The pulmonary metastasis of a transplantable fibrosarcoma in
C3Hf/Bu mice could be reduced by inducing adoptive immunity by
trnasfer of spleen or lymph node cells from the mice bearing
this tumor (Milas 1974). Recently, the role of NK cells in
metastasis has attracted a great interest. It is thought that
NK cells provide cytocidal response long before the T cell
immunity is generated and it should be one of the important
host defence mechanism in the course of metastatic formation.
However, there is also evidences that immune responses of the
host sometimes induce progression of tumor or increase of metastatic potency of tumors. For example, inoculation of B16
melanoma cells together with syngeneic lymphocytes in high

ratio into C57BL/6 mice significantly decreased lung metastasis formation, while with lymphocytes at low ratio, metastatic
foci in the lung seemed to be increased more than the case of
inoculation with the tumor cells alone (Fidler 1974). Phenom-
ena of immunological enhancement of tumor are not the rare
findings in the studies with experimental models, and the
conditions favoring suppression of formation and inhibition
of growth of metastasis should be extensively studied in the
future. Growth of metastatic tumor might be controlled by
immunological conditioning. In addition, another approach
based on a host response was suggested that any agents which
inhibit the activity of tumor angiogenesis factor (TAF) might
retard the growth of a minute metastatic tumor (Folkman 1974,
1982).

Drug sensitivity of tumor cells at metastatic site is
above all a very practical problem in adjuvant chemotherapy.
Advantageous points of chemotherapy of micro-metastasis might
be that the number of tumor cells is limited and the growth
fraction of the cell population might not be samll. On the
contrary, the property of tumor cells in metastatic foci might
be different from the parent tumor owing to selection during
the process of metastasis, or by acquisition of drug resistance by the prior chemotherapy. If the data of the human
tumor stem cell assay is predictable, we can learn the sensitivity of the extirpated parent tumor to drugs, which will
probably be a helpful suggestion in choosing the drug for
treatment of the present metastasis. However, as mentioned
before, there is a possibility that the tumor cells in each
metastatic nodule might exhibit a modified or different sensitivity to drugs from the parent tumor by selection through
the process of metastatic formation. In addition, if the
parent tumor had been treated by some regimens of chemotherapy before resection, the metastatic tumor cells may acquire
drug resistance to the treated drugs. From the experiences
of chemotherapeutic treatment of the human xenografts implanted in nude mice, it is clear that the prior chemotherapy before
removal of the tumor gives a distinct minus effect on the
result of treatment of xenograft with the same drug. Overcoming of drug resistance is of course one of the most important problems in chemotherapy in general, but especially in
adjuvant chemotherapy, we should avoid to use the drugs to
which the tumor cells are resistant, because the patients,
most of whom have received successful surgery, might happen
to suffer only from the side effects of drugs without any
profit.

It has been clarified with Ehrlich carcinoma and P388 leukemia that resistance to some anticancer drugs like anthracyclines, vincristine, and some other intercalators occurs by activation of efflux mechanism of the drugs, resulting in decreased concentration of the drugs inside the cells (Danø 1973; Inaba 1979). Recently, it was found that a resistant line of P388 against vincristine or adriamycin restores its sensitivity to those drugs either in vitro or in vivo in the coexistence of some agents, which have activity of calcium antagonist or calmodulin inhibitor. (Tsuruo 1981) In in vitro study, series of human tumor cells, K562, K562/VCR, Pl2/Ichikawa, CCRF/CEM, Molt-3, RPMI-8402, BALL, and Daudi cells, all increase their sensitivity to vincristine in addition to verapamil in the medium, a calcium antagonist used clinically as a coronal dilator. Without verapamil, sensitivity of these tumor cells to vincristine markedly differs each other, but in addition to 10 to 20 μM of verapamil, all kinds of tumor cells converge to the same sensitivity to vincristine, showing a very small 50% inhibition concentration (IC_{50}) such as a few μM of vincristine. For example, IC_{50} of resistant line, K562/VCR, was 50 nM, while it diminished to 2.5 nM of vincristine in existence of 20 μM of verapamil. Calcium antagonists other than verapamil showed the similar effect and clomipramine, calmodulin inhibitor, also exhibited enhancing activity of cytotoxic action of vincristine. The trials of enhancing sensitivity of tumor cells to drugs or overcoming the resistance will bring an impact in the study of this field.

In purpose of retarding recurrence of tumor after surgery, an intensive but short-term chemotherapy seems to be recommendable, because we want to avoid rewardless side-effects, especially a risk of iatrogenic tumors. Since adjuvant chemotherapy is complicated clinical trials which requires a large number of patients and participation of many doctors and their associate personnels. A long period and a great expenses will be also needed for the practice of treatment or analysis of the results. We hope therefore to have any rational clinical models for confirming the basic hypothesis of adjuvant chemotherapy derived from experimental results with rodent tumors. Desired is a very close cooperation and exchange of information between the clinical and experimental studies to make a rapid progress in adjuvant chemotherapy in the future.

REFERENCES

Danø K (1973): Active outward transport of daunomycin in resistant Ehrlich ascites tumor cells. Biochim Biophys Acta 323:466-483.

Fidler IJ (1974): Immune stimulation-inhibition of experimental cancer metastasis. Cancer Res 34:491-498.

Folkman J (1974): Tumor angiogenesis factor. Cancer Res 34:2109-2113.

Folkman J (1982): Tumor invasion and metastasis. In Cancer Medicine, ed. by Holland JF, Frei E III, Lea & Febiger, pp. 167-177.

Holyoke ED, Frank AL, Weiss L (1972): Tumor thromboplastin activity in vitro. Int J Cancer 9:258-263.

Inaba M, Sakurai Y (1979): Enhanced efflux of actinomycin D, vincristine, and vinblastin in adriamycin-resistant subline of P388 leukemia. Cancer Letters 8:111-115.

Kinsey, DL (1960): An experimental study of preferential metastasis. Cancer 13:674-676.

Milas L, Hunter N, Mason K, Withers HR (1974): Immunological resistance to pulmonary metastasis in C3Hf/Bu mice bearing syngeneic fibrosarcoma of different sizes. Cancer Res 34: 61-71.

Nicolson GL, Winkelhake JL (1975): Organ specificity of blood-borne tumor metastasis determined by cell adhesion. Nature 255:230-232.

Pilgrim HI (1969): The kinetics of the organ-specific metastasis of a transplantable reticuloendothelial tumor. Cancer Res 29:1200-1205.

Sato H (1967): Experimental study on metastasis formation of ascites tumors. Transactions of the Society of Pathologists of Japan 56:9-36 (in Japanese).

Schabel FM (1977): Surgical adjuvant chemotherapy of metastatic murine tumors. Cancer 40:558-568.

Senn HJ (1982): Current status and indications for adjuvant therapy in breast cancer. Cancer Chemother Pharmacol 8: 139-150.

Tsubura E, Yamashita T, Kobayashi M (1977): Inhibitory mechanism of blood-borne pulmonary metastasis by sulfated polysaccharides. Gann Monograph on Cancer Research 20:147-161.

Tsuruo T (1982): Highly metastatic clones of experimental tumor and their organ preference. Oncologia 1:1-11 (in Japanese).

Tsuruo T, Fidler IJ (1981): Differences in drug sensitivity among tumor cells from parental tumors, selected variants, and spontaneous metastasis. Cancer Res 41:3058-3064.

Tsuruo T, Ida H, Tsukagoshi S, Sakurai Y (1981): Overcoming of vincristine resistance in P388 leukemia in vivo and in vitro through enhanced cytotoxicity of vincristine and vinblastine by verapamil. Cancer Res 41:1967-1972.

Yokoro K (1981): Experimental studies on the mechanism of carcinogenesis; factors involved in the development and progression of neoplasia. Annual Report of Research Institute for Nuclear Medicine and Biology, Hiroshima Univ., pp. 107-146 (in Japanese with English abstract).

CONGRESS SYMPOSIA

LATE CONSEQUENCES OF CANCER THERAPY Pihl, A.,
Norway, Chairman; D'Angio, G., USA, Co-Chairman;
Opera House

Late Consequences of Cancer Therapy on the
Endocrine System. *Calman, K. C., Glasgow,
Scotland.

Emotional Effects of Cancer and Cancer Therapy.
*Holland, J. and Rowland, J., New York, NY USA.

Long-Term Effects of Postoperative Adjuvant
Chemotherapy on the Immune System in 100 Cancer
Patients. *Israel, L., Samak, R., Grefft-Alami, A.,
and Edelstein, R., Bobigny, France.

Long-Term Effects of Radiotherapy. *Peckham, M.J.,
London, England. (By Title Only)

Second Malignancies and Chemotherapeutic Agents.
*Kyle, R. A., Rochester, MN USA.

Please note: Papers that are listed as "By Title
Only" were presented at the 13th International
Cancer Congress, but are not included in these
volumes.

13th International Cancer Congress, Part E
Cancer Management, pages 13–20
© 1983 Alan R. Liss, Inc., 150 Fifth Avenue, New York, NY 10011

LATE CONSEQUENCES OF CANCER THERAPY ON THE ENDOCRINE
SYSTEM

KENNETH C. CALMAN

PROFESSOR OF ONCOLOGY
UNIVERSITY OF GLASGOW
GLASGOW, SCOTLAND, UNITED KINGDOM

The increasing use of combined modality therapy in the
management of the cancer patient, together with improved
results of treatment and increased survival rates has highlighted the importance of recognising late effects of cancer
treatment. This recognition has focussed not only on the
physical consequences, but on the psychological and
emotional problems occurring after treatment. From the
point of view of the endocrine system, all forms of cancer
treatment may have an effect, and that these effects themselves may be related to changes in the immune response and
the psychological state, two subjects to be discussed elsewhere in this meeting.

The effects may be early or late, and though this
report will deal with the long term consequences the acute
endocrine problems related to cancer treatment deserve brief
mention. Cancer treatment may effect all endocrine organs
in one way or another and, as the endocrine system as a
whole is interrelated the consequences to one organ may
affect others.

Both adults and children may be affected. In adults
the major consequences are in relation to the reproductive
system, and in children in relation to growth, development
and reproduction. There is also a particularly important
problem in relation to fertility of patients who are in the
child bearing age group. Several recent reviews have
covered these topics (Shalet & Beardwell, 1979/Shalet,1980,
Chapman, 1982).

Surgical Ablative Therapy. Since Beatson removed the ovaries in a series of patients with breast cancer (Beatson, 1896) removal of endocrine organs for the treatment of cancer has been carried out. This has included removal of the ovaries, testes, adrenal,pituitary, thyroid and parathyroid glands. In most instances the acute effects of these procedures are well documented, as are the late consequences (Bajorunas, 1980). Where appropriate hormone replacement therapy is introduced.

Radiotherapeutic Ablation Therapy. Radiotherapy may also affect endocrine organs directly if it is used to decrease hormone synthesis as in ovarian radiation in the management of breast cancer. It may also affect endocrine function if the radiation field takes in a particular organ such as the thyroid in neck irradiation or the ovaries in pelvic irradiation. Recovery of endocrine function depends on the doseage of radio-therapy and the age of the patient, and shielding of the ovaries, for example, reduces the incidence of amenorrhoea (Baker, Morgan, Peckham & Smithers, 1972). Radiation of the head and neck region for non thyroid malignancy does result in thyroid dysfunction(e.g. Fuks, et al, 1976) once again hormone re-placement therapy may be required.

In relation to children, the effects of radiation therapy may be on growth or reproduction and these will be discussed later.

Hormone Therapy. Long term therapy is now used in the treatment of a variety of tumours. This includes the use of thyroid hormone, corticosteroids, progestational agents, oestrogens, androgens and inhibitors of adrenal function, such as aminoglutethimide. The long term effects of these drugs are well recognised, some of which may be related to changes in endogenous hormone synthesis. It is possible that these alterations in hormone balance induced by long term endocrine treatment may have serious consequences such as the cardiovascular effects associated with stilboestrol therapy in prostatic cancer (Blackard, 1975).

Chemotherapy. The increasing use of chemotherapy in cancer management has increased the range and complexity of endocrine effects associated with cancer treatment. The mechanism of action of cytotoxic drugs in DNA synthesis, protein synthesis and steroid biosynthesis inevitably means that these drugs affect endocrine function. In general how-ever the effects are short term and may be reversible.

This will be discussed in more detail later.

Effects on Thyroid Function.   The general effects of
surgery and radiation on thyroid function have been mentioned.
It is interesting to note that this has recently been studied
in patients receiving bone marrow transplantation for acute
leukaemia (Sklar, et al, 1982).   In those receiving chemotherapy alone there was little alteration in function compared to those receiving whole body radiation.   Two reports
have recently appeared indicating that treatment with 5-Fluoro-
uracil may increase serum T_4 levels and that this might be
associated with clinical symptoms (Beex et al, 1977, Breier,
et al, 1982).

Adrenal.   The function of the adrenal gland can be
suppressed by corticosteroid therapy or by the use of aminoglutethimide (Smith et al, 1978).   During treatment with aminoglutethimide, hormone replacement therapy is required.   It
has also been noted (Morgan & O'Hare, 1979) that 5-Fluoro-
uracil, but not other drugs inhibit steroid biosynthesis in
tissue culture.   This may be relevant if long term high dose
5-FU therapy is employed.

Effects on Pituitary Function.   The pituitary gland is
involved in the control of other endocrine organs.   Consequently it is difficult to separate its function from that of
the ovary, testis, adrenal and thyroid.   Several publications
however reported on the effects of chemotherapy on pituitary
function (McFadyen et al, 1979, Wang et al, 1980, Naysmith
et al, 1976, Wilson et al, 1976).   In general these studies
have shown evidence of some effect with chemotherapy though
this was usually associated with effects on other endocrine
organs.

From the point of view of children a major consequence
of interfering with pituitary function relates to growth.
The evidence relates mainly to the effects of radiation in
the treatment of intracranial tumours or in its use in prophylactic treatment of the brain and spinal cord (Shalet &
Beardwell, 1979, Rogers et al, 1982, Serota et al, 1982)
In general the effect of radiation reduces the growth rate
by a small amount but this would appear to be of little
clinical significance.   Long term follow up is required.

A further effect on the pituitary relates to the development of inappropriate ADH secretion after chemotherapy

with the vinca alkaloids, or cyclophosphamide (Ginsberg, Comis, & Fitzpatrick, 1977, Stuart et al, 1975, Harlow et al, 1979). This may be an acute problem or be a longer term recurrent effect. It has been fatal in some instances.

Effect on Gonadal Function. Both the testes and the ovary are affected by chemotherapy and radiotherapy. This affects not only hormone function, but fertility, the development of secondary sexual characteristics, the onset of puberty and timing of the menopause. Treatment also has major effects on the libido and on the psychological response of the patient and relatives. There has been increasing recognition of these effects as the cancer care team strives to improve the quality as well as the quantity of life (Chapman, 1982, Shalet, 1980).

Chemotherapy is well known to cause effects on ovarian and testicular function (Rose & Davis, 1980, Blatt, Poplak & Sherins, 1981, Shamberger, Sherins, Ziegler, Glatstein, Rosenberg, 1981). Hormone synthesis rates are altered and blood levels of trophic hormones modified. Clinically, amenorrhoea is common finding and gynaecomastia may develop (Forbes, 1978, Sherins et al, 1978). In general such effects are reversible. In children given treatment prior to puberty, the evidence seems to point to normal, but delayed menarche and the development of secondary sexual characteristics. When associated with radiotherapy these effects may be much more marked. It is important that prior to treatment with combination chemotherapy and radiotherapy that sperm storeage be considered when appropriate.

Following treatment with chemotherapy alone fertility may be affected, but if hormone levels return to normal then pregnancies have been reported after, and during treatment (Matthews, Wood, 1980, Rostom & White, 1979). A recent report of 13 patients following treatment with chemotherapy for a variety of different types of malignancy suggests that even following intensive chemotherapy normal fertility may occur (Carrol & Case, 1982). The outcome of cancer treatment during pregnancy is more difficult to assess. Recently 78 patients were studied who became pregnant before, during or after therapy (Mulvihill et al, 1982). They found that even during intensive chemotherapy, pregnancy was possible. There was an apparent increase in abnormal outcomes in those patients who conceived after treatment. They suggest that this may be related to altered hormonal patterns.

Effects of Metabolism and Nutrition. Almost all of the hormones mentioned above affect metabolic processes within the cell. Consequently such changes may have an effect on the overall metabolic and nutritional state of the patient. Many cancer patients are nutritionally abnormal prior to treatment (Calman, 1982). The effects of cancer treatment may result in anxiety, anorexia and changes in anabolic and catabolic hormones. The long term consequences of such treatments remain to be defined, but it may take time for individuals who have lost weight to regain it. Insulin or cortisol are two hormones which require special mention. Both are involved in growth and nutritional state and are likely to be affected by cancer treatment.

It might also be worth mentioning other hormones which might be affected in the short term or the long term by cancer treatment. These include the gastrointestinal hormones such as gastrin and secretin and the renal hormone erythro-poietin. There is little evidence at present on the long term effects of treatment on such endocrine organs but it may have clinical relevance.

Psychological Effects. Although it has been stated that the major effects of cancer treatment on the endocrine system relate to growth and reproduction, the psychological effects are equally important. The treatment, diagnosis and investigation of patients with cancer can induce major problems. Endocrine effects of the treatment may enhance them. The loss of libido, amenorrhoea, problems of fertility delay in development of secondary sexual characteristics can all influence the patient's psychological state. Recognition of these problems should lead to an understanding of patient reactions, an effective programme of replacement therapy together with active and early counselling. This latter aspect should receive greater attention

Conclusions. There is increasing awareness of the late endocrine effects of cancer treatment. These late consequences may have not only physical but psychological effects. The major problems are these associated with the reproductive system and on the growth of children. There still remain areas requiring further study both in the long term and the short term. It is hoped that hormone replace-ment therapy together with positive counselling will help to improve the quality of life of these patients.
BAJORUNAS, D.R. (1980) Disorders of endocrine function

following cancer therapies. Clinics.Endocrinol.Metab.9,405.
BAKER, J.W., MORGAN, R.L., PECKHAM, M.J. and SMITHERS, D.W.
(1972). Preservation of ovarian function in patients
requiring radiotherapy for para-aortic and pelvic Hodgkin's
disease. Lancet (i) 1307.
BEATSON, G.T. On the treatment of inoperable cases of
carcinoma of the mammae. Suggestions for a new method of
treatment with illustrative cases. Lancet 2, 104.
BEEX, L., ROSS, A., SMALS, A., KLOPPENBERG, P. (1977).
5-Fluorouracil induced increase of total serum thyroxine
and triiodothyronine. Cancer Treat.Rep. 61, 1291.
BLACKARD, C.E. (1975). The Veterans Administrative Cooperative Urological Research Group studies of carcinoma
of the prostate. Cancer Chemotherapy Reports. 59, 225.
BLATT, J., POLACK, D.G., SHERRINS, R.J. (1981).Testicular
function in boys after chemotherapy for acute lymphoblastic
leukaemia. New Eng.J.Med. 304, 1121.
BREIER, S., KARNER, M., GUINZBURG, R., ROZENFEL, L. (1982).
Variations in thyroid hormones in serum during 5-FU treat-
ment. ASCO Abstracts 30.
CALMAN, K.C. (1982).Cancer cachexia. Brit.J.Hosp.Med. 27,28.
CARROLL, R.J. & CASE, D.C. (1982).Fertility after chemo-
therapy for malignant diseases. ASCO Abstracts 54.
CHAPMAN, R.M., (1982). Effect of cytotoxic therapy on
sexuality and gonadal function. Seminars in Oncol.9, 84.
FORBES, A.P. (1978).Chemotherapy testicular damage and
gynaecomastia: An endocrine blackhole. New Eng.J.Med.299,42.
FUKS, Z., GLATSTEIN, E., MARSA, G.N., BAGSHAW, M.A., KAPLAN,
H.S. (1976). Long-term effects of external irradiation on
the pituitary and thyroid glands. Cancer 37, 1152.
GINSBERG, S.J., COMIS, R.L., FITZPATRICK, A.V. (1977).
Vinblastine and inappropriate ADH secretion. New Eng.J.Med.
296, 941.
HARLOW, P.J., DECLERK, Y.A., SHORE, N.A., ORTEGA, J.A.,
CARRANZA, A., HEUSER, E. (1979). A fatal case of inapprop-
riate ADH secretion induced by cyclophosphamide therapy
Cancer 44, 896.
MATTHEWS, J.H. & WOOD, J.K. (1980). Male fertility during
chemotherapy for acute leukaemia. New Eng.J.Med. 303,1235.
MORGAN, W.E. & O'HARE, M.J. (1979). Cytotoxic drugs and
the human adrenal cortex. Cancer 43, 969.
MULVIHILL, J.J., MCKEEN, E.A., ROSNER, F. & ZARRABI, M.H
(1982). Pregnancy outcomes in patients with cancer.
ASCO Abstracts 50.
MCFADYEN, I.J., RAAB, G., CANT, E., FORREST, A.P.M. GROOM,
G.V. & GRIFFITHS, (1979). The effect of chemotherapy on

pituitary functions in patients with advanced breast cancer.
Clin.Oncol. 5, 153.
NAYSMITH, A., HANCOCK, B.W., CULLEN, D.R., RICHMOND, J.
& WILDE, C.E. (1976). Pituitary function in patients
receiving intermittent cytotoxic and corticosteroid therapy
for malignant lymphoma. Lancet (i) 715.
ROGERS, P., GOSSER, J., SATHER, H., NESBIT, M., ORTEGA, J.,
HAMMOND, D. (1982). Height and growth of children treated
for acute lymphoblastic leukaemia. ASCO Abstracts 130.
ROSE, D.P. & DAVIS, T.E. (1980). Effects of adjuvant
chemotherapy on the ovarian and adrenal function of breast
cancer patients. Cancer Res. 40, 4043.
ROSTOM, A.Y. & WHITE, W.F. (1979). Hodgkin's disease chemo-
therapy and fertility. Lancet (i) 555.
SEROTA, F.T., LUBERTI, A., AUGUST, C.S. (1982). Normal
growth of children after bone marrow transplantation.
AACR Abstracts 121.
SHALET, S.M. (1980). Effects of cancer chemotherapy on
gonadal function of patients. Cancer Treatment Rev.7,141.
SHALET, S.M. & BEARDWELL, C.G.(1979). Endocrine conse-
quences of treatment of malignant disease in childhood.
J.Roy.Soc.Med. 72, 39.
SHAMBERGER, R.C., SHERRINS, R.J., ZIEGLER, J.L., GLATSTEIN,
E., ROSENBERG, S.A. (1981). Effects of postoperative
adjuvant chemotherapy and radiotherapy on ovarian function
in women undergoing treatment for soft tissue sarcoma.
J.Natl. Cancer Inst. 67, 1213.
SHERRINS, R.J., OLENY, C.L.M., ZIEGLER, J.L. (1978).
Gynaecomastia and gonadal dysfunction in adolescent boys
treated with combination chemotherapy for Hodgkin's disease.
New Eng.J.Med. 299,12.
SKLAR, C., KIM, T., RAMSAY, N. (1982). Thyroid dysfunction
among long term survivors of bone marrow transplantation.
AACR Abstracts 157.
SMITH, I.E., FITZHARRIS, B.M., MCKINNA, J.A., FAHMY, D.R.,
NASH, A.G., NEVILLE, A.M., GAZET, J.C., FORD, H.T. POWLES,
T.L. (1978). Aminoglutethimide in treatment of metastatic
breast carcinoma. Lancet (ii) 646.
STUART, M.J., CUASO, C., MILLAR, M., AOSOKI, F. (1975).
Syndrome of recurrent increased secretion of antidiuretic
hormone following multiple doses of vincristine. Blood 45,315.
WANG, C., N.G., R.P., CHAN,T.K.,TODD, D. (1980). Effect
of combination chemotherapy on pituitary-gonadal function
in patients with leukaemia and lymphoma. Cancer 45, 2030.
WILSON, K.S., GRAY, C.E., CAMERON, E.H.D., SETH, J. &
PARKER, A.C.(1976) Hypothalamic/pituitary/adrenal function

in patients treated with intermittent high dose presnisolone
and cytotoxic therapy. Lancet (i) 610.

13th International Cancer Congress, Part E
Cancer Management, pages 21–33
© 1983 Alan R. Liss, Inc., 150 Fifth Avenue, New York, NY 10011

EMOTIONAL EFFECTS OF CANCER AND CANCER THERAPY

Jimmie C. Holland, M.D. and Julia Rowland, M.A.

Psychiatry Service
Memorial Sloan-Kettering Cancer Center
New York, New York 10021

INTRODUCTION

The changing pattern of survival in cancer has resulted in the emergence of new psychosocial problems for patients, their families and physicians. The central issue is frequently no longer adaptation to certain fatal outcome but rather adaptation to the uncertainties of living with apparent (but not assured) cure of cancer. It is reflected by questions of "Am I cured?", "Will it come back?", "What are my chances of a second tumor?", "Can I marry and have normal children?", "Am I different now?" "Must my plans and goals change?" These questions relate to the basic psychosocial concerns associated with cancer: dependency, separation, loss of body integrity and function and ability to meet the demands of normal social and work roles. This paper explores the psychological and social concerns associated with long survival and likely (but not certain) cure of cancer.

A. MODULATING FACTORS

Several key factors modulate the immediate and long term psychological response to cancer and its treatment. Attention to these factors early during treatment will assure integration of psychosocial parameters in patient care; potential problem areas can be anticipated and appropriate management strategies adapted throughout the course of treatment, thereby preventing or minimizing the development of deleterious psychological sequelae. These modulating factors are listed below:

1) age at the time of illness and treatment;
2) type, site and course of disease;
3) treatment modalities (surgery, radiation, chemotherapy);
4) implementation of physical and psychosocial rehabilitation;
5) social supports available;
6) psychological support by the health care team

As the others have been presented elsewhere(Holland 1982), only the first of these modulating factors will be elaborated upon here: Age at Time of Illness.

One factor central to a better understanding of the psychological problems resulting from cancer is the patient's age at onset of disease. Developmental phases throughout the lifecycle each carry age-specific physical and psychological tasks. Rowland and Holland have developed a model to provide a framework for planning of psychosocial rehabilitation. The model recognizes the normal tasks appropriate to each age or stage of development, indicates the usual effects of cancer treatment at that age upon achievement of stage-specific tasks, and outlines specific interventions aimed at reducing interference with normal development which can be implemented. Six stages are presented in schematic form to illustrate how this model is used for psychosocial rehabilitation planning.

DEVELOPMENTAL MODEL FOR PSYCHOSOCIAL REHABILITATION

STAGE	TASKS	DISRUPTION	INTERVENTION
CHILDHOOD (Early)	MOTOR	DEVELOPMENTAL	PHYSICAL/SOCIAL
	SPEECH	SLOWING	STIMULATION
	COGNITION	REGRESSION	STRUCTURED "PLAY"
	FAMILY	SEPARATION	↑ FAMILY
	BONDING	ANXIETY	CONTACT
	SOCIALI-	WITHDRAWAL	CONTINUITY OF
	ZATION	↑ FEARS	STAFF
		(PAIN)	TRUST OF STAFF

STAGE	TASKS	DISRUPTION	INTERVENTION
CHILDHOOD (Late)	PRE-PUBERTAL PEER RELATIONS ↑ INTELLECTUAL ↑ PHYSICAL PROWESS	BEING "DIFFERENT" SCHOOL PHOBIA DEATH FEARS	MAINTAIN APPEARANCE MINIMIZE ABSENCES DISCUSS ILLNESS MONITOR RESPONSES
ADOLESCENCE	MENARCHE/ PUBERTY PEER ACCEPTANCE ↑INDEPENDENCE SEXUAL EXPERIMENTATION IDENTITY	ALOPECIA/AMPUTATION "DIFFERENCES" ↓ SCHOOL/PHYSICAL PERFORMANCE ↑ DEPENDENCE CONFLICTS ABOUT SELF AND SEXUALITY	MAINTAIN APPEARANCES MAINTAIN PEER CONTACT SUPPORT INDEPENDENCE COUNSELING
ADULTHOOD (Early)	INTIMACY MARRIAGE PARENTAL ROLE WORK ROLE	↓ ATTRACTIVENESS STERILITY/ IMPOTENCE ↓ FAMILY ROLE DISRUPTION OF JOB PERFORMANCE	MAINTAIN NORMAL APPEARANCE SEX COUNSELING HOMEMAKER CHILDREN SUPPORTED ↓ JOB INTERRUPTIONS
ADULTHOOD (Middle)	CHANGING HORMONAL STATUS/ MENOPAUSE OLDER CHILDREN "EMPTY NEST" PEAK OF CAREER	ALTERED APPEARANCE DISRUPTED MARITAL/ FAMILY ROLE DISRUPTED ACHIEVEMENTS	MAINTAIN APPEARANCE COUNSELING (PATIENT AND FAMILY) FINANCIAL PLANNING

STAGE	TASKS	DISRUPTION	INTERVENTION
ADULTHOOD (Late)	AGING CHANGES	↑ PHYSICAL/ EMOTIONAL LIMITATIONS	HEALTH-RELATED SERVICES TO MAINTAIN CARE OF SELF
	ADJUSTMENT TO INCRE- SING LOSES	↑ DEPENDENCE ON OTHERS	SOCIAL SUPPORT SYSTEM
	↑ NUTURANCE ↑ AFFECT- TIONAL LOVE	↑ ISOLATION	
	RETIREMENT	↓ FINANCIAL SECURITY	FINANCIAL PLANNING
	↓ INCOME		

B. PSYCHOLOGICAL SEQUELAE IN LONG-TERM SURVIVORS

Psychological problems in long-term survivors reflect a myriad of concerns, from questions of recurrence
and possible delayed effects of treatment, to the emotional and social consequences of surviving a lifethreatening
illness. These common fears and concerns fall into two
major areas:

1. Medical issues:
   a) fears associated with termination of treat
      ment
   b) fears of recurrence and second malignancy
   c) adaptation to "unanticipated" late effects
      (infertility, CNS dysfunction, organ
      failure)

2. Psychological issues:
   a) effects of chronic stress on patient and
      family
   b) development of "survivor" syndrome (guilt)
   c) adaptation to negative societal responses
      (job, friends)

1. Medical issues:

Our observations of patients finishing radiotherapy treatments revealed not a decrease, as might be
expected, but a significant increase in psychological

distress when nearing and ending treatment (Holland et al 1979). The dysphoria of anxiety and depression seemed to be related to fear that the tumor could regrow when treatment was stopped, coupled with the concerns regarding cessation of the almost daily supportive contact with staff and close monitoring of physical state and symptoms. This problem is compounded by the awareness that there is no prescribed number of chemotherapy or radiotherapy treatments which assure total "safety" in stopping; the uncertainty about what is "enough" remains. The even more difficult question of when maintenance therapy should end is a cause for fear in patients and families who seek assurance that cure can be guaranteed.

Patients continue years later to experience anxiety when minor symptoms (which earlier would have been ignored) develop. Return for checkup visits also increases anxiety. Schmale et al (1980) have shown that cured cancer patients experience return to a normal level of well-being, but continue to fear small aches and pains more than others and have less of a sense of control over their health.

Adaptation to delayed side effects of treatment constitutes an additional area of medically-related concerns which may directly effect quality of life. Neurotoxicity, damage to renal and cardiovascular systems, and infertility caused by chemotherapeutic agents and radiation are side effects of therapy which alter normal function and thus cause emotional distress (D'Angio 1978). These compromising effects of treatment are the focus of considerable current retrospective and longitudinal research, especially among populations of patients treated for cancer as children and young adults.

A range of late effects on central nervous system functions has been noted in association with the use of specific chemotherapeutic agents and/or cranial radiation (CRT) (Allen 1978; Weiss 1974; Pizzo et al 1979). The most extensively documented of these effects has been seen among selected groups of childhood ALL patients receiving prophylactic CNS treatment. While preliminary studies reported minimal effects on cognitive function (Soni et al 1975; Obetz et al 1979), subsequent research has revealed that a number of functional deficits as well as structural abnormalities may occur in 25-30% of survivors(Aur et al

1976; Goff Anderson Cooper 1980; Moss Nannik Poplack 1981)
Depending upon the type of prophylaxis used, one or several of these side effects can occur in as many as 80% of
the children involved and lead to transient and in some
instances permanent dysfunction (Freeman 1973). In a recent CALGB study, 106 children who were randomized to one
of three CNS prophylaxis treatment arms, a) intrathecal
methtrexate (IT) alone, b) in combination with CRT or, c)
in combination with intermediate dose systemic methotrexate, were evaluated. A significantly lower mean score on
Full-Scale, Verbal and Performance I.Q.'s was found in the
children who received the CRT + IT combination (Rowland et
al 1982). Children under the age of four at the time
they were diagnosed and received this treatment appeared
to be at greatest disadvantage. These children continue
to be followed longitudinally to assess neurologic, endocrinologic and psychologic sequelae. This data, in conjunction with that from ongoing prospective studies of
similar groups, will provide important answers for patients, physicians and families regarding possible changes
they have or may expect to experience as cured ALL survivors, answers which can guide both treatment and intervention planning.

The psychological problems of fertility are also under closer scrutiny. It appears that neither radiation.
nor chemotherapy has had an oncogenic effect upon progeny,
giving encouragement to couples who want children(Li Jaffe
1974; Meadows et al 1978; Blatt et al 1980). Young women
who have had less than 2000 rads to the pelvis or who have
had ovaries relocated during treatment may remain fertile.
The outlook for all patients, however, is not as positive.
Amenorrhea and ovarian failure related to chemotherapy regimens account for diminished libido and sexual dysfunction in a high percentage of young women following the
MOPP regimen for Hodgkins' disease and chemotherapy for
breast cancer (Chapman et al 1979; Schilsky et al 1980).
Frequently these women have not been prepared for this
early treatment-related menopause; in these cases, an explanation and hormonal therapy can be helpful in adjusting
to the change.

Men who receive pelvic irradiation become aspermic
after 3-4 treatments and remain sterile, if not shielded.
While retroperitoneal node dissection for testicular neoplasms causes no loss in sexual performance, due to inter-
ruption of the sympathetic chain, ejaculation is impaired

and sterility results (von Eschenbach 1980). Adequate planning for sperm banking is an important part of management in anticipation of this long-term effect.

2. Psychological Issues:

Young children who are cured of cancer at an early age (under 5) have few subsequent emotional problems related to illness; they have little recall of having had a potentially fatal disease. Honesty about diagnosis from the beginning appears to be associated with better adaptation at all ages. Children who learn the diagnosis years later often feel betrayed by the lies surrounding their treatment, and often state that they would have preferred to have been told the truth at the time(Slavin et al 1982).

Cancer which occurs in later childhood or adolescence is associated with greater psychological sequelae. In one study, residual mild psychological problems were seen in 59% of children and severe symptoms in 12%(Koocher O'Malley 1981). These children had poorer self-esteem and more anxiety and depression, symptoms which were more pronounced in those who had developed fewer social skills or who had reduced intellectual ability. Holmes and Holmes (1975), however, found cured childhood cancer patients 10 years later to be leading normal lives with completion of education, marriage and parenthood; their study patients appeared to have adapted to considerable handicaps and used denial to cope with problems. For many survivors, a sense of being different, "special", and mature beyond their years is often observed.

Our clincal experience has suggested a similarity in psychological response of some of these survivors to those who survived the Holocaust or a significant castastrophic event(Lifton 1976). Adolescents and young adults express existential concerns, often arising from the question -- "Why was I spared?" They carry on a search for the special meaning or purpose for which their life has been spared, searching for what might be intended for themin the future. They sense having been exempted from the fate of many of their fellow friends and patients who began treatment with them and later died; they often experience severe and prolonged grief for those friends. Their grief tempered by a sense of guilt for having survived, results in a psychological equation that leads them to believe their survival was at the expense of those who died. A need to make some "sense" out of the experience, as a way to master these feelings, leads to lengthy rumination at times. As with the Holocaust survivors, there is a pervasive need to understand why they were allowed to survive.

Reassessment of religious and moral values with exploration of the meaning of life becomes understandable. The reflection that these children and adolescents become "mature beyond their years" and responsible in a way they might not have otherwise appeared, seems to be explained by the impact of surviving this significant life crisis, an event that others did not. The identification with fellow patient-friends becomes part of the need for support with others in the same situation. The sharing of fears about death and use of grieving for others is often used to achieve mastery. Anxiety about death and pondering of its meaning continues, though it diminishes as survival time increases and the assumption of "cure" strengthens.

The survivor from cancer needs to be observed and monitored for early signs of any psychologic decompensation. Ventilation of anxiety, clarification of information and misinformation, especially around issues of survival and whether they can give their illness to others may greatly diminish difficulties associated with "re-entry" into normal life. While many patients appear superficially to be well-adjusted, the possible presence of latent psychologic vulnerabilities, as seen in other survivors, cannot be ruled out in all cases and may later lead to prob-. lems in some patients. The observation of depression and anxiety in some long-term survivors would suggest that they may be more psychologically vulnerable to certain kinds of fears and stress. How many are more vulnerable, how they may be identified early, and how they may be managed to diminish long-term adverse psychologic sequelae remain questions that only more study can supply. Epidemiological studies of the frequency, timing and nature of psychologic problems is needed as well as information about how these problems relate to the presence of other medical sequelae of illness.

Sanders and Kardinal (1977) noted in six patients in remission from leukemia, that they attempted to master the uncertainty by denial of being sick, with resentment toward family for reminding them of illness. They maintained close identification with their "hospital family" and fellow patients, with intense grieving over their loss to disease.

Kennedy et al in a similar study in 1978, found in survivors of five to twenty years, a confidence in recovery, and denial of fears of death, coupled with a reordering of values with increased religious and moral concerns, and increased appreciation of life and others. Smith (1979), studying patients with diseases other than cancer, found the same positive change in goals, values and relationships; a sense of a limited life span and a greater sense of caring and being cared for by others was also seen.

C. INTERVENTION

What can be done from the onset of treatment of cancer to reduce or prevent adverse psychological problems in cured cancer patients? Several guidelines are recommended from studies and clincial observations:

1. Honesty about the diagnosis, coupled with clear communication between the physician, patient and family about diagnosis and treatment, with correction of misinformation.

2. Honesty about possible long-term adverse side-effects. Awareness that a side-effect may occur, has an "immunizing" effect against anxiety when and if the problem does occur; emotional preparation for it enhances ability to adapt. This is particularly true of infertili-. ty which should be discussed before treatment, permiting sperm banking, hormonal replacement, and special shielding as appropriate.

3. Attention to planning for end of active treatment. Such planning must be incorporated in the psychological management so that patients can anticipate the termination of treatment and the consequent decrease in frequency of visits to physician and staff. Informing them of the "normal" increase in fears at this time provides understanding of this emotional reaction and reduces concerns.

4. Continuity of the treating physician and staff.

The longitudinal nature of cancer and the complexity of treatment require that many consultants and specialists be involved in a single patient's care. The continuity of one physician, however, and a nurse or social worker adds greatly to the security of patient and family.

5. Monitoring of the patient in relation to whether development is normal with achievement of appropriate age/stage - specific tasks. The model presented stresses early identification of intellectual, social or emotional problems and early referral for assessment of the nature of the problems. This may entail neurologic, endocrinologic and psychologic evaluation to arrive at a diagnosis and to introduce remediation.

6. Psychological intervention in the patient to treat evidence of anxiety, depression and survivor guilt; any evidence of psychologic decompensation warrants evaluation.

7. Evaluation of maladaptive family interaction around the patient. Parents and siblings of young patients, young children and spouses of the adult group, and children of elderly patients may experience the stress of prolonged treatment; family members as well as the patient require evaluation. Efforts to keeep the patient "sick", to be overprotective, to discourage normal achievements may be cause for intervention.

8. "Veteran" patient support should be encouraged. The psychological gains from ventilation and discussion with others who have had the same tumor and similar treatment has proven increasingly valuable.

SUMMARY

Prevention of adverse psychological sequelae of cancer begins at the time of diagnosis (D'Angio 1975). By proper management, in which accurate information is given in a positive way, misinformation is corrected and a supportive continuous relationship to a physician and staff is established. Information should similarly be given about when termination of therapy is anticipated and re--entry to normal life can be expected. Attachment to the hospital, staff and fellow patients is expected and can be used as a positive force by development of "veteran" and

"fellow" patient groups. When symptoms of psychological
distress do occur in a long-term survivor, they warrant
immediate attention and a workup that takes into account
the vulnerability to endocrine and neurologic delayed effects, as well as psychological. Interventions should be
based on diagnostic findings and include consideration of
maladaptive patterns of interaction within the family and
the patient's social setting.

More clinical studies of long-survivors are needed to
clarify the interaction of medical and psychological variables which contribute to quality of life of the cured
cancer patient.

BIBLIOGRAPHY

Allen JC (1978). The effects of cancer therapy on the
nervous system. J Peds 93:903.
D'Angio GJ (1975). Pediatric cancer in perspective: cure
is not enough. Cancer 35:866.
D'Angio CJ (1978). Complications of treatment encountered
in lymphoma-leukemia long-term survivors. Cancer 42:1015.
Aur R, Husto O, Simone J (1976). Leukoencephalopathy in
children with acute lymphocytic leukemia receiving
preventive central nervous system therapy. Proc AACR
17:97.
Blatt J, Mulvihill JJ, Ziegler JL, Young RC, Poplack DG
(1980). Pregnancy outcome following chemotherapy: the
national cancer institute experience. Proc ASCO 21:381.
Chapman RM, Sutcliffe SB, Malpas JS (1979).
Cytotoxic-induced ovarian failure in women with hodgkin's
disease. 1. Hormone function. JAMA 242:1877.
von Eschenbach AC (1980). Sexual dysfunction following
therapy for cancer of the prostate, testis, and penis.
Front Radiat Ther Onc 14:42.
Freeman JE, Johnston PG, Voke JM (1973). Somnolence after
prophylactic cranial irradiation in children with ALL. Br
Med J 4:523.
Goff JR, Anderson HR, Cooper PF (1980). Distractibility
and memory deficits in long-term survivors of acute
lymphocytic leukemia. Devel Behav Peds 1:158.
Holland JC (1982). Psychologic aspects of cancer. In
Holland JF, Frei E III (eds): "Cancer Medicine, Edition
2," Philadelphia: Lea and Febiger, p 1175.

Holland JC, Rowland J, Lebovits A, Rusalem R (1979).
Reactions to cancer treatment: assessment of emotional
responses to adjuvant radiotherapy as a guide to planned
intervention. Psychiat Clin N Am 2:347.

Holmes HA, Holmes FF (1975). After 10 years, what are the
handicaps of life styles of children treated for cancer?
Clin Peds 14:819.

Kennedy BJ, Tellegen A, Kennedy S, Havernick N (1978).
Psychological response of patients cured of advanced
cancer. Cancer 38: 2184.

Koocher GP, O'Malley JE (1981). "The Damocles Syndrome."
New York: McGraw-Hill.

Li FP, Jaffe N (1974). Progeny of childhood cancer
survivors. Lancet 2: 707.

Lifton RJ (1976). "History and Human Survival." New York:
Vantage Books.

Meadows AT, D'Angio GJ, Evans AG, Harris CC, Miller RW,
Mike V (1978). Oncogenesis and other late effects of
cancer treatment in children. Radiology 114:175.

Moss HA, Nannis ED, Poplack DG (L981). The effects of
prophylactic treatment of the central nervous system on
the intellectual functioning of children with acute
lymphocytic leukemia. Am J Med 71:47.

Obetz SW, Smithson WA, Groover RV, Houser OW, Klass DW,
Ivnik RJ, Colligan RC, Gilchrist GS, Burgert EO (1979).
Neuropsychologic follow-up study of children with acute
lymphocytic leukemia; a preliminary report. Am J Ped
Hematol/Oncol 1:207.

Pizzo PA, Poplack DG, Bleyer WA (1979). Neurotoxicities of
current leukemia therapy. Am J Ped Hematol/Oncol 1:127.

Rowland J, Glidewell O, Sibley R, Holland JC, Brecker M,
Tull B, Berman A, Glicksman A, Forman E, Harris M,
McSweeny J, Jones B, Black M, Cohen M, Freeman A (1982).
Effect of cranial radiation on neuropsychologic function
in children with acute lymphocytic leukemia. Proc ASCO
1:123.

Sanders J, Kardinal C (1977). Adaptive coping mechanisms
in adult leukemia patients in remission. JAMA 238:952.

Schilsky RL, Lewis BJ, Sherins RJ, Young RC (1980).
Gonadal dysfunction in patients receiving chemotherapy
for cancer. Ann Int Med 93:109.

Schmale A, Morrow G (1980). Psychosocial well-being in
cancer survivors. Paper presented at the Annual American
Psychosomatic Society Meeting, April 1980, Boston.

Slavin LA, O'Malley JE, Koocher GP, Foster DJ (1982). Communication of the cancer diagnosis to pediatrtic patients: impact on long-term adjustment. Am J Psychiat 139:179.

Smith DW (1979). Survivors of serious illness. Am J Nursing 79:441.

Soni S, Marten GW, Pitner SE, Duenas DA, Powazek M (1975). Effects of central nervous system irradiation on neuropsychologic functions of children with acute lymphocytic leukemia. NEJM 293:113.

Weiss HD, Walker MD, Wiernik PH (1974). Neurotoxicity of commonly used antineoplastic agents. NEJM 291:75.

13th International Cancer Congress, Part E
Cancer Management, pages 35–44
© 1983 Alan R. Liss, Inc., 150 Fifth Avenue, New York, NY 10011

LONG-TERM EFFECTS OF POSTOPERATIVE ADJUVANT CHEMOTHERAPY ON
THE IMMUNE SYSTEM IN 100 CANCER PATIENTS.

Lucien ISRAEL, Raymond SAMAK, Abdelmoumen
GREFFT-ALAMI, Richard EDELSTEIN.
Medical Oncology Service. Chair of Oncology
Laboratory of Human Tumors Immuno-Biology
CHU Avicenne. Bobigny. 93000 France.

INTRODUCTION

   This study was undertaken to investigate the possible
long-term effects of adjuvant chemotherapy on immune parameters. One hundred patients with solid tumors who had all
received adjuvant chemotherapy more than 12 months previously were studied. To the best of our knowledge there is no
such study in the literature so this one appears to be
the first of its kind. The preliminary results (26 months
median follow-up after completion of chemotherapy) look
reassuring.

MATERIAL AND METHODS

Patient Population and Controls

   One hundred patients (73 women, 27 men ; mean age :
52.7 ± 13.62 years) treated by chemotherapy following
"complete" surgical resection of their tumor were included
in this study. The breakdown of this population according
to cancer type and treatment administered is shown in
table 1.

TABLE 1

Distribution of patients according to cancer type
and treatment administered.

Primary	Nb of patients	Treatment administered	Mean duration of treatment (months)
Breast Ca	64	44 LPAM-5FU	24
		20 CTX-MTX-5FU	
Melanoma	10	10 CCNU-DTIC-DAC-VCR	16
Ca of testis	8	1 VLB-BLM-HOL-MTH	18
		7 DDP-BLM-MTH-VLB	
Lung Ca	6	1 5FU-CTX-MTX	10
		4 MITO-ADM-MTX	
		1 CTX	
Ovarian Ca	4	2 CTX-MTX-5FU	19
		1 DAC-BLM-VLB-MTH	
		1 LPAM	
Large Bowel Ca	3	1 CTX-5FU	12
		2 MITO-5FU	
Osteosarcoma	2	2 ADM-VCR-BLM-CTX	16
		CCNU-LPAM-RUFO	
Uterine leiomyosarcoma	1	1 CTX-VCR-RUFO-BLM	16
Malignant schwanoma	1	1 CTX-5FU-MTX-VCR	18
Thymic seminoma	1	1 ADM-VCR-BLM-HXML	18

All immunological tests for any given patient were
performed on the same day and at least one year after
chemotherapy had been stopped. None of the patients had any
signs of recurrent disease at the time of testing.

The control group was composed of 30 healthy blood
donors from the "Centre de Transfusion Sanguine" of the
Hôpital Avicenne who underwent the same tests.

Immunological Parameters Studied.

The number of peripheral blood monocytes was determined
by counting May-Grunwald-Giemsa stained smears under the
light microscope.

In vitro monocyte chemotaxis was studied in a modified
Boyden chamber using the technique described by Mc Vie et
alii (Mc Vie 1977) : after separation of mononuclear cells
on a Ficoll-Hypaque gradient (lymphocyte separation medium -
Flow Laboratories), the cells were washed three times and
adjusted to a final concentration of 0.5×10^6 monocytes/ml
in Mc Coy's medium containing 20 % human AB serum and 50 mcg
of streptomycin. 650 µl of this cell suspension were placed
in the first compartment of a modified Boyden chamber. The
second compartment was filled with a 1 mg/ml casein solution
(Merck Laboratories) in Mc Coy's medium. The two compartments were separated by a millipore filter (Millipore S.A.,
Molsheim, France) of 0.8 µm pore size. The chambers were
incubated for 90 minutes at 37°C, after which the filters
were recovered, dehydrated by a graded series of ethanols,
stained with hematoxylin and eosin, washed, dried and fixed
to glass slides with Depex (Serlabo, Paris, France). The
slides were examined using a Leitz, Dialux 20 microscope
equipped with a micrometer scale on the fine adjustment.
Monocyte migration was determined by measuring the distance
on the micrometer scale between the surface of the filter
and the two cells that had migrated furthest. Twenty fields
were examined for each sample.

In vivo nonspecific macrophage chemotaxis was tested
using a previously described technique (Samak 1980a ;
Samak 1980b ; Israël 1982). Briefly, a hairless area of the
forearm was cleaned with ether and abraded with a spherical
rotating bit of standardized diameter mounted on a minia-
ture drill. The abrasion (skin window) was covered with a
sterile glass coverslip protected by a gauze dressing and
maintained in position on the forearm by adhesive tape.
The coverslips were changed at precise intervals : 3, 6 and
12 hours after the start of the test, and the last coverslip
was withdrawn 24 hours after the abrasion had been made.
The coverslips were air-dried, mounted on glass-slides
(cell-surface uppermost), and stained with May-Grunwald-
Giemsa and examined under the light microscope (magnifica-
tion x 500). All the cells on the coverslips were counted
and for the purposes of analysis, the absolute number of
macrophages at 24 hours was considered.

The number of peripheral blood lymphocytes was

determined by light microscope counts of May-Grunwald-Giemsa stained smears.

Lymphocyte subpopulations were studied by marking surface membrane antigens in direct or indirect immuno-fluorescence assays. After separation of mononuclear cells on a Ficoll-Hypaque gradient and adjustment to the final appropriate concentration, the following subpopulations were characterized :

B lymphocytes. The mononuclear cell suspension was incubated for 30 minutes at +4° C with fluorescein-labelled goat anti-human IgG, A, M and D Fab$_2$ fragments. The number of fluorescent cells was counted under a Leitz Dialux microscope using epifluorescence and phase contrast.

T lymphocytes. The percentage of peripheral blood T lymphocytes was determined using OKT3 monoclonal antibodies (Ortho Diagnostic System) (Kung 1979). After incubation of the cells for 30 minutes at +4°C with the OKT3 antibody, the cells were washed and reincubated for 30 minutes at 4°C with fluorescein-labelled goat anti-mouse immunoglobulin antibodies. The cells were then washed three times and examined under a fluorescence microscope. The percentage of fluorescent cells was determined on 500 cells.

Helper/inducer T lymphocytes. The percentage of helper/inducer T lymphocytes was determined using the same indirect immunofluorescence technique described above. In this case, the monoclonal antibody was OKT4 (Ortho Diagnostic System).

Suppressor/cytotoxic T lymphocytes were characterized by the OKT8 monoclonal antibody using the same technique as above.

Lymphocyte response to mitogens. Lymphocyte blastogenic response to the mitogens phytohemagglutinin (PHA) and poke-weed mitogen (PWM) was studied using the technique described by Hirschhorn (1963). Briefly, mononuclear cells were separated and adjusted to 2×10^6 cells/ml. 100 µl aliquots were distributed in the wells of a microtiter plate. 50 µl of optimal concentration PHA or PWM were added to the wells and the plates were then pulsed with 0.5 µCi of tritiated thymidine and re-incubated for a further 18 hours. The cells were then harvested, lysed and deposited on filters by an automatic cell harvester. The filters were immersed in vials containing scintillation liquid and blastogenesis was determined by measuring the number of counts per minute recorded on a Kontron β-scintillation counter.

Delayed cutaneous hypersensitivity was studied using a disposable multipuncture device (Multitest-Institut Mérieux, Lyon. France) which delivers 7 antigens simultaneously :

tetanus, diphteria, streptococcus, tuberculin, proteus, trichophyton and candida albicans.

Serum immunoglobulin G, A and M levels were determined by nephelometry. These assays were done in the "Laboratoire de Biochimie" Hôpital Avicenne, Bobigny, France, by P. Cornillot and F. Fabia.

STATISTICAL ANALYSIS

Statistical comparison of mean values was performed using Student's t test for unpaired values.

The analysis of the correlation coefficients was performed by the method of Fisher and Yates, controlled by the t test.

RESULTS

The means and standard deviations for each of immunological parameters studied are shown in table 2, together with the significance of the difference between the patient and control groups.

1. The patient group exhibited a significantly lower number of peripheral blood lymphocytes than the control group (1511 ± 661 vs 2088 ± 663). The number of peripheral blood monocytes was comparable in the two groups.

The decreased number of peripheral lymphocytes was due selectively to a drop in the T lymphocyte population which was significantly lower than in the control group, and particularly to the T4 (helper/inducer) lymphocyte subset, also lower than in the controls. The B and T8 (suppressor/cytotoxic) lymphocyte subpopulations were comparable in the two groups.

This alteration in the distribution of the T4 subpopulation accounted for a significantly decreased T4/T8 ratio is the patient group.

2. The patient group had a significantly weaker blastogenic response to the two mitogens tested, phytohemagglutinin and pokeweed mitogen.

TABLE 2

Means ± standard deviations for each immunological parameter
studied in the control and patient populations. Significance
of the comparison of these two groups.

	Controls	Patients	Significance of comparison
Nb of Per. blood lymphocytes	2088 ± 663	1511 ± 661	p = 0.01
Nb of T cells	1503 ± 475	922 ± 466	p < 0.001
Nb of T help/ind.	1006 ± 347	537 ± 319	p < 0.001
Nb of T sup/cyt.	541 ± 252	414 ± 247	NS
Ratio T4/T8	2.16 ± 1	1.43 ± 0.8	p < 0.05
Nb of B cells	291 ± 169	248 ± 142	NS
Blastogenic response to PHA (log CPM)	4.72 ± 0.19	4.3 ± 0.57	p < 0.02
Blastogenic response to PWM (log CPM)	4.4 ± 0.2	3.86 ± 0.59	p < 0.001
Skin tests	> 10	17.9 ± 9.2	NS
Nb of Per. blood monocytes	382 ± 167	347 ± 186	NS
In vivo monocyte chemotaxis (Nb of monocytes à 24 h)	3112 ± 864	2605 ± 1792	NS
In vitro monocyte chemotaxis	23.6 ± 8.4	25.9 ± 10.6	NS
IgG	11.5 ± 1.7	12.27 ± 2.5	NS
IgA	2.7 ± 0.9	2.4 ± 1.3	NS
IgM	1.5 ± 0.5	1.6 ± 0.8	NS

3. Monocyte-macrophage chemotaxis, both in vitro and in vivo, showed comparable values in the patient and control groups.

4. Delayed cutaneous hypersensitivity to recall antigens were normal (a score above 10) in 93 of 100 patients.

5. No alterations were noted in either group for immuno-globulin levels.

Analysis of individual values showed that although there was no difference in the mean values for in vivo macrophage migration, 47 of the 100 patients had values that were less than the mean control value minus one standard deviation.

A study of combined parameters showed : 1) A simultaneous decrease of the number of helper/inducer lymphocytes and in vivo nonspecific macrophage chemotaxis in 38 patients out of 100. 2) An increased number of suppressor/cytotoxic lymphocytes in only 6 patients, combined with a decreased number of helper/inducer lymphocytes in 4 cases (one of them has recurred 5 months after testing). 3) Five patients had all tests within normal limits. 4) The other patients showed an alteration of a single parameter : decreased in vivo macrophage migration (9 patients) ; decreased number of T helper/inducer lymphocytes (33 patients).

No difference was observed when patients were analyzed as a function of the post chemotherapy interval. The study of the degree of relationship between these various parameters by paired correlations and using the test of independance of Fisher and Yates, controlled by Student's t test, showed that there was a relationship between : the number of peripheral helper/inducer lymphocytes and the blastogenic response to PHA ($p < 0.01$) and pokeweed mitogen ($p < 0.05$) ; the number of peripheral helper/inducer lymphocytes and the in vivo macrophage migration response ($p < 0.05$).

A number of patients reported increased susceptibility to infections, though no correlation could be established between this reported susceptibility and the immunological abnormalities observed.

DISCUSSION

This study investigated 15 immunological parameters in 100 cancer patients who received postoperative adjuvant chemotherapy for 18 to 24 months, terminated at least 12 months previously. We noted a significant decrease of several parameters, namely the number of peripheral T helper /inducer lymphocytes and blastogenic response to the mitogens phytohemagglutinin and pokeweed mitogen. Almost half of the patients also showed decreased in vivo macrophage chemotaxis.

These abnormalities were documented after a mean post-chemotherapy interval of 25.7 ± 16 months. It must be noted that these results emerge from a comparison with a control group of healthy subjects, and it may be argued that a more appropriate control group would have been post operative cancer patients who did not receive adjuvant chemotherapy. Because healthy subjects were used as the controls, it cannot be firmly concluded that the immunological abnormalities noted were indeed due to postoperative chemotherapy. Some of the "disease-free" patients may have had microscopic metastases responsible for the abnormalities noted. However, some indication that these abnormalities were chemotherapy-related can be derived from a study performed simultaneously (Samak 1982) in which the same immunological parameters were studied in two different groups of patients, namely patients with metastatic tumors and patients with localized operable tumors. In neither of these two groups of patients was there any significant decrease in the number of total lymphocytes, T lymphocytes or helper/inducer T lymphocytes. It was noted however in this study that 30 % of patients with either metastatic or localized operable tumors had an increased number of suppressor/cytotoxic lymphocytes, combined with a decrease in the number of T helper/inducer lymphocytes. This increase in suppressor/cytotoxic T cells is not found in the patients included in the present study.

From these data there appears to be a strong probability that the T helper/inducer deficiency observed in patients following adjuvant chemotherapy is due to the chemotherapy rather than to the underlying disease.

It is important to mention that the vast majority of patients were treated with an alkylating agent. It has not been possible so far to show any relationship between the immune deficiencies observed, tumor recurrence or onset of a second malignancy. Obviously, longer follow-up of these patients will be necessary to detect such a relationship if it exists.

We are not suggesting however, that the immune deficiencies seen in these patients should discourage adjuvant chemotherapy. It must be remembered that these patients are at high risk for recurrence. This risk must be weighed against the potential consequences of chemotherapy induced immune depression.

CONCLUSION

In summary this study tends to support the conclusion that the two main long term immunological effects of prolonged chemotherapy are : a) a decrease in T helper cells without increase in the numbers of suppressor/cytotoxic T cells ; b) a decrease in in vivo nonspecific macrophage chemotaxis. These effects were not correlated with any susceptibility to infection.

We would like to thank particularly Martine Samak and Odile Scemama for considerable help in the in vitro studies and in analyzing the data.

REFERENCES

Hirschhorn K, Bach F, Kolodny RL (1963). Immune response and mitosis of human peripheral blood lymphocytes "in vitro". Science 142:1185.

Israël L, Samak R, Edelstein R, Amouroux J, Battesti JP, de Saint Florent G (1982). In vivo non specific macrophage chemotaxis in cancer patients and its correlation with extent of disease, regional lymph node status, and disease-free survival. Cancer Research 42:2489.

Kung PC, Goldstein G, Reinherz E, Schlossman SF (1979). Monoclonal antibodies defining distinctive human T cell surface antigens. Science 206:347.

Mc Vie JG, Logan EM, Kay AB (1977). Monocyte function in cancer patients. Europ J Cancer 13:351.

Samak R, Edelstein R, Bogucki D, Samak M, Israël L (1980a). Testing the monocyte macrophage system in human cancer. Biomedicine 32:165.

Samak R, Israël L, Edelstein R (1980b). Influence of tumor burden, tumor removal, immune stimulation, plasmapheresis or monocyte mobilisation in cancer patients. In Escobar ME and Friedman RE (ed) : "Macrophages and Lymphocytes" part B, New York, Plenum Publishing Corporation, p 411.

Samak R, Grefft A, Edelstein R, Israël L (1982). Study of T lymphocyte subpopulations, characterized by monoclonal antibodies in the peripheral blood of patients with solid tumors. 8th Annual Meeting of the European Society for Medical Oncology. Nice. Abstract (in press).

This work was supported in part by grants from the "Association pour le Développement de la Recherche sur le Cancer" Villejuif, 94800 France and by the "Caisse Nationale d'Assurances Maladies d'Ile de France" Paris, 75019 France.

13th International Cancer Congress, Part E
Cancer Management, pages 45–54
© **1983 Alan R. Liss, Inc., 150 Fifth Avenue, New York, NY 10011**

SECOND MALIGNANCIES AND CHEMOTHERAPEUTIC AGENTS*

Robert A. Kyle, M.D.

Division of Hematology and Internal Medicine
Mayo Clinic and Mayo Foundation
Rochester, Minnesota 55905

The association of acute leukemia with chemotherapy for hematologic neoplasms, solid tumors, and nonneoplastic diseases has become a significant problem. The development of lymphoma, myeloma, and other tumors after chemotherapy also has been recognized.

ACUTE LEUKEMIA ASSOCIATED WITH CHEMOTHERAPY

Multiple Myeloma

Since the first report suggesting the possible role of alkylating agents administered for multiple myeloma in the subsequent development of acute leukemia (Kyle et al. 1970), more than 150 cases have been recognized (Casciato, Scott 1979; Rosner, Grünwald 1980a).

Of 908 patients with multiple myeloma diagnosed at the Mayo Clinic from 1965 through 1975, 17 developed acute leukemia. The actuarial rate was 10.1% at 10 years. Of these 17 patients, 12 were men and 5 were women. Their ages ranged from 40 to 79 years (median 56). In this group, chemotherapy consisted of melphalan, given orally every day to eight patients, orally and intermittently to six, and intravenously to one; BCNU to one; and cyclophosphamide to one. Five of the patients also received radiation therapy. The median

*Supported in part by NIH Research Grants CA-16835 and CA-4646.

duration of chemotherapy was 54 months (range 30 to 142).
Sixteen patients had acute myelocytic or myelomonocytic leukemia, and the 17th patient had erythroleukemia. All but
three patients had minimal evidence of multiple myeloma at
the time acute leukemia was diagnosed. Antileukemic therapy
with cytosine arabinoside and doxorubicin or daunorubicin was
instituted in four cases, but no complete remissions were obtained. Survival ranged from 1 to 5 months (median 1 month).

During this same period, there were seven additional patients with myeloma who had pancytopenia and bone marrow abnormalities consistent with an evolving myeloproliferative
process (preleukemia). These abnormalities developed at a
median of 43 months after multiple myeloma was diagnosed.
All seven patients required multiple transfusions and all
ultimately died from complications of the pancytopenia but
did not develop overt acute leukemia. Median survival after
recognition of pancytopenia was 10 months (range 2 to 18
months).

The incidence of acute leukemia and multiple myeloma in
patients treated with alkylating agents has varied from 0.2
to 7%, and the reported actuarial rates at 4 to 5 years have
ranged from 4.8 to 19.6%. The age at onset (about 60 years)
and the sex incidence (about 60% male) are similar to those
of patients with multiple myeloma who do not have acute
leukemia.

Pancytopenia frequently precedes the development of
overt acute leukemia; in our experience, discontinuation of
chemotherapy when pancytopenia appears does not prevent the
development of acute leukemia.

Most patients have acute myelocytic or myelomonocytic
leukemia. Acute erythroleukemia as well as acute lymphocytic leukemia has been described. Involvement of the erythroid cells and megakaryocytes in addition to granulopoie-
sis (panmyelosis) is frequent (McKenna et al. 1981). The
differentiation of acute myelocytic leukemia from plasma
cell leukemia may be difficult, but immunoperoxidase and
nonspecific esterase stains and electron microscopy are
helpful in the diagnosis. The incidence of acute leukemia
has been reported to be less when the drugs are given
intravenously as a pulse dose than when given in a continuous fashion (McIntyre et al. 1981).

Abnormal karyotypes are found in the cells of peripheral blood or in the bone marrow in most patients who develop acute leukemia after chemotherapy or radiation. In 1981, Rowley et al. reported that 25 of 26 patients with acute non-lymphocytic leukemia or dysmyelopoietic syndrome after treatment of a primary malignancy had an abnormal karyotype in myeloid cells. They also found loss of part or all of chromosome 5 or chromosome 7 (or both chromosomes) in 23 of 25 patients with aneuploidy.

The acute leukemia progresses rapidly, and most patients die within a few weeks or months. Remissions are infrequent and survival is short in acute leukemia compared with de novo acute myelocytic leukemia. Therapy during the preleukemic phase is not recommended. We have been impressed with the absence of symptomatic myeloma at the time of diagnosis of acute leukemia (Kyle et al. 1975).

Multiple myeloma and acute leukemia have been recognized simultaneously in a number of instances (Rosner, Grünwald 1980b). But without the evidence of lytic bone lesions and significant amounts of Bence Jones proteinuria and with only moderately increased serum monoclonal protein, it is difficult to distinguish acute leukemia and multiple myeloma from acute leukemia with monoclonal gammopathy of undetermined significance (MGUS).

Waldenström's Macroglobulinemia

Rosner and Grünwald (1980b) described 18 patients with Waldenström's macroglobulinemia and acute leukemia. In six of the patients, both diseases occurred simultaneously or within a few months of each other.

Hodgkin's Disease

Rosner et al. (1975, 1979) collected a total of 93 cases of acute leukemia with Hodgkin's disease. The mean age at the diagnosis of Hodgkin's disease was 34 years (range 4 to 74). The two diseases occurred simultaneously or within 6 months in seven cases. The mean interval from the diagnosis of Hodgkin's disease to the diagnosis of acute leukemia was 6 years. The leukemia was myeloblastic, myelomonocytic, or monocytic in 70 cases and acute lymphoblastic in 7. All but three patients had received radiation for the Hodgkin's disease.

In a 1980 review emphasizing methodologic considerations in studies of multiple primary cancers, Brody and Schotten- feld estimated that the crude risk of acute nonlymphocytic leukemia occurring with Hodgkin's disease reported since 1960 was 3.14 per 1,000 person-years. In 1982, Valagussa et al. reported that the actuarial risk of developing acute non- lymphocytic leukemia was 6.5% for 249 patients given MOPP (nitrogen mustard, Oncovin, procarbazine, prednisone) plus irradiation, compared with 0% for 84 patients given ABVD (Adriamycin, bleomycin, vinblastine, and decarbazine). This is a most interesting finding but needs to be confirmed with a study of more patients and longer observation.

Non-Hodgkin's Lymphoma

Rosner et al. (1979) reported on 45 patients with non- Hodgkin's lymphoma and acute leukemia. In five, the two diseases occurred simultaneously. Among the 40 patients in whom leukemia developed later, 22 had received both radio- therapy and chemotherapy, 8 had had chemotherapy only, and 10 had had radiotherapy only. Acute myeloblastic or myelomono- cytic leukemia was identified in 23 patients and erythroleu- kemia in 5.

Chronic Lymphocytic Leukemia

In 1977, Zarrabi et al. reviewed the reports of 41 pa- tients with chronic lymphocytic leukemia in whom acute leu- kemia developed. In 10, however, the two diseases occurred simultaneously or within 4 months of each other. The mean age of the patients was 64.6 years, and the mean interval from the diagnosis of chronic lymphocytic leukemia to the recognition of acute leukemia was 5.6 years. Ten patients had lymphoblastic leukemia and five had myeloblastic or mye- lomonocytic leukemia.

The significance of the association of acute leukemia with chronic lymphocytic leukemia is not clear. At the pres- ent time, one cannot definitely implicate chemotherapy; acute leukemia may represent the natural course of chronic lympho- cytic leukemia.

Acute Lymphocytic Leukemia

In a 5-year review, Mosijczuk and Ruymann (1981) found 33 patients with acute lymphocytic leukemia in whom a second malignant lesion had developed. Histiocytic medullary reticulosis occurred in seven, Hodgkin's disease in four, another acute leukemia in nine, and chronic myelocytic leukemia in four. In the remaining nine patients, a nonhematologic malignancy developed.

Carcinoma of the Breast

In a 1979 review of 78 patients with cancer of the breast and acute leukemia, Rosner et al. found 8 in whom the diseases occurred simultaneously. Of the other 70, 45 had received radiotherapy, 8 chemotherapy, 10 both radiotherapy and chemotherapy, 7 excision, and 6 endocrinologic ablation. The mean interval from the diagnosis of carcinoma to the development of leukemia was 7 years. Most patients in whom leukemia developed after cancer of the breast have received radiation or chemotherapy (or both).

Carcinoma of the Ovary

In a survey of 70 institutions participating in a study of alkylating agent therapy in advanced ovarian carcinoma, Reimer et al. (1977) found 13 patients with acute nonlymphocytic leukemia among the 5,455 patients. The expected number of cases was 0.62 (relative risk was 21). Nine of the 13 patients had received radiation therapy, and all 9 had been treated with various alkylating agents, including phenylalanine mustard, chlorambucil, cyclophosphamide, thiotepa, and uracil mustard.

Other Malignancies

In a double-blind study of 726 patients with bronchogenic carcinoma, 4 of the 243 patients treated with busulfan developed acute leukemia, but none of those given cyclophosphamide or placebo did so. Acute leukemia also has been noted with carcinoma of the bladder, carcinoma of the tonsil, malignant melanoma, and leiomyosarcoma.

Chlorambucil appears to have a role in acute leukemia associated with polycythemia vera. In a prospective random- ized study, the risk of acute leukemia among patients treated with chlorambucil was 2.3 times greater than that among those treated with radioactive phosphorus and 13.5 times greater than that among those treated with phlebotomy alone (Berk et al. 1981).

Nonneoplastic Diseases

In 1979, Grünwald and Rosner described 61 patients with nonneoplastic disease whose treatment with chemotherapeutic agents terminated in acute leukemia. The mean age of the pa- tients at primary diagnosis was 42 years (range 6 months to 71 years). One-third of the patients had rheumatoid arthri- tis, and another third had nephropathy or had undergone renal transplantation. The remainder of the patients had multiple sclerosis, psoriasis, Wegener's granulomatosis, amyloidosis, scleroderma, systemic lupus erythematosus, pyoderma gangreno- sum, cold agglutinin disease, malignant exophthalmos, chronic active hepatitis, scleromyxedema, and temporal arteritis. More than two-thirds of the patients had acute myeloblastic or myelomonocytic leukemia. Thirty patients received only alkylating agents (chlorambucil 17, cyclophosphamide 8, mel- phalan 4, and busulfan 1), and 10 were given only antimetabo- lites (azathioprine 8, mercaptopurine 1, and aminopterin 1). Eighteen patients were treated with multiple agents selected from those listed above as well as mechlorethamine hydrochlo- ride, methotrexate, uracil mustard, dactinomycin, or radia- tion. Two patients received total-body radiation. Two pa- tients were given intra-articular radioisotopes, and one pa- tient was treated with iodine-131 for hyperthyroidism $4\frac{1}{2}$ years before the appearance of acute leukemia. The mean du- ration of chemotherapy was 40 months (range 4 to 45). The mean interval from the onset of chemotherapy to the develop- ment of acute leukemia was 4.8 years (range 9 months to 18 years).

NON-HODGKIN'S LYMPHOMA AFTER CHEMOTHERAPY

In 1979, Krikorian et al. described six patients with non-Hodgkin's lymphoma who had been treated for Hodgkin's disease. Five of the six were from a group of 579 patients with Hodgkin's disease treated at Stanford University Medical

Center. All six had received chemotherapy and radiation for the Hodgkin's disease, and none had evidence of that disorder when the non-Hodgkin's disease was recognized. Four had diffuse, undifferentiated lymphoma, and two had a diffuse histiocytic lymphoma. The 10-year actuarial risk of non-Hodgkin's lymphoma in Hodgkin's disease was 4.4%, whereas the risk of acute leukemia was 2.0%.

Non-Hodgkin's lymphoma has been diagnosed in a number of patients with dermatomyositis, systemic lupus erythematosus, and rheumatoid arthritis. However, the chemotherapy may not have affected the development of non-Hodgkin's lymphoma in these patients.

OTHER TUMORS DEVELOPING AFTER CHEMOTHERAPY

Although the incidence of acute leukemia among patients given chemotherapy is elevated, there is no evidence that the incidence of solid tumors in patients treated with various chemotherapeutic agents is increased except for bladder cancer.

Bladder cancer after the administration of cyclophosphamide was found in 22 patients (Durkee, Benson 1980; West 1976). Most of the patients had transitional cell carcinoma, but squamous cell, epidermoid, and anaplastic carcinomas have been reported. In two patients, multiple myeloma was diagnosed after radiation therapy for carcinoma of the breast (Yeh, Axelrod 1979). In two patients, osteogenic sarcoma was recognized after long remission of Hodgkin's disease (Niebrugge et al. 1981).

DISCUSSION

The relationship between the use of chemotherapeutic agents and the development of a second unrelated malignant lesion is not well understood. There is no question that the incidence of acute leukemia is increased in patients with multiple myeloma or Hodgkin's disease who have been given chemotherapy.

The cause of the second malignancy is not known. Alkylating agents are potent mutagens and can damage DNA, similar to radiation. The acute granulocytic or myelomonocytic type

of leukemia that usually appears as the second malignancy is
the kind that would be expected from radiomimetic agents.
Immunosuppression from alkylating agents also may have a
role, as suggested by the increased incidence of lymphoma
among recipients of organ transplants who have been treated
with immunosuppressive drugs. Chemotherapy may activate a
normal oncogene. There is also the possibility that retro-
viruses have a role in the leukemic transformation of normal
cells. However, prolongation of survival by chemotherapy for
malignant disease may permit patients with myeloma or other
tumors to develop acute leukemia or malignant lymphoma. Yet,
the infrequency of acute leukemia with multiple myeloma or
Hodgkin's disease before the advent of alkylating agent therapy makes that possibility unlikely. The development of
acute leukemia in patients receiving long-term chemotherapy
probably is related to the use of alkylating agents. The incidence is relatively low, however, and in patients with multiple myeloma and Hodgkin's disease, the risk of chemotherapy
is well justified.

The physician must carefully weigh the risk of leukemia
or lymphoma in patients with malignant diseases who are
treated with adjuvant chemotherapy in an effort to reduce the
incidence of metastatic disease. The ultimate value of adjuvant chemotherapy can be determined only from a long-term
assessment of improved survival, balanced against the side
effects of chemotherapy. Great caution must be exercised in
giving adjuvant chemotherapy to patients at low risk of relapse, such as those with carcinoma of the breast and negative axillary lymph nodes. The long-term risks of iatrogenic
cancer in children also must be carefully assessed.

Another matter of great concern is the use of alkylating
agents in the treatment of nonmalignant diseases such as
rheumatoid arthritis, systemic lupus erythematosus, nephrop-
athies, and dermatologic diseases. The increasingly frequent
diagnosis of acute leukemia in these cases almost certainly
reflects increasing incidence of this fatal complication.
Consequently, alkylating agents should not be used for benign
conditions.

Perhaps better recognition of preleukemic states would
be helpful. Limiting chemotherapy to as short a duration as
possible may reduce the incidence of leukemia. Combination
chemotherapy and radiation seems to have a significant part
in the development of acute leukemia and should be avoided if

possible. Various combinations of chemotherapeutic agents having lesser potential for the development of malignancies should be sought. In the final analysis, one must weigh carefully the benefits and the long-term toxicity--including development of a second malignancy--before embarking on a course of chemotherapy.

REFERENCES

Berk PD, Goldberg JD, Silverstein MN, Weinfeld A, Donovan PB, Ellis JT, Landaw SA, Laszlo J, Najean Y, Pisciotta AV, Wasserman LR (1981). Increased incidence of acute leukemia in polycythemia vera associated with chlorambucil therapy. N Engl J Med 304:441.
Brody RS, Schottenfeld D (1980). Multiple primary cancers in Hodgkin's disease. Semin Oncol 7:187.
Casciato DA, Scott JL (1979). Acute leukemia following prolonged cytotoxic agent therapy. Medicine (Baltimore) 58:32.
Durkee C, Benson R Jr (1980). Bladder cancer following administration of cyclophosphamide. Urology 16:145.
Grünwald HW, Rosner F (1979). Acute leukemia and immunosuppressive drug use: a review of patients undergoing immunosuppressive therapy for non-neoplastic diseases. Arch Intern Med 139:461.
Krikorian JG, Burke JS, Rosenberg SA, Kaplan HS (1979). Occurrence of non-Hodgkin's lymphoma after therapy for Hodgkin's disease. N Engl J Med 300:452.
Kyle RA, Pierre RV, Bayrd ED (1970). Multiple myeloma and acute myelomonocytic leukemia: report of four cases possibly related to melphalan. N Engl J Med 283:1121.
Kyle RA, Pierre RV, Bayrd ED (1975). Multiple myeloma and acute leukemia associated with alkylating agents. Arch Intern Med 135:185.
McIntyre OR, Pajak TF, Wiernik P, Glowienka LP, Cornwell GG, Harley J, Leone L (1981). Delayed acute leukemia in myeloma patients receiving pulsed vs. continuous treatment (abstract). Blood 58 Suppl 1:167a.
McKenna RW, Parkin JL, Foucar K, Brunning RD (1981). Ultrastructural characteristics of therapy-related acute non-lymphocytic leukemia: evidence for a panmyelosis. Cancer 48:725.
Mosijczuk AD, Ruymann FB (1981). Second malignancy in acute lymphocytic leukemia: review of 33 cases. Am J Dis Child 135:313.

Niebrugge D, Monzon C, Perry MC, Hakami N (1981). Osteogenic sarcoma following Hodgkin's disease. Cancer 48:416.

Reimer RR, Hoover R, Fraumeni JF Jr, Young RC (1977). Acute leukemia after alkylating-agent therapy of ovarian cancer. N Engl J Med 297:177.

Rosner F, Grünwald H (1975). Hodgkin's disease and acute leukemia: report of eight cases and review of the literature. Am J Med 58:339.

Rosner F, Grünwald HW (October 1980a). Cytotoxic drugs and leukaemogenesis. Clin Haematol 9:663.

Rosner F, Grünwald HW (1980b). Multiple myeloma and Waldenström's macroglobulinemia terminating in acute leukemia: review with emphasis on karyotypic and ultrastructural abnormalities. NY State J Med 80:558.

Rosner F, Grünwald HW, Zarrabi MH (1979). Acute leukemia as a complication of cytotoxic chemotherapy. Int J Radiat Oncol Biol Phys 5:1705.

Rowley JD, Golomb HM, Vardiman JW (1981). Nonrandom chromosome abnormalities in acute leukemia and dysmyelopoietic syndromes in patients with previously treated malignant disease. Blood 58:759.

Valagussa P, Santoro A, Fossati Bellani F, Franchi F, Banfi A, Bonadonna G (1982). Absence of treatment-induced second neoplasms after ABVD in Hodgkin's disease. Blood 59:488.

West WO (1976). Acute erythroid leukemia after cyclophosphamide therapy for multiple myeloma: report of two cases. South Med J 69:1331.

Yeh GK, Axelrod MR (1979). Development of multiple myeloma in long term survivors of breast cancer. Clin Oncol 5:175.

Zarrabi MH, Grünwald HW, Rosner F (1977). Chronic lymphocytic leukemia terminating in acute leukemia. Arch Intern Med 137:1059.

CONGRESS SYMPOSIA

DESIGN AND EVALUATION OF CLINICAL TRIALS
Bonadonna, G., Italy, Chairman; Taylor, W.,
USA, Co-Chairman; Opera House

Adaptive Randomization Using the Biased Coin
Design: Evaluation in a Cooperative Group
Clinical Trial. *Hannigan, J. F., Jr. and
Brown, B. W., Jr., Palo Alto, CA USA.
(By Title Only)

Guidelines for Publishing Papers on Cancer
Clinical Trials: Responsibilities of Editors
and Authors. *Zelen, M., Boston, MA USA.

Methods for the Analysis of Time to Failure
Date. *Prentice, R. L., Seattle, WA USA.

Improved Approaches to Randomization in Clinical
Trials. *Bailar, J. C., III, Boston, MA USA.
(By Title Only)

Principles of the Organization of Trials in
Adjuvant Chemotherapy. *Garin, A. M., Moscow,
USSR. (By Title Only)

Please note: Papers that are listed as "By Title
Only" were presented at the 13th International
Cancer Congress, but are not included in these
volumes.

13th International Cancer Congress, Part E
Cancer Management, pages 57– 68
© **1983 Alan R. Liss, Inc., New York, NY 10011**

GUIDELINES FOR PUBLISHING PAPERS ON CANCER CLINICAL TRIALS:
RESPONSIBILITIES OF EDITORS AND AUTHORS

Marvin Zelen[1], Ph.D.

Harvard School of Public Health and the
Sidney Farber Cancer Institute
Boston, Massachusetts 02115

INTRODUCTION

One of the most important modern advances in experimental therapeutics is the development and widespread adoption of the use of the clinical trial to evaluate the benefits of new therapies as well as to confirm the utility of
therapies which have long been used. We define a clinical
trial as a scientific experiment to generate clinical data
for the purpose of evaluating one or more therapies on a
patient population. The main distinction between a clinical
trial and an observational study is that a clinical trial
will have a study design describing the patient population
and the manner in which the therapies will be allocated to
the patients, whereas in an observational study one is
simply noting a phenomenon. Clinical trials may be randomized, nonrandomized, multi-institution or single institution.

Cancer refers to many different disease sites, each
with different etiologies and natural histories. Therapeutic decisions may not only differ for each disease site,
but are critically dependent on whether the disease is local, regional, or metastatic. Decisions for secondary and
tertiary treatment of disease are particularly difficult,

1. This paper was written as part of the author's partici-
    pation in the Committee on Controlled Therapeutic Trials
    of the International Union Against Cancer and was sup-
    ported in part by grants from the U.S. Public Health Ser-
    vice CA-23415, CA-06516 from the National Cancer Institute.

due to the conflicting opinions of "experts" and the lack of unequivocal scientific evidence. Even decisions on primary treatment can be difficult. For example, consider the problems faced by the surgeon, radiation therapist, and medical oncologist in treating breast cancer. How should one choose optimal primary treatment? -- A mastectomy (radical or simple), lumpectomy followed by suitable radiotherapy? In addition to the problems of selecting optimal primary therapy, they must decide on the potential benefit of adjuvant chemotherapy. Is there unequivocal evidence that adjuvant chemotherapy significantly prolongs survival? Do postmenopausal women have the same potential benefit as premenopausal women? If the medical oncologist recommends adjuvant chemotherapy, what treatment should be chosen? How long should it be administered? Should the dose(s) be reduced as toxicity is observed? Should the recommendation depend on the patient's age and axillary node status? -- etc. etc.

The practicing oncologist must rely heavily on the published literature to help him make therapeutic decisions. There are too many cancer sites and the current views on the systemic treatment of disease may appear to be moving too quickly for most oncologists to have personal experience with "latest treatments". Furthermore, the reliance on the published literature by oncologists is likely to increase in the next decade. It is for this reason that editors of medical journals bear a special responsibility to insure that the clinical papers published in these journals be of high quality and not be misleading or ambiguous. The purpose of this paper is to propose guidelines to journal editors for the publication of results of clinical trials in cancer. Although these guidelines are put forth in the concept of cancer investigations, they apply equally to clinical trials in every disease. The adoption of these or similar guidelines will help raise the scientific quality of clinical trials by providing authors with an outline of what is expected by editors. Although these guidelines imply a focus on publication, it is hoped that adoption by editors will have major implications for the design, conduct, and analysis of clinical trials.

Editors of journals share a responsibility which many had not envisioned. Today, publication of papers on clinical investigations promptly affects the current practice of medicine. Unfortunately, even in the best journals, the normal standards for reporting clinical trials may not be entirely suitable. The upgrading of standards of publication is most important for eliminating those clinical papers which can do positive harm.

THE EFFECT OF THE 5% FALSE-POSITIVE RATE

In nearly all medical journals, it is necessary to make a minimum statistical analysis before editors and referees will accept the conclusion that a treatment is "better" than or the "same" as another treatment. This requirement is usually carried out by using conventional statistical tests. The use of these statistical tests involves adopting a significance level which is commonly chosen as 5%. This 5% significance level is the false-positive rate, i.e., on the average, among 100 trials where there are no differences between the therapies, five trials will be reported as a positive.

The impact of the five-percent false positive rate can only be assessed if one knows how many clinical trials are currently in progress. The most recent NCI Compendium of Clinical Trials, published in 1982 (1), lists 1,544 Phase II and III studies currently accruing patients. This listing is composed mainly of trials from cooperative groups, comprehensive cancer centers, and other NCI funded clinical trials. If the time for accrual takes three years and there is a steady-state situation, one would expect approximately 500 new trials to be started per year. Thus, if the rate of reporting on trials was the same (500/year), then we would expect 5% of them (25) to be reported as positive if all 500 were null studies.

However, the false-positive rate is actually higher than 5%. The discussion in the previous paragraph assumed one statistical test per trial. Usually the statistical analysis of a clinical trial makes subgroup comparisons with many of the prognostic factors associated with the natural history of the disease. These factors usually include disease stage, pathology, demographic factors, etc. If two independent statistical tests are made, each with a 5% false-positive rate, the false-positive rate of the two is 10%. Thus, if one conservatively assumes two subgroup comparisons per trial, one would expect approximately 50 false-positive reports if all five hundred new trials which are analyzed are null trials.

Finally, one should note that the NCI Compendium is far from complete, and only represents a fraction of clinical trials currently being carried out. Also, these calculations do not take into account clinical trials which are biased because of poor experimental design and those for which improper conclusions are inadvertently made. Consequently, the expected number of false-positive therapies reported in the literature may be much higher.

One way to sift the true- from the false-positive results is to have independent confirmation of the clinical results. In nearly all scientific endeavors, a new experimental finding is regarded as tentative until it can be confirmed independently by other investigators. Unfortunately, independent confirmation of clinical investigations usually requires several years, and in some instances may not be feasible. Nevertheless, it should be done for clinical findings having major therapeutic impact.

Many journal editors are reluctant to publish articles which are confirmations of earlier published clinical trials. Confirmatory trials are not regarded as being as exciting or innovative as the first report of a therapeutic advance. If one is ever going to be able to sift out the true positive from the false-positive clinical findings, it is important for editors to take a more favorable attitude toward the publication of a well conducted confirmatory clinical trial. The publication of such confirmatory papers has an important impact on the everyday practice of oncology.

THE REPORTING OF CLINICAL TRIALS

While authors should make certain that the published report of a clinical trial is clear, journal editors and referees must be prepared to enforce this discipline. The paper by Der Simonian et al. (2) surveyed 67 clinical trials published in four leading medical journals with respect to the frequency of reporting of eleven important aspects of a clinical trial. They concluded that only 56 percent of these eleven items were clearly reported among the 67 published trials examined. In this section, a set of detailed guidelines is proposed for the guidance of authors, editors, reviewers, and readers.

1. Population Under Study. There should be clear statements describing the population under study. Major subgroups of patients who are excluded should be mentioned; e.g. "patients over age 65 were not eligible for the study".

2. Therapy. The reporting of the protocol therapy (especially chemotherapy) should be outlined in sufficient detail so that the therapy can be duplicated by another physician. Not only the contents of the written protocol, but also the therapy actually received by patients. This is especially important for chemotherapy, where full doses as written in a protocol may not often be given to patients. Summary measures such as: average dose per course, proportion of patients receiving incomplete courses, proportion of patients receiving full doses, average number of courses, etc. should be provided. If the written protocol provided for a de-escalation or escalation of dose(s) as a function of toxicity, details should be given. Also, information should be given on the toxicity criteria used to lower doses.

3. Study Design. The study design should be outlined. A schema, which is a pictorial display of the study design, is helpful to the reader. If the study is randomized, it is not sufficient to simply state that it was a randomized study. A statement should indicate how the randomization was carried out, e.g. central randomization, closed envelope, etc. The actual randomization scheme should be described. Occasionally a randomization schedule or procedure may be changed during the course of the study. If this was done, details should be given regarding the reasons for the change. If there is institutional balancing or other kinds of stratification, it should be so stated. The randomization schedule should be described, e.g. "permuted blocks of size four for each stratum". The source from which the randomization schedule was constructed should be given. Random number tables are preferred, but some studies use assignment procedures based on day of the month (even or odd days dictating treatment). There are many ways of executing a randomized trial, many of which are poor and often defeat the purposes of randomization. The paper should contain sufficient detail on this aspect of the trial so that the reader can verify whether indeed the randomization was carried out and designed properly.

4. Patient Accounting. There should be a detailed
accounting of all patients registered for the study. Registration should be carefully defined. How is a patient officially registered? Are all patients officially registered
prior to first day of treatment, within one week, one month,
etc? It is surprising to learn that in many single institution studies, nonrandomized registration may take place
months after the first day of teatment. This leaves open
the possibility that not all patients on a protocol are
registered. In a randomized study, patients are registered
from the moment of randomization. Nonrandomized studies
should have similarly precise rules for registration. Failure of any study to have a stated registration system should
be an automatic rejection of the paper for publication.

The number of patients who are classified as cancelled
or unevaluable should be given by treatment. A cancelled
patient is defined as a registered patient who withdrew
from the study before the first day of treatment. An
unevaluable patient may be one who has incomplete information. Some studies classify an unevaluable patient as one
who has major deviations from the protocol. If the reasons
for patients being classified as cancelled or unevaluable
are related to the treatment assignment, then it is mandatory that all patients be included in the treatment comparisons. Otherwise the selective inclusion of patients
may result in wrong conclusions being drawn from the study.

5. Follow-up. The follow-up period for the patients
should be given separately for each treatment. Statistics
should be included on the average follow-up time, number
followed for one, two years, etc., and maximum and minimum
follow-up times. The number of patients lost to follow-up
and the reasons should be reported for each treatment. If
a relatively large number of patients is lost to follow-up
(say 10%), then statements about long-term effects may not
be correct.

6. Data Quality. There should be a discussion of the
quality control methods used for the data. Was there
Second Party Review? A Second Party Review is defined as a
patient data review by individuals other than the investigator generating the patient record. This could be carried
out by the study chairman or a special committee. If there
were a central data management, it should be mentioned.
The review should be centered on answering three major

questions for each patient. -- Was the patient eligible?
-- Was the protocol followed? -- Was there objective documentation of the major endpoints? There should be statements about the quality control of surgery if these treatment modalities were involved in the study. Such quality
control can be carried out using panels. Similar remarks
hold for pathology panels. The names of the individuals
involved in independent quality control efforts should be
mentioned. The editor and readers are relying on these
individuals' scientific integrity attesting to the quality
control of the patient data. They should not be anonymous.
Editors should encourage authors to have a mechanism for
Second Party Review of patient data. This is a characteristic of a high quality study.

7. Endpoints and Censored Data. Trials in which the
endpoints of evaluating therapy are survival and disease-
free survival may often have patients with incomplete data.
This happens if patients are still alive or in the disease-
free state at the time of analysis. Such observations are
called censored observations. Several situations arise in
defining censored observations which could seriously skew
the results. We mention only two which are in widespread
use and could lead to incorrect conclusions. The first of
these is when a patient dies from a cause other than cancer, e.g. cardiovascular disease, suicide, etc. The other
arises when a patient is switched off the therapy protocol
onto some other therapy which may be more beneficial. When
there are appreciable numbers of patients dying from competing causes of death, it could seriously alter the conclusions of a study if these patients were treated as censored observations. The cancer may have been an important
contributing factor. Also, there is little need to demonstrate that a relatively poor therapy can be made to look
outstanding if, just before the endpoint is likely to be
reached, the patient is taken off study. It is unfortunate
that such practices are widespread. It is for this reason
that the report of a clinical trial should indicate the
reasons for classifying patients as censored when the classification arises other than the usual situation where not
enough follow-up time has elapsed to have a complete observation.

NONRANDOMIZED STUDIES

Nonrandomized studies require special discussion. The
evaluation of the experimental therapy is usually made by
comparing the results to an historical control group. In
order for the analysis to be valid, the control group must
be comparable to the experimental therapy group with regard
to all major factors which affect the outcome. In making
the comparison, one must be aware that there may be biases
in one group not found in the other. These biases may be
of such magnitude that they could obviate any confidence in
conclusions drawn from the study. However, there may be
some diseases in which the prognosis is so predictably poor
that any significant improvements can easily be associated
with the intervention rather than possible sources of bias;
e.g. the successful cure of rabies in a single nonrandom patient. Unfortunately, very few trials are of this kind.
The great bulk of nonrandomized studies requires comparison
with an historical control group.

Publications on nonrandomized studies should include a
discussion of the possible sources of bias which have the
potential for altering the main conclusions of the study.
Here we list six such common potential sources of bias, but
this list is incomplete.

  (i)   Physician Selection Bias. Physicians can bias
        results by selecting patients for entry into
        study. If there is physician selection bias,
        it would be important to have a discussion as
        to how this selection could bias results.

  (ii) Patient Bias. Patients who do give patient
        consent constitute a subgroup of patients who
        are self-selected. This bias is not present
        in the historical control group.

  (iii) Diagnosis and Staging Bias. Methods and cri-
        teria must be the same for both treatment and
        historical control groups. If not, how do devi-
        ations affect conclusions?

  (iv) Supportive Care and Patient Management. It is
        doubtful whether this would be the same for both
        the treatment and historical groups. A discus-
        sion should bring out the main differences and

state how important the differences are with
respect to the main conclusions of the study.

(v) <u>Patient Evaluation and Quality of Follow-up.</u>
What effect do different methods of patient
evaluation and follow-up have on the use of the
historical control group?

(vi) <u>Prognostic Factor Bias.</u> The patient population
for both the historical and experimental therapy
groups should be approximately the same. Details should be given comparing major prognostic factors for each group.

THE STATISTICAL ANALYSIS OF CLINICAL TRIALS

The report on therapeutic benefit should be presented
so that there is no ambiguity if a treatment difference refers to the entire patient population or to special subgroups of patients. It is necessary that the analysis consider all known major prognostic factors which can affect
the outcome. Otherwise there may be disappointment when the
therapy is applied in practice. The comparison of proportions, survival curves, etc. must be made using objective
statistical procedures. If a complicated statistical model
is used, it should be described in the paper or in an appendix. The description of the statistical methods must be
adequate enough so that another statistician could reproduce
the analysis if the source data were available.

When the paper uses a new statistical technique which
was derived for the clinical trial paper being reviewed,
brief details must be presented in the text of the paper or
in an appendix. Otherwise it may be impossible for anyone
to substantiate the results.

The outcome of statistical tests depends on both the
existence of a true difference and the number of patients
in the study. If the number of patients is small, then the
study will have low sensitivity (power) to detect small or
moderate treatment differences. Failure to find statistical
significance may be due to small numbers, rather than lack
of a difference. It is for this reason that every paper
should have a discussion of statistical power and how it can
influence the conclusions of the paper.

The analysis should also contain a discussion relating to the termination of patient entry to the study. For example, was the trial (or part of the trial) stopped because of an unusual outcome associated with a treatment -- a very good or poor treatment? Was patient accrual terminated after a predetermined number of patients entered the trial? All of these affect the reader's interpretation of the study conclusions.

EARLY REPORTING OF STUDIES

It is not uncommon for a study to be published with inadequate follow-up time. This arises when the investigators believe they have demonstrated a therapeutic advance and wish to communicate their findings promptly. Such papers should only be accepted for publication if the study chairman or senior author agrees to continue to follow the patients. He should be obligated to review the new data to make certain that the initial conclusions have not changed with additional follow-up information.

An early significant result can occur due to statistical fluctuations or because of large real differences between treatments. It is only with additional follow-up that one can determine whether the initial reported conclusions are sustained and are not attributed to unusual statistical fluctuations. Furthermore, questions of long-term survival or delayed toxicity can only be answered with longer follow-up.

It is recommended that editors make an agreement with the senior investigator or study chairman of the submitted paper that the patients in the study will be followed for a reasonable period of time. The senior investigator will be obligated to review the new information with regard to its impact on the conclusions of the original paper. At designated periods, the senior author must communicate to the editor a brief summary of his review. If the conclusions change significantly with follow-up, the editor could publish a letter or a brief communication from the principal investigator. Otherwise the editor need take no action. Failure of the senior author to write the editor at the prescribed times would require the editor to publish a brief note that no communication has been received. Of course, the editor would use discretion in allowing for lateness due to unforeseen delays.

If this recommendation is adopted by medical journals, it will make clear to all investigators that early reporting of clinical trials carries responsibility for longer term reporting. Failure to have such a strong requirement will perpetuate the widespread practice of early and often premature reporting of dramatic findings. Many of these early dramatic findings may disappear with additional follow-up, but the readers of the journal in which the original paper was published could well be unaware of the change.

A. B. Miller, commenting on an earlier draft of this paper, suggested that an early report of a clinical trial must be accompanied by a clear statement that the results are preliminary and a more definitive analysis must await longer follow-up time. The authors should be specific about the number of years of follow-up required with a statement that a paper will be submitted for publication after sufficient follow-up time has elapsed.

CONCLUSIONS

This paper has laid out guidelines for editors (and their referees) in accepting papers on cancer clinical trials for publication. The adoption of these or similar guidelines will substantially aid editors in their selection process. It undoubtedly would delay publication of many studies but the delays would be for studies that should not be published in their original form anyway. An expectation is that substandard trials would not even be submitted to journals adopting the guidelines in this paper. Perhaps the most important result is that practicing physicians would be better able to decide when they should adopt new therapies. Their decision to use new therapies will depend in part on the confidence they have in the journals which publish these therapeutic advances.

ACKNOWLEDGEMENT

The author is grateful to Drs. John Bailar, Robert Flamant, Anthony Miller, John Simes, Don Switz, and Emmanuel van der Schueren, who read an earlier draft of this paper and made many constructive suggestions.

REFERENCES

1. International Cancer Research Data Bank, <u>Compilation</u>
    <u>of Cancer Therapy Protocol Summaries</u>, 6th edition,
    1982. NIH Publication No. 80-1116.
2. Der Simonian, R et al. Reporting Methods in Clinical
    Trials, New England Journal of Medicine 306:1332-
    1337 (1982).

13th International Cancer Congress, Part E
Cancer Management, pages 69–79

METHODS FOR THE ANALYSIS OF TIME TO FAILURE DATA

R.L. Prentice

Fred Hutchinson Cancer Research Center, 1124
Columbia Street, Seattle, Wa., 98104 and
Department of Biostatistics, University of Wash.

1. INTRODUCTION

The past decade has seen very substantial developments
in the methodology for the analysis of time to 'failure'
data. 'Failure' is used generically and may, for example,
represent remission, relapse, major infection incidence or
death in a cancer therapy trial, or may represent disease
diagnosis in a cancer prevention trial or in an epidemiologic
cohort study. Distinguishing features of failure time data
include the usual presence of right censoring, as occurs
when a subject is without failure throughout the study
follow-up period or is lost to follow-up, and the fact that
various study subject characteristics (e.g., blood cell
counts, immune function measures, performance status, or
cumulative exposure estimates) may be monitored over the
follow-up period. Classical statistical procedures are not
well suited to the accommodation of such data features.

An important stimulus to the development of powerful
and flexible failure time data methods was provided by the
paper by Cox (1972). This paper proposed a regression method
for failure time data that will, here, be referred to as the
relative risk regression method, though it is sometimes referred to as the Cox regression method, or as the proportional
hazards regression method in view of an important special
case. The purpose of this paper is to describe and illustrate the use of the relative risk regression method. A
number of desirable properties and flexibilities will be
brought out. In particular it is the author's point of view
that such methodology provides the best currently available

approach to the quantification of treatment effects and toward the explanation of treatment differences in terms of 'intermediate' response variables or patient characteristics. Furthermore, the relative risk regression method provides a unified approach to the analysis of failure time data from clinical studies, from animal follow-up studies, from epidemiologic cohort studies and even from time-matched case-control studies.

2. ESTIMATION AND COMPARISON OF SURVIVAL CURVES

Let $T > 0$ denote a failure time random variable, with survivor function $F(t) = pr(T \geq t)$ and failure rate (hazard) function

$$\lambda(t) = \lim_{\Delta t \to 0} (\Delta t)^{-1} pr(T < t + \Delta t | T \geq t)$$

$$= - d \log F(t)/dt .$$

Suppose now that a group of subjects are followed forward from some time origin $t = 0$ (e.g., time of entry into a clinical trial) and that distinct failures occur at times $t_1 < t_2 < \cdots < t_k$. Suppose further that d_i failures occur at t_i, $i = 1, \ldots, k$ and that n_i subjects are at risk (i.e., under follow-up and without failure) just prior to time t_i. Based on such data the Kaplan-Meier (1958) survival curve estimator is given by

$$\hat{F}(t) = \prod_{i | t_i < t} \left(\frac{n_i - d_i}{n_i} \right)$$

assuming an independent censoring mechanism; that is, assuming, at any t, that the failure rate for subjects without censoring is equal to that for the study population as a whole.

In addition to the graphical display of estimated survivor functions one is frequently interested in formal comparisons of two or more survival curves. Censored data rank tests are most frequently used for this purpose. Tests in common usage, for the comparison of two survival curves, can be written

$$v = \sum_{i=1}^{k} w_i (d_{1i} - d_i n_{1i} n_i^{-1})$$

where, continuing the above notation, d_{1i} and n_{1i} are the number of failures and the number of subjects at risk at t_i, respectively, in the first of the two groups, $i=1,\ldots,k$ and w_i is a weighting factor associated with the ith failure time that may depend on the failure and censoring data prior to t_i. The special case in which $w_i \equiv 1$ has come to be known as the logrank test (Mantel, 1966; Peto and Peto, 1972) while a suitable censored data generalization of the Wilcoxon statistic (Peto and Peto, 1972; Prentice, 1978) is given by

$$w_i = \prod_{i|t_i < t} \left(\frac{n_i - d_i + 1}{n_i + 1} \right) .$$

Note that, under the hypothesis of equality of the two survival curves, $d_i n_{1i} n_i^{-1}$ is the expected number of failures in the first group given the risk set sizes and the total number of failures at t_i. The statistic v is therefore a weighted sum, over the k distinct failure points, of the observed minus the (conditionally) expected number of failures in the first group. A corresponding 'hypergeometric' variance estimator can be written

$$V = \sum_{i=1}^{k} w_i^2 \frac{n_{1i}}{n_i} \left(1 - \frac{n_{1i}}{n_i} \right) \left(d_i \frac{n_i - d_i}{n_i - 1} \right) ,$$

whence $v'V^{-1}v$ can be compared to χ^2 tables in order to test the hypothesis of survival curve equality. A natural generalization exists for the comparison of more than two survival curves.

   The comparison of two survival curves may be adjusted for potential confounding factors by stratifying the study population into a fixed number, m, of strata, by calculating the value of a censored rank test v_s and its corresponding variance estimator V_s in each stratum, $s = 1,\ldots,m$, and by comparing

$$\left(\sum_{1}^{m} v_s \right)' \left(\sum_{1}^{m} V_s \right)^{-1} \left(\sum_{1}^{m} v_s \right)$$

to χ^2 tables. The stratified logrank test is often referred to as the Mantel-Haenszel (see Mantel and Haenszel, 1959) test. The reader is referred to Latta (1981) for a study of the small sample properties of these and related tests and to Peto, et al (1977) for a detailed discussion of the application of the logrank test to the analysis of clinical trials.

3. REGRESSION ANALYSIS OF FAILURE TIME DATA

3.1 Motivation

A number of topics arise in the analysis of follow-up studies that cannot be readily addressed using only survival curve estimators or censored data rank tests. For example, sample sizes may not permit a detailed stratification on confounding factors in survival curve comparisons; quantification of treatment or exposure variable effects on failure time (or failure rate) may be an important study objective; identification of prognostic factors (or risk factors) and assessment of their relationship to failure rate may be of interest; the explanation of treatment effects on cancer patient survival (or exposure variable effects on cancer incidence or mortality) in terms of intermediate response variables (e.g., immune function, relapse status, major infection incidence) may be a worthy objective; similarly, the ability to study time-varying predictive variables in relation to cancer survival or incidence may be important; and finally, failure time data methods should be able to accommodate such special features as competing risks, multivariate failure times, nonstandard sampling designs and multiple testing procedures (e.g., sequential tests).

3.2 Approaches to Regression Modelling

Much of the early work on the regression modelling of failure time involved the use of parametric models such as Weibull and lognormal regression models. Most such models specify a linear relationship between log T and a fixed regression vector $z = (z_1, \ldots, z_p)$. Limitations of such an approach include the strong assumptions implicit in a fully parametrized model for T given z, and the lack of ability (except in very special cases) to accommodate time-varying regression variables and multivariate failure times. See Kalbfleisch and Prentice (1980, Chts. 2 and 3) and Lawless (1982) for details on such parametric regression models. Toward the detailed control of potential confounding factors epidemiologists frequently use discriminant analysis or related techniques in order to define a univariate score upon which strata can be defined for use in conjunction with a Mantel-Haenszel procedure. The relative risk regression method discussed below permits confounding factor control either by means of stratification or regression modelling

or both. It relaxes the modelling assumptions of the parametric regression approach in an important manner by allowing
an unrestricted 'baseline' failure rate function in each
stratum while modelling only the ratio of the failure rate
function to the baseline failure rate function; that is, while
modelling only the relative risk function. Furthermore, the
relative risk regression method provides a comprehensive,
unified and efficient approach to virtually all of the topics
mentioned in Section 3.1.

3.3 Relative Risk Regression

First consider a fixed regression vector $z=(z_1,...,z_p)$,
defined for each study subject. For example components of
z may be treatment indicators or prognostic factor levels.
Denote by $\lambda(t;z)$ the failure rate at time t for subjects with
regression vector z. Since primary interest usually centers
on comparison of failure rates (or, equivalently, comparison
of survival curves) one may select a 'baseline' regression
vector $z_0 = (z_{10},...,z_{p0})$ to serve as a standard for comparison. Let $\lambda_0(t) = \lambda(t;z_0)$ denote the corresponding 'baseline'
failure rate function. The relative failure rate, or more
simply the relative risk, at time t for a subject with
regression vector z, compared to a subject with the standard
regression vector z_0 is then defined by

$$RR(t,z) = \lambda(t,z)/\lambda_0(t) \quad .$$

More generally each study subject may have a time-varying
regression variable. Let $z(u) = \{z_1(u),...,z_p(u)\}$ denote the
regression vector value at follow-up time u. For example,
in a cancer clinical trial involving immunosuppressive drugs,
components of $z(u)$ may include blood counts, immune response
measures, infection occurrence indicators or performance
status measurements. Let $Z(t) = \{z(u); 0 \le u < t\}$ denote
the subject's entire covariate history from time 0 up to time
t. The failure rate, $\lambda\{t;Z(t)\}$, at time t for a subject with
covariate history $Z(t)$, relative to that for a subject with a
'baseline' history $Z_0(t) = \{z_0(u); 0 \le u < t\}$ will be denoted
$RR\{t,Z(t)\}$, whence

$$\lambda\{t;Z(t)\} = \lambda_0(t) \; RR\{t,Z(t)\}$$

where, as before, $\lambda_0 = \lambda\{t;Z_0(t)\}$.

Modelling assumptions now enter through the specification of a parametric form for $RR\{t,Z(t)\}$. The most commonly used parametrization, and the form used in Cox's (1972) key paper, specifies

$$RR\{t,Z(t)\} = \exp\{x(t)\beta\}$$

where $x(t) = \{x_1(t),\ldots,x_q(t)\}$ is a data-analyst defined function of t and $Z(t)$, and β is a corresponding column q-vector of parameters to be estimated. In some applications a linear relative risk form

$$RR\{t,Z(t)\} = 1 + x(t)\beta$$

may lead to a simpler or more readily interpreted description of the data. Various other parametric forms, $r\{x(t)\beta\} \geq 0$ with fixed function $r(\cdot)$, can also be entertained. Note that it is unnecessary to place any restrictions on the baseline failure rate function $\lambda_0(\cdot)$. Note also that with the exponential relative risk form, the interpretation of the regression parameter β is entirely independent of the choice of baseline covariate Z_0.

Consider now estimation of the regression parameter β. Continuing the notation of Section 2, denote by F_i the set of d_i subjects failing at t_i while R_i denotes the set of subjects at risk just prior to t_i. A partial likelihood function (Cox, 1975) for β can then be written

$$L(\beta) = \prod_{i=1}^{k} \frac{\prod_{\ell \in F_i} RR_\beta\{t_i, Z_\ell(t_i)\}}{\left(\prod_{\ell \in R_i} RR_\beta\{t_i, Z_\ell(t_i)\} \right)^{d_i}}$$

upon applying an approximation (Breslow, 1974) to accommodate tied failure times. In this expression $RR_\beta\{t,Z(t)\}$ denotes some parametric specification of the relative risk function with parameter β. Much recent work has been devoted to showing that standard asymptotic likelihood methods may be applied to $L(\beta)$. For the exponential relative risk form, $\exp\{x(t)\beta\}$, notable recent efforts include Tsiatis (1981) and particularly Andersen and Gill (1982) while Prentice and Self (1982) have generalized these results to include other parametric regression forms $r\{x(t)\beta\} \geq 0$. Other important work (e.g., Efron, 1977; Oakes, 1977) show that inferences based on $L(\beta)$ generally have good efficiency properties. The book by Kalbfleisch and Prentice (1980) provides a detailed discussion of the theory and application of the relative risk regression method and describes other generalizations.

3.4 Application

In order to illustrate the data analysis methods outlined above consider the survival of severe aplastic anemia patients receiving bone marrow transplants at the Fred Hutchinson Cancer Research Center. The author is grateful to Dr. Rainer Storb for permission to use these data for this illustration. Most of the analyses described below are extracted from the submitted manuscript by Storb et al (1982).

The analyses given below involve 130 aplastic anemia patients who received bone marrow grafts from HLA matched sibling donors and who achieved sustained engraftment. The follow-up periods for these patients ranges from 1 year to over 11 years. A total of 33 of the 130 patients have died. Consider the relationship between the randomized placement into the protective environment of a laminar air flow (LAF) room and patient survival. Figure 1 shows Kaplan-Meier survival curves for the 39 patients (5 deaths) placed in LAF rooms and the 91 patients (28 deaths) not so placed. The sum of conditionally expected numbers of deaths among LAF patients is 11.1 under the null hypothesis giving rise to a logrank test with (asymptotic) significance level p=0.03.

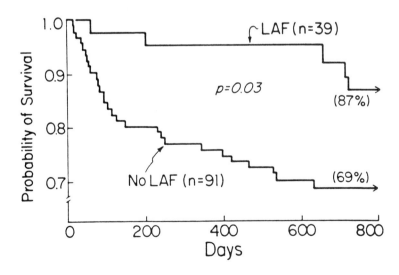

Figure 1. Estimated Survival of Patients Treated Inside
   Laminar Air Flow Rooms Compared to That of Patients
   Treated Outside. 'Days' Represents Days from Bone
   Marrow Transplantation.

    Relative risk regression analyses were conducted in
order to quantify the apparent survival improvement among LAF
patients and in order to 'adjust' the survival curve comparison of Fig. 1 for possible prognostic factors. Table 1
gives results of two such analyses. In each the failure time
variate is days from bone marrow transplantation while the
fixed regression vector consists of binary variates for LAF
assignment, for whether or not patients are refractory to
platelet transfusions from random donors (pre-transplant),
whether or not patient and donor are sex matched, whether the
patient has been previously transfused and whether or not
donor-derived buffy coat cells were infused with the bone
marrow. The regression vector also includes patient age in
10-year units. The analysis labelled Model 1 involves a
single stratum. The model presumes that each of the factors
listed exercises at most a multiplicative effect on the failure
rate. Table 1 lists these estimated multiplicative relative
risk factors. Note that patients in LAF rooms have an estimated 30% death rate compared to those not so assigned (p=0.01)
according to this model, while refractoriness to random
platelets and patient age appear to be very strong survival
predictors (e.g., death rate is estimated to increase by a
factor of 1.86 with each increase of 10 years in patient age).
The patient accrual period for this study is over 10 years in
duration. More recent patients tend to be a shorter time
from diagnosis and to be less likely to be transfused. It
then seems important to accommodate calendar time in such
analysis. The analyses listed under Model 2 extend the Model 1
analyses by stratifying on transplant date in two-year intervals. Relative risk estimates are wholly based on comparisons among patients transplanted within two years of each
other. It is evident that such stratification does not
noticeably affect either the relative risk estimates or their
corresponding significance levels.

Table 1. Relative Risk (RR) Regression Analysis of LAF and
   Other Factors in Relation to Patient Survival. Significance
   Levels Test the Hypothesis RR=1.

Regression Variable	(codes)	MODEL 1		MODEL 2	
		RR Estimate	(Sig. Level)	RR Estimate	(Sig. Level)
Laminar Air Flow	(0-no, 1-yes)	0.30	(0.01)	0.26	(0.01)
Refractory to Random Platelets	(0-no, 1-yes)	3.06	(0.0004)	2.91	(0.009)
Patient Age	(Yrs./10)	1.86	(<0.0001)	1.86	(0.0004)
Sex Matched	(0-yes, 1-no)	1.66	(0.18)	1.56	(0.26)
Previous Transfusions	(0-yes, 1-no)	0.77	(0.62)	0.95	(0.93)
Added Donor Buffy Coat	(0-yes, 1-no)	1.25	(0.57)	1.36	(0.57)

   This regression model framework can now be used to
systematically examine, and to generalize as necessary, the
modelling assymptions involved in Table 1. For example, the
assumption that relative risks for each factor are constant
over follow-up time can be relaxed by defining the regression
vector x(t) to consist of the sum of the fixed vector z times
an indicator variable for day zero to day 120 from bone marrow
transplantation plus the same regression vector times an
indicator for day 120 or later. Such modelling merely allows
each of the relative risks of Table 1 to differ before and
after day 120; day 120 was chosen to give approximately equal
numbers of deaths before and after. Without showing the full
results of these analyses it can be commented that the estimated relative risk corresponding to LAF is 0.10 (p=0.03)
before day 120 as opposed to 0.58 (p=0.35) after day 120. One
might anticipate such a pattern since patients are isolated
for a minimum of 50 days and rarely for more than 100 days
following grafting. Similarly the presumed constancy of the
relative risk for LAF over other patient or treatment elements
could be examined by including product terms in the regression
vector. If all the relative risks in Table 1 are permitted to

differ between younger and older patients one obtains a relative risk estimate for LAF of 0.19 (p=0.13) for the 72 patients (13 deaths) under 20 years of age and, in close agreement, a relative risk estimate of 0.24 (p=0.03) for 57 older patients (20 deaths).

Now consider the use of time-dependent regression variables in an attempt to gain insight into the mechanism whereby LAF isolation apparently gives rise to improved patient survival. The major complication experienced by patients with sustained engraftment is the possible occurrence of severe acute graft-versus-host-disease (GVHD). One might ask whether the LAF placement gives rise to reduced incidence, or delayed incidence of acute GVHD. A relative risk regression analysis with the same predictor variables as in Table 1, but with days to severe acute GVHD as failure time variable gives rise to an estimated relative risk of 0.46 (p=0.02) for LAF placement (p=0.05 for corresponding logrank test). One might, however, proceed further to examine whether reduced GVHD incidence wholly accounts for the survival improvement or whether, for example, patients with severe GVHD are protected by LAF placement from the major or minor infections that are frequently the proximate cause of death for patients in the first few months following marrow transplantation. For this purpose a time-dependent component is added to the regression analysis of Table 1 (Model 1). This component took value zero until severe acute GVHD was diagnosed and value one thereafter. After such inclusion the relative risk estimate corresponding to LAF assignment was 0.29 (0.02) overall with the even smaller value of 0.12 (p=0.04) for the first 120 days from transplant. One may conclude that the beneficial role for LAF is not restricted to the apparent reduction in acute GVHD incidence. It is worth noting that the death rate increases by an estimated factor of 6.46 (p<0.0001) upon diagnosis of severe GVHD.

This work was supported by NIH grants GM-28314, GM-24472 CA-15704, CA-30924 and CA-18221.

References

Andersen PK and Gill RD (1982). Cox's regression model for counting processes: a large sample study. To appear, Ann Statist, December 1982.
Breslow NE (1974). Covariance analysis of censored survival data. Biometrics 30:89.
Cox DR (1972). Regression models and life tables (with discussion. J Roy Statist Soc B 34:187.

Cox DR (1975). Partial likelihood. Biometrika 62:269.

Efron B (1977). Efficiency of Cox's likelihood function for censored data. J Amer Statist Assoc 72:557.

Kalbfleisch JD and Prentice RL (1980). "The Statistical Analysis of Failure Time Data." New York: Wiley.

Kaplan EL and Meier P (1958). Nonparametric estimation from incomplete observations. J Amer Statist Assoc 53:457.

Latta RB (1981). A Monte Carlo study of some two-sample rank tests with censored data. J Amer Statist Assoc 76:713.

Lawless J (1982). "Statistical Models and Methods for Lifetime Data." New York: Wiley.

Mantel N (1966). Evaluation of survival data and two new rank order statistics arising in its consideration. Cancer Chemo Rep 50:163.

Mantel N and Haenszel W (1959). Statistical aspects of the analysis of data from retrospective study of disease. J Natl Cancer Inst 22:719.

Oakes D (1977). The asymptotic information in censored survival data. Biometrika 64:441.

Peto R and Peto J (1972). Asymptotically efficient rank invariant test procedures (with discussion). J Roy Statist Soc A 135:185.

Peto R, Pike MC, Armitage P, Breslow NE, Cox DR, Howard SV, Mantel N, McPherson K, Peto J and Smith PG (1977). Design and analysis of randomized clinical trials requiring prolonged observation on each patient. Part 2. Analysis and examples. Br J Cancer 35:1.

Prentice RL (1978). Linear rank tests with right censored data. Biometrika 65:167.

Prentice RL and Self SG (1982). Asymptotic distribution theory for Cox-type regression models with general relative risk form Submitted.

Storb R, Prentice RL, Buckner CD, Clift RA, Appelbaum F, Deeg J, Doney K, Hansen JA, Mason M, Sanders JE, Singer J, Sullivan K, Witherspoon RP, Thomas ED (1982). Graft-versus-host disease and survival in patients with aplastic anemia treated by marrow grafts from HLA-identical siblings. Submitted.

Tsiatis AA (1981). A large sample study of Cox's regression model. Ann Statist 9:93.

CONGRESS SYMPOSIA

IMMUNOPHARMACOLOGY OF CANCER THERAPY Mathe, G.,
France, Chairman; Papermaster, B., USA,
Co-Chairman; Playhouse

Human Interferon as a Therapeutic in Cancer.
*Merigan, T. C., Stanford, CA USA.
(By Title Only)

Effects of Lymphokines in Tumour-Bearing Patients:
Clinical and Laboratory Studies. *Dumonde, D. C.,
Pulley, M., Southcott, B. and den Hollander, F. C.,
London, England and Oss, The Netherlands.

Role of Thymosin in Cancer Immunotherapy and
Neuroendocrine Regulation. *Goldstein, A. L.,
Low, T. L-K., Zatz, M., Hall, N. R., Schulof, R. S.
and McClure, J. E., Washington, DC USA.
(By Title Only)

The Immunopharmacology of Synthetic Immunomodulators. *Wybran, J., Brussels, Belgium.

Immunosuppression in Cancer. *McKhann, C.,
New Haven, CT USA. (By Title Only)

Please note: Papers that are listed as "By Title
Only" were presented at the 13th International
Cancer Congress, but are not included in these
volumes.

13th International Cancer Congress, Part E
Cancer Management, pages 83–93
© 1983 Alan R. Liss, Inc., 150 Fifth Avenue, New York, NY 10011

EFFECTS OF LYMPHOKINES IN TUMOUR-BEARING PATIENTS:
CLINICAL AND LABORATORY STUDIES

D C Dumonde, Melanie S Pulley

Department of Immunology, St Thomas' Hospital
London SE1, United Kingdom

Barbara M Southcott
Department of Radiotherapy, Charing Cross
Hospital, London W6, United Kingdom

F C den Hollander
Organon Scientific Development Group
Organon International BV
Oss, The Netherlands

Lymphokines are non-antibody proteins, generated by lymphocyte activation, that act as intercellular mediators of the immunological response. By virtue of their multiple actions related to inflammation and host defence, there is increasing interest in the therapeutic potential of lympho-kines in human cancer. This paper summarizes our experience of short-term and long-term administration of human lymphoid cell line lymphokine (LCL-LK) to some 30 patients with advanced cancer resistant to other therapeutic modalities. The study showed that local or systemic injection of LCL-LK was well tolerated and that no toxicity was observed over a 2-year period of systemic administration. Analysis of the acute-phase response to intravenous LCL-LK reveals criteria on which to base strategies and protocols for the evaluation of lymphokines in cancer research therapy.

I. BACKGROUND AND RATIONALE OF THE STUDY

Investigation of the role of lymphokines in inflammation, host defence and immunoregulation has become a field of intense research activity in molecular and cellular immunology (Dumonde *et al*, 1969; Cohen *et al*, 1979; de Weck *et al*, 1980; Khan and Hill, 1982). Lymphokines produced by the culture of lymphocytes with specific antigen are biologically potent but are obtainable in minute quantities and present technical difficulties in standardization, bioassay and purification. However, human lymphoid cell lines in continuous culture generate biologically active proteins with a range of lymphokine-like activities (Schook *et al*, 1981); in this way it is possible to recover large amounts of materials whose ability to activate granulocytes, lymphocytes and mononuclear phagocytes closely resemble that of antigen-induced lymphokines. Sustained interest in the role of different leucocyte classes in resistance to neoplasia (Herberman, 1981) coupled with growing interest in the immunopharmacological augmentation of white cell function (Hersh *et al*, 1981) has invited serious consideration of the therapeutic potential of LCL-LK in human cancer (Goldstein and Chirigos, 1981).

The rationale of giving LCL-LK to advanced cancer patients has been reinforced by several lines of investigation. Thus patients with progressive neoplasia characteristically develop depression of cell-mediated immunity and some patients have serum factors blocking lymphocyte function or lymphokine activity (Favila *et al*, 1978). Lymphokines can inhibit tumour cell metabolism and migration *in vitro* (Cohen *et al*, 1978) and can activate cultured macrophages to tumouricidal capacity (Fidler and Raz, 1981). Systemic injection of lymphokines into mice augments tumour regression induced by chemotherapy (Papermaster *et al*, 1982) and intralesional injection of lymphokine in mouse or Man induces local tumour regression (Papermaster *et al*, 1976). Moreover, certain bacterial preparations or pharmacological agents which enhance resistance to tumours may well act by augmenting lymphokine production (Hersh *et al*, 1981).

Beginning in 1976 we have studied the response of some 30 advanced cancer patients to intra-lesional or systemic injection of LCL-LK derived from the lymphoblastoid B-cell line RPMI-1788 (Hamblin *et al*, 1978; Dumonde *et al*, 1981). Most patients have had advanced cancer of the breast or prostate; and by virtue of unresponsiveness to other

therapeutic modalities, all were considered to have
irreversible neoplastic disease. With ethical permission,
informed consent and individual patient care (Southcott
et al, 1982) we have set out to extend knowledge of the
histopathological response to the intralesional and intradermal injection of LCL-LK and to investigate the clinical,
haematological, biochemical and immunological responses of
patients to single and repeated systemic injections of LCL-LK.

II. LYMPHOKINE PREPARATIONS AND PATIENT MANAGEMENT

LCL-LK are prepared at Organon Laboratories, Holland
by large scale culture of the RPMI-1788 cell line. The
processing of culture supernatants by hollow-fibre filtration has been fully described (Verheul *et al*, 1982).
Lymphokine preparations are dispensed in a freeze dried
state and sterility, pyrogenicity and safety tests are done
on the final products. Quality control of lymphokine
activity is monitored by reference to a standardized LIF
assay (den Hollander *et al*, 1981; Hamblin *et al*, 1982) but
a wide variety of lymphokine activities are represented in
the preparations (Verheul *et al*, 1982) which have very little
endotoxin-like activity as judged by the *Limulus* lysate test
(5-15 ng/mg dry weight). Some preparations have contained
a small amount of α-interferon activity but the most
frequently studied batch (LK-5792) was devoid of interferon
(Pulley *et al*, 1982a). In order to exclude the participation
of serum proteins or of small amounts of endotoxin in the
observed responses, control protein (CP) preparations were
made in an identical way from culture medium only (Pulley
et al, 1982b).

Intralesional injection of LCL-LK was undertaken in
dermal metastases of breast carcinoma and by direct injection
into carcinomatous prostate (Dumonde *et al*, 1981; 1982a;
Paradinas *et al*, 1982). The dose range for intralesional
injection was judged by reference to the amount of LCL-LK
which, when injected intradermally, would induce 24-hour
skin test reactions of 30 mm diameter erythema (ED_{30}-doses).
On this basis 1-6 intralesional injections were given,
ranging from 2-76 ED_{30} skin test doses over a period of
2-12 days, with excision biopsy (of breast nodules) or
needle biopsy (of prostate) 1-7 days after the last
injection (Dumonde *et al*, 1981; 1982a).

Systemic administration of LCL-LK was given intravenously and also by intramuscular injection. Patients
were kept recumbent for up to 8 hours after a single
(intravenous) injection and fever index charts were plotted
from half-hourly temperature recordings. Full blood counts
were usually done at 0, 4 and 24 hours and in some patients
were done hourly for the first six hours. Likewise, time-
course studies were made of hormone levels, of plasma
concentrations of zinc and iron, and of acute phase proteins
(Pulley *et al*, 1982a,b). Some patients were maintained on
daily, alternate day or weekly lymphokine injections for
courses of up to one month duration; and four of the patients
received repeated courses of intravenous LCL-LK for up to
2 years. Further details of clinical management have been
published (Dumonde *et al*, 1981; Southcott *et al*, 1982;
Pulley *et al*, 1982a,b).

III. RESPONSE TO INTRADERMAL AND INTRALESIONAL INJECTION OF LCL-LYMPHOKINE

Intradermal injection of active LCL-LK preparations
led to the development of dose-related skin reactions,
characterized by erythema and induration, appearing within
the first hour, lasting for up to 72 hours and being
characteristically maximal between 12-18 hours. Histologically,
an early polymorph exudation (at 30-60 mins) was followed by
progressive mononuclear cell infiltration; and at 48 hours
the more intense skin reactions closely resembled the tuberculin reaction, with perivascular mononuclear cell infiltration and endothelial hypertrophy of post-capillary
venules. No such effects were produced by comparable injections of control protein (Dumonde *et al*, 1982a,b). Intralesional injection led to clinical regression of the injected
dermal metastases, sometimes accompanied by ulceration. The
histological appearances of such nodules revealed intense
infiltration of tumour by lymphocytes, macrophages and poly-
morphs together with large areas of tumour cell necrosis,
though no clear evidence of macrophage contact cytotoxicity
could be observed by electron microscopy (Dumonde *et al*,
1982a; Paradinas *et al*, 1982).

These findings lend strong support to the view that
lymphokines are mediators of delayed hypersensitivity in the
human and indicate that both skin testing and intranodular

injection may be of value in the screening of batches of lymphokine for clinical activity.

IV RESPONSE TO INTRAVENOUS INJECTION OF LCL-LYMPHOKINE

A single intravenous injection of LCL-LK produces a dose-dependent acute phase reaction characterized by pyrexia and neutrophil leucocytosis as well as a lymphopenia and increases in plasma ACTH, cortisol and serum growth hormone, all maximal between 2-6 hours after injection. Plasma, zinc and iron levels start to decrease during this time and reach a trough between 5-12 hours; and acute-phase proteins (CRP and α_1AG) peak later at 24-48 hrs (Pulley *et al*, 1982a). Analysis showed that there was insufficient *Limulus*-reactive material in the lymphokine preparations to account for the response on the basis of endotoxin contamination; and a special study was undertaken, using control-processed plasma protein (CP), which showed that these responses could not be attributed to endotoxin (Pulley *et al*, 1982b). Furthermore, the haematological and biochemical changes were not related to the stress of pyrexia itself; and pyrexia and leucocytosis still occurred in patients receiving steroids whose cortisol responses were suppressed.

Repeated daily injection of LCL-LK intravenously results in some degree of tolerance, as judged by both haematological and pyrexial responses. However, injection of LCL-LK on alternate days or at less frequent intervals did not lead to tolerance, and predictable acute-phase responses occurred. In a first series of 20 patients reported (Southcott *et al*, 1982), four received intravenous courses of LCL-LK for 9-25 months; six were given LCL-LK for 2-4 months and ten were studied acutely (for 1-3 weeks). All patients volunteered feelings of well being; and two patients were of particular interest in that an objective response of partial remission by the tumour to the lymphokine was observed (Southcott *et al*, 1982).

We have concluded that RPMI-1788 lymphokine preparations are safe for clinical use, for no adverse short-term or long-term toxicity has been evident in our experience. These findings reinforce the growing view that lymphokines may well have a place in cancer research therapy amongst other biological response modifiers (Goldstein and Chirigos, 1981).

V.   IMMUNOLOGICAL IMPLICATIONS

The sequence of events which follow intravenous injection of LCL-LK into Man are compatible with a direct early effect of lymphokine upon host macrophages and secondary effects resulting from release of interleukin 1 or endogenous pyrogen (Dinarello,1982). Systemic reactions of delayed hypersensitivity are characterized by fever, lymphopenia, neutrophil leucocytosis and depression of plasma levels of iron and zinc (Uhr and Brandriss, 1958; Kampschmidt and Pulliam, 1974), events which can also be produced by injection of endogenous pyrogen (EP) itself (Kampschmidt and Upchurch, 1970). It seems likely that the LCL-LK preparations contain an EP-inducing factor (Atkins *et al*, 1980) which then acts on the hypothalamus to induce pyrexia and to activate the pituitary-adrenal axis. On this basis the lymphopenia would be due to effects of cortisone on lympho-cyte compartmentation (Cox and Ford, 1982); the acute phase protein response, together with changes in Zn and Fe levels, to effects of EP (IL-1) upon hepatocytes (Selinger *et al*, 1980; McAdam and Dinarello, 1980); and the polymorph leuco-cytosis to effects of EP (IL-1) upon cell mobilization from bone marrow (Kampschmidt *et al*, 1972).

Recent evidence therefore supports the view that lymphokines are mediators of both local and systemic reac-tions of delayed hypersensitivity. Detailed cellular immunological studies on patients receiving LCL-LK have yet to be undertaken though there is some evidence for enhance-ment of polymorph phagocytic capacity and NK cell activity (Rodes *et al*, 1982; Gouveia *et al*, 1982). Our findings also support the view that lymphokine release *in vivo* may provide a link between the immune and neuroendocrine systems (Besedovsky *et al*, 1981) and so activate immunoregulatory mechanisms extrinsic to the immune system itself. The identity of these biologically active materials in the LCL-LK preparation has yet to be established and is an objective of our current work.

VI. CLINICAL IMPLICATIONS

Although this preliminary study was not designed to
examine clinical efficacy of LCL-LK in tumour bearing
patients, it seems worthwhile and ethically justifiable to
continue this work in advanced cancer, against the background of informed consent and of careful and compassionate
management of individual patients. In establishing a formal
phase I study of LCL-LK we are aware of the complexities
of strategy and design implicit in the use of a 'biological
response modifier' (Carter, 1980; Oldham, 1981). In
characterizing further the acute-phase and longer-term
responses to LCL-LK we can investigate the hypothesis that
certain components of a patient's acute response will be of
value in predicting whether longer-term administration of
LCL-LK results in a favourable outcome. It seems plausible
to suggest that recurrent stimulation of an acute-phase
response by intravenous injection of LCL-LK may favourably
diminish the side effects of irradiation or chemotherapy.
On this basis the 'lymphokine strategy' is aimed at improving
the ability of a tumour bearing host to tolerate existing
treatment modalities rather than being aimed at killing the
tumour by virtue of the cytotoxic or cytostatic action of
lymphokines themselves.

In order to pursue this, we have set ourselves the
following objectives: (a) to determine the relationship
between individual components of the acute phase response
and the dose and specific activities of injected lymphokines;
(b) to establish whether stimulation of white-cell function
is more readily achieved by dose schedules which avoid
acute-phase tolerance or by schedules which lead to selective tolerance of an acute response (eg pyrexia); and (c)
to determine whether longer-term administration of LCL-LK
results in a greater ability to tolerate or recover from the
depressive effects upon white-cell function of extensive
radiotherapy or chemotherapy. We appreciate that working
in advanced cancer with biological preparations containing
a mixture of lymphokines will have its difficulties; however, we hope that the results will be of value in the
design of future studies in less advanced cancer with more
purified lymphokine preparations, as these may become
possible.

Acknowledgments We thank Prof. A Fleck, Dr G Carter and Dr B Muller, Dept of Chemical Pathology, Charing Cross Hospital, London; and Prof. Lesley Rees, Dept of Endocrinology, St Bartholomew's Hospital, London, for hormone, acute phase protein, Zn and Fe assays.

REFERENCES

Atkins E, Askenase PW, Francis L, Bernheim HA (1980). Release of an endogeneous pyrogen from guinea pig leucocytes: the role of T lymphocytes and correlation with suppression (desensitization) of delayed hypersensitivity. J Immunol 125:2069.

Besedovsky HO, Del Rey A, Sorkin E (1981). Lymphokine-containing supernatants from ConA-stimulated cells increase corticosterone blood levels. J Immunol 126:385.

Carter SK (1980). Biological response modifying agents: what is an appropriate Phase I-II strategy ? Cancer Immunol Immunother 8:207.

Cohen M, Goss A, Yoshida T, Cohen S (1978). Inhibition of migration of tumor cells in vitro by lymphokine-containing supernatants. J Immunol 121:840.

Cohen S, Pick E, Oppenheim JJ (eds) (1979). "Biology of the lymphokines". New York: Academic Press.

Cox JH, Ford WL (1982). The migration of lymphocytes across specialized vascular endothelium. Prednisolone acts at several points on the recirculation pathways of lymphocytes. Cell Immunol 66:407.

De Weck AL, Kristensen F, Landy M (eds) (1980). "Biochemical characterization of lymphokines". New York: Academic Press.

Den Hollander FC, van Lieshout JI, Schuurs AHWM (1981) Statistically designed assay of migration-inhibitory activity in lymphokine preparations. Int J Immunopharmacol 3:161.

Dinarello CA (1982). Leukocytic Pyrogen. Lymphokines 7:23.

Dumonde DC, Wolstencroft RA, Panayi FS, Matthew M, Morley J, Howson WT (1969). "Lymphokines": Non-antibody mediators of cellular immunity generated by lymphocyte activation. Nature 224:38.

Dumonde DC, Pulley MS, Hamblin AS, Singh AK, Southcott BM, O'Connell D, Paradinas FJ, Robinson MRG, Rigby CC, den Hollander F, Schuurs A, Verheul H, van Vliet E (1981). Short-term and long-term administration of lymphoblastoid cell-line lymphokine (LCL-LK) to patients with advanced cancer. In Goldstein AL, Chirigos MA (eds):

"Lymphokines and Thymic factors: their potential utilization in cancer therapeutics". New York: Raven Press, p 301.

Dumonde DC, Pulley MS, Paradinas F, Southcott BM, O'Connell D, Robinson MRG, den Hollander F (1982a). A histological study of intradermal and intralesional injection of human lymphoid cell line lymphokine (LCL-LK) in patients with advanced cancer. In Khan A, Hill NO (eds): "Human Lymphokines: the Biological Immune Response Modifiers". New York: Academic Press, p 665.

Dumonde DC, Pulley MS, Paradinas FJ, Southcott BM, O'Connell D, Robinson MRG, den Hollander F, Schuurs AH (1982b). Histological features of skin reactions to human lymphoid cell line lymphokine in patients with advanced cancer. J Path 138 (4): in press

Favila L, Jimenez L, Castro ME, Garcia-Garcia G, Guiterrez A, Pulida I (1978). Blocking factors of migration inhibition factor production in patients with cervical carcinoma. A possible role in vivo. J Nat Canc Inst 60:1279.

Fidler IJ, Raz A (1981). The induction of tumoricidal capacities in mouse and rat macrophages by lymphokines. Lymphokines 3:345.

Goldstein AL, Chirigos MA (eds) (1981). "Lymphokines and thymic factors: their potential utilization in cancer therapeutics". New York: Raven Press.

Gouveia J, Riband P, Goutner A, Mathé G (1982) Phase 1 study of systemic lymphokine (LCL-LK) administration in advanced cancer patients. In Khan A, Hill NO (Eds): "Human lymphokines: the Biological Immune Response Modifiers". New York: Academic Press, p 633.

Hamblin AS, Wolstencroft RA, Dumonde DC, den Hollander FC, Schuurs AHW, Backhouse BM, O'Connell D, Paradinas F (1978). The potential of lymphokines in the treatment of cancer. Develop Biol Stand 38:335.

Hamblin AS, Zawisza B, Shipton U, Dumonde DC, den Hollander F, Verheul H, Schuurs A (1982). Standardization of the indirect LIF test by reference to lymphoid cell line lymphokine (LCL-LK) as a standard material. In Khan A, Hill NO (eds): "Human Lymphokines: the Biological Immune Response Modifiers". New York: Academic Press, p 85.

Herberman RB (1981) Overview of role of macrophages, natural killer cells and antibody-dependent cellular cytotoxicity as mediators of biological response modification. In: Chirigos MA, Mitchell M, Mastrangelo MJ, Krim M (eds): "Mediation of cellular immunity in cancer by immune modifiers". New York: Raven Press, p 261.

Hersh EM, Chirigos MA, Mastrangelo M (1981) (eds) "Augmenting agents in cancer therapy". Progr Canc Res Ther, 16, New York: Raven Press.

Kampschmidt RF and Pulliam LA (1974). Effect of delayed hypersensitivity on plasma, iron and zinc concentration and blood leukocytes. Proc Soc Exp Biol Med 147:242.

Kampschmidt RF and Upchurch HF (1970). The effect of endogenous pyrogen on the plasma zinc concentration of the rat. Proc Soc Exp Biol Med 134:1150.

Kampschmidt RF, Long RD, Upchurch HF (1972). Neutrophil releasing activity in rats injected with endogenous pyrogen. Proc Soc Exp Biol Med 139:1224.

Khan A, Hill NO (eds) (1982). "Human Lymphokines: the Biological Immune Response Modifiers". New York: Academic Press.

McAdam, KPWJ, Dinarello, CA (1980). Induction of serum amyloid A synthesis by human leucocytic pyrogen. In Agarwal MK (ed): "Bacterial Endotoxins and Host Response". Amsterdam: Elsevier/North Holland, p 167.

Oldham RK (1981) Biological reponse modifier therapy - an overview. The Cancer Bulletin 33:244.

Papermaster BW, Holtermann OA, Klein E, Djerassi I, Rosner D, Dao T, Costanzi JJ (1976). Preliminary observations on tumour regressions induced by local administration of a lymphoid cell line supernatant fraction in patients with cutaneous metastatic lesions. Clin Immunol Immunopathol 5:31.

Papermaster BW, McEntire JE, Gilliland CD (1982). Lymphokine adjuvant therapy: Bioassay of human lymphokine fractions in a mouse tumour model. In Khan A, Hill NO (eds) "Human Lymphokines: The Biological Immune Response Modifiers". New York: Academic Press, p 459.

Paradinas FJ, Southcott BM, O'Connell D, den Hollander F, Schuurs AH, Pulley MS, Dumonde DC (1982). Changes induced by local injection of human lymphoid cell line lymphokine into dermal metastases of breast carcinoma: a light and electron microscopical study. J Path 138 (4): in press.

Pulley MS, Dumonde DC, Carter G, Muller B, Fleck A, Southcott BM, den Hollander F (1982a). Hormonal, haematological and acute phase protein responses of advanced cancer patients to the intravenous injection of lymphoid cell line lymphokine (LCL-LK). In Khan A, Hill NO (eds): "Human Lymphokines: the biological immune response modifiers". New York: Academic Press, p 651.

Pulley MS, Dumonde D, Carter G, Muller B, Southcott B, den Hollander F (1982b). Lymphokines as mediators of extrinsic immunoregulatory circuits. In Cohen S, Oppenheim JJ (eds): "Interleukins, Lymphokines and Cytokines: Proceedings of the Third International Lymphokine Workshop". New York: Academic Press, in press.

Rodes ND, McEntire JE, Dunn PA, Gay C, Decker M, Kardinal CG, Gilliland CD, Oxenhandler RW, Papermaster BW (1982). Phase 1 clinical studies with lymphoblastoid lymphokine preparations from the RPMI-1788 cell line. In Khan A, Hill NO (eds): "Human Lymphokines:the Biological Immune Response Modifiers". New York: Academic Press, p 699.

Schook LB, Otz U, Lazary S, de Weck A, Minowada J, Odavic R, Kniep E, Edy V (1981). Lymphokine and monokine activities in supernatants from human lymphoid and myeloid cell lines. Lymphokines 2:1.

Selinger MJ, McAdam K, Kaplan MM, Sipe JD, Vogel SN, Rosenstreich DL (1980). Monokine-induced synthesis of serum amyloid A protein by hepatocytes. Nature 285:498.

Southcott BM, Dumonde DC, Pulley MS, van Vliet E, den Hollander F, Schuurs A (1982). Systemic lymphokine treatment of selected cancer patients. In Khan A, Hill NO (eds): "Human Lymphokines: the Biological Immune Response Modifiers". New York: Academic Press, p 641.

Uhr JW, Brandriss MW (1958). Delayed hypersensitivity IV. Systemic reactivity of guinea pigs sensitized to protein antigens. J exp Med 108:905.

Verheul HAM, den Hollander FC, Dijkhuizen DM, Gijzen JWL, Kessels JGM, Schuurs AHWM (1982). Production and biological characterization of lymphoid cell line lymphokine (LCL-LK) preparations. In Khan A, Hill NO (eds): "Human lymphokines: the Biological Immune Response Modifiers". New York: Academic Press, p 343.

13th International Cancer Congress, Part E
Cancer Management, pages 95–103
© 1983 Alan R. Liss, Inc., 150 Fifth Avenue, New York, NY 10011

THE IMMUNOPHARMACOLOGY OF SYNTHETIC IMMUNOMODULATORS.

Joseph Wybran, M.D.

Department of Immunology and Hematology
Erasme Hospital
Université Libre de Bruxelles, 1070 Brussels,
Belgium.

The place of synthetic immunomodulators in the treatment of cancer is, at the present time, not clearly understood. However, since both the understanding of the immune reaction against tumor cells and the mode of action of immunomodulators are now better known, one can probably formulate certain guidelines useful in this field.

It is, however, clear that the current data are not sufficient to have a final answer regarding the place of these drugs in the treatment of cancer. Indeed, it was taken as a dogma that immunostimulation alone can not eliminate important tumor masses. Clearly, there are now some indications that bladder carcinoma can respond to BCG and that metastases of hypernephroma may partially respond to thymic extracts. Therefore, at this time, one should be more descriptive than dogmatic.

The immune system will mount an immunological response against cancer cells by multiple means. Although the existence of specific tumor antigens have not yet been clearly shown, their existence is postulated. They probably act as neo antigens and thus elicit a specific immune response, mainly by T cells. These immune cells will be cytotoxic and kill the tumor cells. Killing and inhibition of tumor cell division can also be achieved non specifically by activated macrophages and by natural killer (NK) cells. These latter may have a more important role in the prevention of metastases. Other cells, called K cells (or killers), will destroy the tumor cells with the help of a specific antibody (antibody dependent cellular cytotoxicity or ADCC). Humoral immunity can also be involved by the action of speci-

fic antibodies cytotoxic in the presence of complement. Finally, some products of the immune response like lymphokines and interleukins can directly or indirectly destroy the
tumor cells. Nonetheless,all these defense mechanisms are
sometimes overcome without necessarily representing a failure of the immune system. Indeed the immune response may
generate humoral products or cells which will send to suppress the positive immune response. For instances, blocking
antibodies, free antigen and antigen-antibody complexes can
inhibit some cellular cytotoxic response. Furthermore, one
has described cells with suppressive activities. These
cells belonging to the macrophage lincage or to T cells can
prevent specific and non specific cellular cytotoxicity.

In consequence, any manipulation of the immune system
should try to increase the positive cytotoxic immune mechanisms and decrease the suppressive mechanisms. The ideal
immunomodulatory drug should thus increase specific T cell
cytotoxicity, non specific NK activity and macrophage functions. It should decrease suppressor function and prevent
the formation of inhibitory humoral substances. It should
also tend to increase the non specific and specific immune
response to higher levels perhaps by enhancing tumor antigenicity. Since most of the immunomodulatory drugs do not
have all these properties, one can theorically postulate
that multiple drugs will be necessary to achieve this goal
and postulate that polyimmunotherapy will be used in the
future rather than monoimmunotherapy.

In this short review, regarding the immunopharmacology
of synthetic immunomodulators, only the major drugs with a
potential impact upon cancer treatment will be presented.
Since only very limited data have been obtained using these
agents, the emphasis will not be necessarily stressed upon
this point.

1) LEVAMISOLE
Formula: 6 phenyl-2,3,5,6-tetrahydro-imidazol (2,1) thiazole

This agent is the first synthetic drug which was used
as an immunomodulator. It appears to decrease the intracellular content of cyclic AMP and increase the cyclic GMP
in the lymphocytes. It restores to normal value the immunologic system of cancer patients acting mainly on T cells
and macrophages. It increases the activity of polymorph
neutrophils. Beneficial clinical results have been obtained

in chronic viral infections and rheumatoid arthritis. There
are about 40 controlled trials in cancer. It appears that
levamisole is best effective in the case of advanced disease before or associated with conventional therapy. These
controlled trials suggest a moderate increase in survival
and prolongation of disease free interval (the results with
levamisole are about 10% better than without the drug). The
optimal dosage for levamisole is 2.5 mg/Kg/day 2 days every
week. (Amery 1978).

2) BESTATIN
Formula : 3 amino-2 hydroxy-4 phenylbutanoyl-L-leucine.

It is an inhibitor of aminopeptidase B and leucine aminopeptidase, isolated from a fungus Actynomyces species.
It appears to be able to modify tumor antigenicity towards
a greater recognition by the immune system. It immunoresto-
res cancer patients as judged by enhancement of lymphocyte
response, blood T cells and skin response to antigens. It
increases NK as well as ADCC cytotoxicity. This restorati-
ve effect has been observed in breast cancer (associated
with radiotherapy), lymphomas and laryngeal cancer. Preliminary studies also suggest a beneficial effect of bestatin
upon the survival of melanoma patients. The optimal dosage
is around 30 mg daily taken orally. (Schorlemmer, Bosslet,
Sedlacek 1982).

3) DTC (Imuthiol)
Formula : sodium diethylcarbamate.

This non toxic agent has been shown to recruit functional T cells from precursors. It restores the immunosuppression caused by chemotherapy or surgical trauma. It
regulates blood T cell subsets (T4/T8 ratio). It augments
NK activity. It possesses also a direct in vitro killing
activity upon some tumor cells. Among its other interesting activities, one can mention the inhibition of cispla-
tinin nephrotoxicity and of some of UV irradiation toxicity. (Roumantzieff, Charbonnier, Armand, Renoux, Renoux 1982)

4) AZIMEXON
Formula : 2 cyanaziridinyl-2 carbomoylaziridinyl-1-propane.

In cancer patients, azimexon will increase the blood
active T rosettes and restores their immunosuppressive state (mitogen response, skin anergy). It regulates, in vitro,

T cell subsets (T4/T8 ratio). It increases macrophage activity and NK function. This drug can induce hemolytic ane-
mias and is positive in the Ames test. Some direct beneficial effects have been observed in melanoma. The usual dosage is around 100 mg (Bicker 1978).

5) GLUCANS

The glucans are fungal polysaccharides (β glucans) with
high molecular weights. Some of them have already been investigated for many years mainly in Japan. The best known
are Crestin (PSK), Lentinan and Schizophyllan (SPG). They
increase macrophage activity as well as cytotoxicity. Apparent good results have been obtained in association with
chemotherapy, mainly in gastric cancer.

6) MDP (muramyldipeptide)

It is the smallest active component of the mycobacte-
rium cell wall having adjuvant activity. Perhaps by acting
upon the intracellular levels of cyclic nucleotides, it
activates macrophage function as well as T cells and B cells.
Many analogs have been synthesized. It has been mainly studied in animals where it enhances survival in some tumor
models. It can also protect from various bacterial infections. One of the current most developed application is
the demonstration of an adjuvant effect during immunization
(Chedid, Carelli, Audibert 1979).

7) THERAFECTIN (SM 1213)
Formula : isopropylidine-3-0-3-N,N-dimethylamino-n-propyl-D-
            glucofuranose.

It acts by increasing macrophage activity and NK activity. It could increase interleukin 1 production. The animal data suggest a potential effect in the field of viral
infections, rheumatoid arthritis as well as in tumor models
where delay of deaths have been recorded.

8) INTERFERON INDUCERS

Interferon can be induced by a variety of natural
agents like viruses, some fungi, some bacterias and their
products (endotoxins, lipopolysaccharides), antigens and
mitogens. A monoclonal antibody directed against T cells
(OKT3) also stimulates the production of interferon.

However, very interestingly, the industry has now synthesized a variety of interferon inducers: anionic polymers (pyrans) like MVE-2 (maleic anhydride divinyl ether copolymer), polynucleotides (poly-IC and the more stable poly ICLC), tylorone, pyrazolo-quinolines (atabrine, acridones), lipoidalamines (CP 20, 961) and pyrimidones (like ABPP or 6 phenylpyrimidones).

Indeed, much work is now being done on the interferons which are the prototypes of the modifyiers of the biological response. They are able to increase macrophage activity, NK activity and at high doses have some direct antitumor activity. It is not yet clearly demonstrated whether the transient beneficial effects seen in cancer patients treated with interferon are due to the immunological effects.

The advantages of some of the interferon inducers are the following : orally active, minimal hyporeactivity, economical preparation and prophylactical or therapeutical activity (Chirigos, Stylos 1980; Stringfellow 1980).

9) LYNESTRENOL

Lynestrenol is a well established synthetic progesteron drug. It increases phagocytic activity and T cell function. It restores depressed cellular immunity in cancer patients (skin test and lymphocyte response). In animals, it delays tumor growth. Since its immunological activity is only seen at high doses (1-2 mg/Kg/day), it may well be that the beneficial effects observed with high doses of progesteron like substance in hypernephroma or metastatic breast cancer are due to a stimulation of the immunological system (Wybran, Thiry 1978).

10) INDOMETHACIN

This drug may perhaps, in the future, qualify as an immunomodulator since it suppresses the activation of suppressor cells.

11) CIMETIDINE

Perhaps by its action on the histamine H_2 receptor present on suppressor T cells, cimetidine increases some cell mediated immune mechanisms. Conflicting data suggest some immunorestorative activity. Finally, non confirmed data indicate that cimetidine is active in some animal tumor systems.

12) ENDORPHINS

Natural and synthetic endorphins and enkephalins have shown that they can increase the response to mitogens and the NK activity. This is probably due to the presence of endorphin and enkephalin receptors on B and T lymphocytes. Leucine enkephalins increase the survival of mice bearing tumors (Wybran, Appelboom, Famaey, Govaerts 1979).

13) INOSIPLEX (Isoprinosine,methisoprinol)
Formula : complex of inosine with the p-acetamidobenzoic salt of N-N-dimethylamino-2-propanol (DIP-PAcBA) in a molar ratio of 1:3.

This synthetic drug has probably been the most intensively studied these last years in the field of immunomodulators. Its molecular mechanism of action is not well understood: one hypothesis is that the DIP-PAcBA moiety allows a better metabolic utilization of the inosine into the purine pathway of the cell.

Isoprinosine increases in vitro T cell function and macrophage activity. It induces the appearance of T cell markers and enhances the lymphocyte response to mitogens and antigens. This property appears to be due to the synthesis of a mitogenic helper factor, probably interleukin 2, by isoprinosine-treated lymphocytes. In vivo, it also increases antibody formation, T cell functions and macrophage activity. Isoprinosine has also been shown to increase both interleukin 1 and interleukin 2 production. It restores T cell immunosuppression in post-radiotherapy cancer patients and the lymphocyte response to mitogens in cancer. It increases NK activity in vivo in animals. The action upon NK is further demonstrated by the observation that isoprinosine inhibits the suppression of NK activity induced by Concanavalin A in vitro and thus enhances such NK activity in this system. In vivo, Talpaz, Mavligit and Hersh have shown that cancer patients receiving either 1 gr or 4 gr of Isoprinosine daily for one week will be immunorestored as judged by the increase of ability of their blood T cells to mount a xenogeneic graft-versus-host assay. Isoprinosine potentiates the antiviral and antitumor activity of interferon. It delays the early appearance of autoimmu-

nity and the early tumor development of interferon treated
NZB-NZW mice suggesting a potential benefit in auto immune
syndromes.

Clinically, isoprinosine, in non-blind studies, has
been shown to be beneficial in various viral diseases like
subacute sclerosing panencephalitis, cutaneous herpes and
aphtous stomatitis, influenza challenge, cytomegalovirus
hepatitis, Reiter's syndrome and possibly warts. Isoprinosine also shows promising results in rheumatoid arthritis;
clinical improvement was observed two to six weeks after
the onset of treatment. Immune monitoring performed in patients receiving isoprinosine suggests the modification of
the inducer-suppressor/cytotoxic phenotypes of blood lymphocytes.

In summary, isoprinosine, a synthetic immunomodulatory
agent, has activities meeting to the criteria of a biological response modifier. It is likely that its immunological
properties explain at least in part its clinical beneficial
effects. The usual dosage is 50 mg/Kg/day taken orally.
The only side effect of the drug can be a moderate increase
in the serum level of uric acid. In view of its multiple
effects on the immunological system, lack of toxicity (some
patients take this drug for more than two years without any
adverse reaction), isoprinosine represents an ideal synthetic immunomodulator (Wybran, Famaey, Appelboom 1981; Wybran,
Famaey, Görtz, Dab, Malfroot, Appelboom 1982).

14) NPT 15392
Formula : eythro 9-(2 hydroxy-3 nonyl) hypoxanthine.

This drug, like isoprinosine, possesses a purine moiety
in its structure. It is thus likely that it acts on the purine metabolic pathway of the lymphocyte.

NPT 15392 markedly increases the percentages of active
T rosettes without affecting other T rosette assays. This
property seems due to the synthesis of a rosetting factor
by mononuclear cells incubated with the drug. It also enhances T cell induced cytotoxicity in mixed lymphocyte culture. NPT 15392 markedly increases the polymorph neutrophil phagocytosis of yeast particles. In cancer patients,
a unique oral dose of 0.4 mgr or 0.7 mgr increases blood T
rosette percentages in systems like active, autologous and
total T rosettes. Twenty cancer patients also received 0.4

or 0.7 mgr of NPT 15392 every 3 days for 10 days. Although
skin tests were not modified by the drug, other T cell
assays showed a significant increase : number of blood T
lymphocytes, percentages of E rosettes, percentages of autologous T rosettes and PHA stimulation. NK function was
increased to normal values in patients with low NK cytotoxicity before treatment. It can be concluded that NPT
15392 possesses neutrophil, T cell and NK immunostimulato-
ry properties (Wybran 1982).

CONCLUSIONS

    This short review indicates that the industry now syn-
thesizes a variety of agents able to modulate the immune
functions. Most of the results in cancer patients are preliminary. In a phase 1- phase 2 study in cancer patients,
various doses of these drugs are given and the immunological parameters are studied. In a first step, it is observed whether these drugs can restore cellular functions like the lymphocyte response to mitogens, the increase in
blood T cells or the modifications of T cell subsets and
the modification in T, K and NK cellular cytotoxicity.
Restoration of skin reactivity is also evaluated. In rare
instances, a direct effect of the immunomodulatory drug
upon the tumor mass has been observed. Although the place
of synthetic immunomodulators in cancer treatment is not
clearly proved, it is likely that a drug may find its place perhaps as adjuvant therapy to classical treatment after
or during tumor mass reduction. Since most of the drugs
do not possess all the properties required for an ideal
immunomodulator, one can postulate the use of polyimmunotherapy in the future.

REFERENCES

Amery MA (1978). Final results of a multicenter placebo-
controlled levamisole study of resectable lung cancer.
  Cancer Treat. Rep. 62:1677.
Bicker U. (1978). Immunomodulating effects of BM 12.531
  (Azimexon) in animals and tolerance. Cancer Treat. Rep.
  62:1987.
Chedid L, Carelli C., Audibert F. (1979). Recent development concerning muramyl dipeptide, a synthetic immunoregulating molecule. J. Reticuloendothel. Soc. 26:631.
Chirigos MA, Stylos WA (1980). Immunomodulatory effect of
  various molecular weight maleic anhydride divinyl ethers
  and other agents in vivo. Cancer Res. 40:1967.

Roumantzieff M., Charbonnier C., Armand J., Renoux M. and Renoux G. (1982). DTC, an immunopotentiator specific for T cells. Int. J. Immunopharmacol. 4:286.

Schorlemmer HU, Bosslet KA and Sedlacek HH (1982). Activation of macrophages for killing of tumor cells by the immunomodulator bestatin. Int. J. Immunopharmacol. 4:278.

Stringfellow DA (ed) (1980). Interferon and interferon inducers. Marcel Dekker, N.Y.

Wybran J. (1982). Immunological properties of NPT 15392: a review. In "New immunomodulatory agents and biological response modifiers". In Human Cancer Immunology vol.3. Eds. J. Wybran, G. Mayer, B. Serrou and C. Rosenfeld. Elsevier Biomedical, Amsterdam. 89.

Wybran J., Appelboom T., Famaey J.P. and Govaerts A.(1979). Suggestive evidence for morphine and methionine-enkephalin receptors-like on normal human blood T lymphocytes. J. Immunol. 123:1068.

Wybran J., Famaey J.P. and Appelboom T. (1981). Inosiplex, a novel treatment in rheumatoid arthritis ? J. Rheumatol. 8:643.

Wybran J., Famaey J.P., Görtz R., Dab I., Malfroot A. and Appelboom T. (1982). Inosiplex (Isoprinosine): a review of its immunological and clinical effects in disease. In Advances in Pharmacology and Therapeutics II. Ed. by Y. Yoshida, Y. Hagihara and S. Ebashi, Pergamon Press, 6:123.

Wybran J., Thiry L.(1978). Delay of tumor growth in hamsters treated with lynestrenol and effect of staphylococcus aureus Cowan A. J. Nat. Cancer Inst. 61:173.

CONGRESS SYMPOSIA

APPLICATION OF BASIC CONCEPTS TO CLINICAL
CHEMOTHERAPEUTIC DESIGN Tanneberger, S., GDR,
Chairman; Chabner, B., USA, Co-Chairman;
Rainier Room

Biochemical Basis of Clinical Drug Testing.
*Myers, C., Bethesda, MD USA. (By Title Only)

Determinants of ARA-C Action: Biochemical
Consideration. *Rustum, Y. M., Slocum, H. K. and
Li, Z. R., Buffalo, NY USA

Potentials of Pharmacokinetic Studies in
Cancer Chemotherapy. *Pinedo, H. M. and
Keizer, H. J., Amsterdam, The Netherlands.

Cell Biological Systems for Prediction of
Individual Human Tumor Drug Sensitivity.
*Tanneberger, S. and Nissen, E., Berlin,
German Democratic Republic.

Clinical Application and Limitation.
*Eckhardt, S., Budapest, Hungary.

Please note: Papers that are listed as "By Title
Only" were presented at the 13th International
Cancer Congress, but are not included in these
volumes.

13th International Cancer Congress, Part E
Cancer Management, pages 107–120
© 1983 Alan R. Liss, Inc., 150 Fifth Avenue, New York, NY 10011

DETERMINANTS OF ARA-C ACTION: BIOCHEMICAL CONSIDERATION

Y.M. Rustum[1], H.K. Slocum and Z.R. Li[2]

Department of Experimental Therapeutics and
Grace Cancer Drug Center, Roswell Park Memorial
Institute, 666 Elm Street, Buffalo, NY   14263

INTRODUCTION

1-β-arabinofuranosylcytosine (Ara-C) is a pyrimidine nucleoside analog active against a variety of mouse and human tumors. In order for this agent to exert its activity, the drug must be phosphorylated by a series of enzymes to the level of the active moeity, Ara-C triphosphate (Ara-CTP). At the target cell level, although the activity of this agent is associated primarily with its ability to inhibit DNA polymerase, recent results by Kufe et al (1981) suggested that Ara-C incorporation into DNA is another critical factor in the action of this agent. In an in vivo situation where the whole organism is involved, both pharmacokinetic and target cell factors are involved in determining the selective action of this agent. Although pharmacokinetic considerations of Ara-C will not be discussed in detail herein, suffice it to say that in order for Ara-C to exert its effect it must be delivered to target cell in a sufficient concentration for a sufficient period of time. Once this is achieved it is likely that target cell factors will determine the selective action of this agent.

Studies from this laboratory demonstrated that the lack of intracellular activation of Ara-C is sufficient for prediction of Ara-C resistance (Rustum et al 1981). In sensitive cells, however, differential intracellular retention of Ara-CTP between tumor and normal cells is the critical determinant of Ara-C action in leukemic patients (Rustum and Preisler, 1979) and in mice bearing transplantable tumors as shown by Rustum (1978) and Chou et al (1975).

In this presentation, results of studies conducted to evaluate factors that are critical to the action of this agent are reported.

METHODS

High Performance Liquid Chromatography (HPLC)

The methods developed previously by Rustum and Higby (1978) were utilized here for analysis of intracellular Ara-C anabolites. Radiolabeled fractions in the area of the mono-, di, and triphosphates of Ara-C were collected and counted in a Packard-Tricarb Liquid Scintillation Counter with 35% efficiency for ^{3}H. Ara-CTP were also quantitated by 280 nm absorption and radioummunoassay developed by Pailer (1979) and adapted by Rustum et al (1982).

In Vivo Ara-C Metabolism and Retention

Mice bearing tumors (L1210 in female DBA2/J, P1798 lymphosarcoma in Balb-C) were given ^{3}H-Ara-C i.v. and at various times thereafter, 3 mice/time point were sacrificed and tumor cells were removed for analysis of Ara-C anabolites found in the acid-soluble fractions. For mice bearing i.p. L1210 cells, ^{3}H-Ara-C was administered i.v. 3 days after tumor transplant of 1.0×10^6 cells. For s.c. tumors, treatments were initiated when tumor sizes were >100 mg. In case of solid tumors, mice were anesthesized and tumors were excized rapidly and dropped into liquid nitrogen. Tumor tissues were then homogenized with 6% PCA, and the neutralized acid-soluble fractions were then analyzed by HPLC for Ara-C anabolites.

Antitumor Activity

Mice bearing tumors were treated with Ara-C and the survival times were calculated following saline and drug treatments. Day of tumor transplant was considered day zero. Average survival tines for 1×10^6 L1210 cells transplanted i.p. or s.c. were 7.5 ± 0.5 (S.D.) and 6.5 ±

0.8 days, respectively. For mice bearing s.c. P-1798, the average survival time was 35 ± 3.0 days.

RESULTS AND DISCUSSION

Antitumor activity of Ara-C

The data in Table 1 outline the antitumor activity of Ara-C in mice bearing leukemic L1210 or lymphosarcoma P-1798 tumor cells. In mice bearing i.p. or s.c. tumors, although the pharmacokinetic parameters of ara-C were similar with an α and β phases t 1/2 of 0.18 hr and 2 hr, respectively (data not shown), these tumors responded differently to treatments with ara-C. In case of i.p. tumors, treatments by either continuous infusion and/or fractionated doses yielded comparable increase in the life span and long term survivals. Mice transplanted with s.c. tumors, however, had marginal increase in life span, and no long term survivals. In mice bearing P-1798 lymphosarcoma, treatment with Ara-C produced significant increase in life span and cure rate. This schedule showed marginal activity against L1210 cells whether transplanted i.p. or s.c.

Table 1

Antitumor activity of Ara-C in mice bearing tumor cells with differential sensitivity to Ara-C. For L1210 (s.c.) and Lymphosarcoma P-1798, treatments were initiated when tumor size was >100mg and for all others, treatments were initiated 24 hr following the transplant of 1×10^6 tumor cells. All treatments were via the i.v. route.

Tumor (%)[+]	Schedule	Dosage (mg/kg)	Increase in life span (% control)	Cure
L1210,i.p.	5d. cont. infusion	2.5	120	20
L1210,i.p.	q 4hrx6	15.0	130	30
L1210,i.p.	dailyx5	100.0	40	0
L1210,S.C.	5d infusion	2.5	30	0
	q 4hrx6	15.0	50	0
P-1798,S.C.	dailyx5	100.0	60	60

[+] Cured mice bearing L1210 and P1798 survived greater than 30 and 90 days, respectively.

The data in Table 1 also indicate that the sensitivity of L1210 tumor cells is dependent on the site of tumor transplant. Although this may be a reflection of differences in drug delivery to the i.p. vs solid tumor cells, the results in P-1798 tumor suggest that metabolic sensitivity of target tissues to a drug and the intracellular retention of a critical concentration of the active moeity of the drug at target site are more important factors in determining tumor cell response in vivo.

L1210/Ara-C is resistant to Ara-C in vitro and in vivo due to the deletion of deoxycytidine/cytidine kinase, the enzyme responsible for the activation of Ara-C to Ara-CMP. In leukemic patients, the intracellular retention of Ara-CTP better predicted the duration rather than the probability of complete remission (Rustum, 1979).

The data in Fig. 1 demonstrate further that the activity of Ara-C is schedule dependent, as demonstrated by
Skipper, 1967, 1979, Rustum, 1978. In earlier studies by
Rustum, 1978 and Chou, 1975 it was demonstrated that in
L1210 cells the critical determinant of Ara-C action was
the differential retention of Ara-CTP between tumor cells
and normal host tissues. It was found that while L1210
cells appear to retain sufficient Ara-CTP for up to 8 hr
following drug administration, normal bone marrow cells and
intestinal tissues eliminated the drug more rapidly. Thus
it was suggested that administration of the drug every 4 hr
should spare normal tissues, while the cytotoxic action
against tumor cells remains. Indeed the data in Fig. 1
indicate that the optimal schedule of ara-C therapy is
every 4 hr for 24 hr.

Data in Fig 1 also indicate that when mice bearing leukemia
L1210 cells were treated with Ara-C 10mg/kg every 2 hr for
24 hr, mice died of toxicity. A possible explanation is
that at the time when the second dose of Ara-C was administered, the ara-CTP pools in tumor and normal cells were
comparable. The 12 hr schedule probably failed due to insufficient maintenance of drug level.

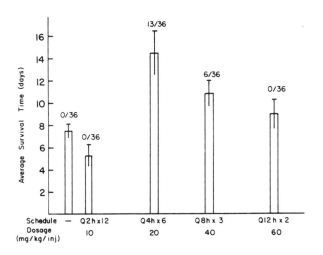

Figure 1   Schedule dependence of the antitumor activity of
Ara-C in mice bearing leukemia L1210 cells. Mice were inoculated i.p. with 1×10^6 cells and treatments were initiated 24hr thereafter.

Ara-C metabolism and retention results in Table 2 and 3 suggest a possible basis for the sensitivity of L1210 cells when treatment was repeated every 4 or 8 hr.

Table 2

Ara-C metabolism and retention by tumor and normal cells.

Cell: at 4hr[+]	Peak Ara-CTP[+] (pmol/10[6]cells)	% Retention[+]
L1210/0	250	50
L1210/Ara-C	3	48
P-1798	85	100
Small intestine	200	10
Bone marrow	150	15

[+] - initial values represent the peak intracellular ara-CTP pools achieved after an i.v. administration of therapeutic doses of the drug. Retention at 4hr was calculated as the percent of the peak ara-CTP values.

Table 3

Intracellular retention of Ara-CTP by tumor cells. Mice bearing tumors were treated i.v. with 100mg/kg ara-C containing 5 mCi/kg 5-^{3}H-ara-C(15Ci/mmol), and at various times thereafter, 3 mice/group were sacrificed and acid-soluble fractions were analyzed for Ara-CTP pools by HPLC. Ara-CTP retention was calculated as the percent of the values for each tumor type obtained at 30 min after drug administration.

| Tumor | Tumor Transplant | Ara-CTP Retention (% of 30 min value) at | | | |
		1	4	8	16hr
L1210	i.p.	89	43	28	6
L1210	S.C.	78	11	7	5
P-1798	S.C.	100	100	92	48

In case of P-1798, the data in Table 3 indicate that at 16 hr following i.v. administration of the drug, about 50% of the drug remained intracellular with no detectable level in bone marrow cells. Thus, although the initial level of ara-CTP achieved intracellularly in P-1798 was lower than that achieved in L1210 cells (Table 2), P-1798 cells were exposed to ara-CTP for a longer period of time.

Relationship between Ara-CTP pools and Ara-C incorporation into DNA. The data in Fig. 2 demonstrate that more ara-C was incorporated into the DNA of P-1798 cells than of L1210 cells. These data also demonstrate a relationship between the amount of ara-CTP found in the acid-soluble fractions and the amount of drug incorporated into DNA of L1210 and P1798 cells. P-1798 cells incorporated more drug into DNA at any given intracellular concentration of ara-CTP.

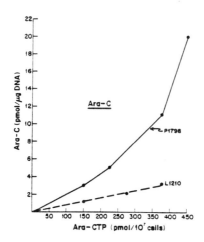

Figure 2 Relationship between Ara-CTP pools and the amount of Ara-C incorporated into DNA by P-1798 lymphosarcoma and L1210 leukemia cells. Animals bearing these tumors were treated i.v. with different doses of Ara-C and the amount of Ara-CTP in the acid-soluble fractions and amount of Ara-C incorporated into DNA were determined in each sample.

Recent studies by Kufe et al. (6) demonstrated a relationship between the amount drug incorporated into DNA and inhibition of L1210 growth in vitro. It is possible, therefore, that the sensitivity of L1210 and in particular P-1798 could be due not only to a higher pool and retention of Ara-CTP, but also to a higher and more prolonged inhibition of synthesis of macromolecules through drug incorpration into DNA.

The results in Table 4 demonstrate that at 4 and 8 hr following administration of a therapeutic dose of Ara-C to mice bearing L1210, thymidine incorporation into DNA was inhibited by about 86 and 72%, respectively. In contrast, 24 hr following drug administration, thymidine incorporation was still inhibited by 80% in P1798 cells. From the data presented in Fig 1 and Tables 2-4, inhibition of DNA synthesis must be maintained at greater than 80% to obtain maximum therapeutic efficacy.

Table 4

Inhibition of Thymidine incorporation into the DNA of Leukemia L1210 and P-1798 Lymphosarcoma cells by Ara-C. Ara-C was administered i.v. at 15mg/kg and various times thereafter ^{3}H-TdR was administered. Thirty minutes later, mice were sacrificed and the amount of thymidine incorporated into DNA was determined in control and in drug treated animals.

Tumor	% inhibition at				
	2	4	8	16	24h
L1210	98	86	72	30	20
P-1798	98	96	95	85	80

In L1210/Ara-C the lack of sensitivity of this tumor in vitro and in vivo is due to deletion of the deoxycytidine/cytidine kinase, the enzyme responsible for activiting Ara-C to Ara-CMP. In leukemia patients, however, the intracellular retention of ara-CTP was critical to the duration of complete remission rather than the induction of complete remission. These data are consistent with the principle that in order for a drug to exert its lethal effect it must be delivered to the target tissue in sufficient concentrations for a sufficient period of time, and that target tissue must be metabolically sensitive.

The data in Fig 1 demonstrate further that the therapeutic effect of Ara-C is schedual dependent (1,2,3,4). In an earlier studies (2,5) it was demonstrated that in L1210 cells the critical determinant of Ara-C action was the differential retention of Ara-CTP. It was found that while L1210 cells appear to retain critical concentrations of Ara-CTP for up to 8 hr following drug administration, normal bone marrow cells and intestinal tissues eliminate the drug more rapidly; thus on the basis of these findings it was suggested that administration of the drug every 4 hr should spare toxicity of normal tissues to Ara-C.

In Vitro Ara-C metabolism by human leukemic cells.

Treatment of acute myelocytic leukemia patients during the last years has been advanced through the administration of Ara-C by 24 hr contineous infusion for 7 or 10 days in combination with anthracycline (Preisler, 1979). Bone marrow removed from these patients and incubated with using Ara-C indicates direct relationship was found between the 4 hr retention of Ara-CTP and the duration of complete remission (Rustum, 1979). In recent years, attempts have been made to modify both the intracellular concentration of Ara-CTP and its retention. This has included the use of metabolic modulators such as thymidine (Danhauser, 1981 and Rustum, 1981), deazauridine and 5-azacytidine (Li, 1982) and high dose ara-C (Early, 1982, Rudnick, 1979, Schwartz, 1982).

Studies were conducted in vitro under conditions mimiking the conditions of high and low dose regimens of Ara-C in an attempt to modify its metabolism. The results in Table 5 indicate that a siginficant increase in the ara-CTP pools did not occur in all cases. In nearly all cases, however, high dose Ara-C (50 g/ml) caused proportionally a much greater increase in the Ara-CMP pools. This suggests that the conversion of Ara-CMP to Ara-CTP is limiting the achievable Ara-CTP concentration in the cells under these conditions.

Table 5

In vitro Ara-C metabolism by human bone marrow leukemic myeloblasts. Cells were incubated with 1, and 50μg/ml for one hour, washed, centrifuged, and extracted with PCA. Acid soluble fractions were analyzed for Ara-C anabolites using the HPLC method.

Patient	Drug Concentration (μg/ml)	Ara-CMP (pmol/107 cells)	Ara-CTP
1	1	24	160
	50	96	310
2	1	82	289
	50	72	283
3	1	15	137
	50	197	428
4	1	24	173
	50	342	347
5	1	15	85
	50	91	407
6	1	10	50
	50	97	178
7	1	14	40
	50	120	120
8	1	3	60
	50	380	230

These preliminary data suggest that by increasing the intracellular pools of Ara-CTP and possibly its incorporation into DNA, it may be possible to improve on the therapeutic efficacy of Ara-C. These studies are now in progress.

In summary, the data presented here demonstrate that retention of Ara-CTP, its incorporation into DNA, and subsequent inhibition of DNA synthesis are associated with sensitivity of P-1798 and L1210 cells to this agent. Since retention of adequate pools of Ara-CTP is the prerequisite of the other effects, the observation that this predicts therapeutic effects at the clinical level seems logical. The endpoint effect in the animal models, however, seems to be inhibition of DNA synthesis, and this may ultimately prove to be the most dependable determinant of the efficacy of this agent.

SUPPORT

This work was supported in part by a clinical biochemical Pharmacology Program Grant CA-21071 and Project Grant CA-18420 from the National Cancer Institute.

[1]To whom reprint requests should be addressed
[2]Visiting scientist from the People's Republic of China

ACKNOWLEDGEMENT

The authors acknowledge the support of Dr. H. Preisler, Department of Medical Oncology, Leukemic Service, for providing leukemic bone marrow cells. We wish to thank G. Wang, J. Goranson, E. Kelly and C. Wroszek for their excellent technical assistance.

REFERENCES

Chou T-C, Hutchinson DJ, Schmid FA, Philips FS (1975). Metabolism and selective effect of 1-β-D-aribonu- furanosylcytosine in L1210 and host tissues in vivo. Cancer Res 35:225.
Danhauser L, and Rustum YM (1980), Effect of thymidine on the toxicity, antitumor activity and metabolism of 1-β-D Arabinosylcytosine in rats bearing a chemically induced colon carcinoma. Cancer Res. 40, 1274.
Early AP, Preisler HD, Slocum H, Rustum YM (1982). A pilot study of high dose 1-β-arabinosylcytosine for acute leukemia and refractory lymphoma: Clinical response and pharmacology. Cancer Res 42:1587.
Karanes C, Wolff SN, Herzig GP, Phillips GL, Lazarus HM and Herzig RH (1979). High dose Ara-C in the treatment of patients with refractory acute non-lymphocytic leukemia, Blood 54, 191a.

Kufe DW, Major PP, Egan EM, Beardsley GP (1981).
Correlation of cytotoxicity with incorporation of ara-C
into DNA. J Biol Chem 255:8997.
Li ZR and Rustum YM (1982). Effects of 3 deazauridine on
the subsequent metabolism, toxicity and antitumor
activity of 5-azacytidine against mice bearing leukemia
L1210 sensitive and resistent to 1-β-D arabinofuranosylcytosine. Cancer Treat. Rept. in press.
Paile EM, Aherne GW and Marks VM (1979). A Radioimmunoassay
for cytosine arabinoside. Br. J. Cancer, 40, 548.
Preisler HD, Rustum YM, Henderson ES (1979). Treatment of
acute nonlymphocytic leukemia: Use of anthracycline in
cytosine arabinoside induction therapy and compariton
of two maintenance regimens. 53:464.
Rudnick S, Cadman EC, Capizzi RL, Skeel RT, Bertino JR,
McIntosh S (1979). High dose cytosine arabinoside in
refractory acute leukemia. Cancer (Phila), 44:1189.
Rustum YM (1978). Metabolism and intracellular retention
of 1-β-D-archinofuronosylcytidine as predicted of re-
sponse of animal tumors. Cancer Res 38:543.
Rustum YM, Danhauser L, Luccioni C, Au JL (1981).
Determinant of response to and metabolites and their
modulation by ara-C purine and pyrimidine metabolites.
Cancer Treat Rept 65(suppl 3):73.
Rustum YM, Higby D (1978). Biochemical and clinical
studies of chemical lymphocytic leukemia, Europ. J
Cancer 14:5.
Rustum YM, Mayhew E, and Campbell J (1981). Inability of
Liposome encapsulated 1-β-D-Arabinofuranosylcytosine
Nucleotides to overcome drug resistance in L1210 cells,
Europ. J. Cancer and Clinical Oncology 17, 809.
Rustum YM, Preisler HD (1979). Correlation between
leukemic cell retention of 1-β-D-arabinofuranosylcyto-
sine 5'-triphosphate and response to therapy. Cancer
Res 39:42.
Rustum YM, Slocum HR, Wang G, Bakshi D, Kelly E, Buscaglia
D, Wrzosek C and Preisler H (1982). Relationship be-
tween plasma Ara-C and intracellular Ara-CTP pools un-
der conditions of continuous infusion and high dose
Ara-C treatment, Medical and Pediatric Oncology, in
press.
Schwartz S, Horgenstern B, Capizzi RL (1982). Schedule
dependent synergy and antagonism between high dose
1-β-D arabinofuranosylcytosine and asparaginase in the
L51784 murine leukemia. Cancer Res. 42, 2191.

Skipper HE, Schabel FM Jr, Mallett LB, Montgomery JA, Wilkoff LT, Lloyd HH, Brochman RW (1979). Implication of biochemical cytokinetics pharmacologic and toxicologic relationship in the design of optimal therapeutic schedules. Cancer Chem. Rept 54:431.

Skipper H, Schabel FM Jr, Wilcox WS (1967).Experimental evaluation of potential anticancer agents XXI scheduling or arabinosylcytosine to take advantage of S phase specifically against leukemia L1210 cells. Cancer Chem Rept 51:125.

13th International Cancer Congress, Part E
Cancer Management, pages 121–128
© 1983 Alan R. Liss, Inc., 150 Fifth Avenue, New York, NY 10011

POTENTIALS OF PHARMACOKINETIC STUDIES IN CANCER CHEMOTHERAPY

Herbert M. Pinedo, M.D., Ph.D. and
H. Jan Keizer, M.D., Ph.D.
Netherlands Cancer Institute and
Free University Hospital,
Amsterdam, The Netherlands.

INTRODUCTION

Pharmacokinetic studies have acquired a central place
in many fields of medicine and are being used routinely for
anti-arrythmic drugs and antibiotics. The main reasons for
monitoring plasma drug concentrations are 1) wide inter-
individual variations in case of metabolism, 2) the
occurrence of saturation kinetics, 3) low therapeutic ratio,
4) when clinical toxicity is difficult to identify at an
early stage, 5) the presence of gastro-intestinal, hepatic
or renal dysfunction, and 6) when drug interactions are
suspected. Indeed, many of these circumstances are often
present in the case of anti-neoplastic drug treatment. Up
to now guidelines for dose adjustment in case of specific
organ toxicity have been developed mostly empirically for a
variety of drugs. Pharmacokinetic studies have had
relatively little impact on cancer chemotherapy. For a
limited number of drugs they have helped the clinical
oncologist in designing safe dose schedules but most drug
schedules presently used have also been developed empirically. This is partly due to the fact that sensitive
analytical techniques were not available which limited
pharmacokinetic studies to the use of radiochemicals. The
latter have severe limitations, such as impurity, lability
of the radiolabel and the difficulties to identify metabolic
products. The development of new, sensitive and more
practical assays has recently triggered studies on pharmacokinetics of anti-neoplastic agents. In the future the

ultimate purpose of clinical pharmacokinetics should be to design safe and effective treatment for individual patients. Some basic aspects of pharmacokinetic studies, their potential and limitations will be discussed.

ABSORPTION, DISTRIBUTION, METABOLISM AND EXCRETION

The initial goal of pharmacokinetic studies is to define absorption, tissue distribution, and elimination by metabolism and excretion of drugs. This information has recently been collected for many anti-neoplastic drugs from animal studies and clinical phase I trials, and has been useful for selected compounds in determining dose, schedule and route of administration for further clinical investigations.

Many attempts have been made to describe the four pharmacological processes mentioned above by mathematical models. As with many other agents the fate of most anti-cancer agents can be described by two compartment open model (Wagner 1975), consisting of a central and a peripheral compartment (Fig. 1). The drug is initially distributed from the central compartment to the peripheral compartment after which an equilibrium is established. The central compartment corresponds to the plasma and highly-perfused organs of biotransformation and excretion, including liver and kidneys. The peripheral compartment constitutes less well perfused tissues such as muscle, skin, fat and most solid tumors. The properties of a drug will determine to which particular compartment i.e. central or peripheral, specific body tissues will be associated. For example, although being a well-perfused tissue, for most anti-cancer drugs the brain will pertain to the peripheral compartment. There are three possible types of two-compartment systems. They differ in that elimination occurs either from the central compartment, from the peripheral compartment or from both.

PHARMACOKINETIC PARAMETERS

Which are the most important pharmacokinetic parameters resulting from the processes described above? After intravenous injection of a drug the peak plasma concentration will be reached almost immediately. Thereafter two more

phases can be distinguished. The distribution phase (α)
(Fig. 2) corresponds to the drug distribution from the
central compartment to the peripheral compartment. Although
the central compartment is kinetically considered a common
homogeneous unit, this does not necessarily imply that at
a given time the drug concentration is similar in all
tissues. However, it assumes that any change which occurs
in the plasma level of a drug quantitatively reflects a
change which occurs in the central compartment tissue levels.

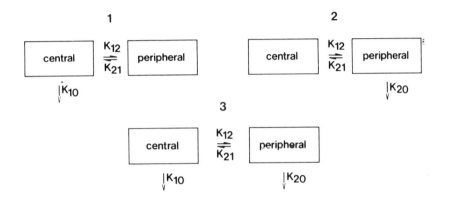

Fig. 1. Schematic representation of three types of two-
compartment open systems consisting of a central and a peripheral compartment. The three types differ in the elimination of drug occurring from one or both of the compartments.
k_{12}, rate constant for transfer of drug from central to
     peripheral
k_{21}, rate constant for the reverse transfer
k_{10}, k_{20}, elimination rate constant

The second phase which can be identified is the β-phase,
which is longer and represents elimination of the drug from
the central compartment. The elimination of the major part
of the drug is assumed to occur by first-order processes,
i.e. the rate of elimination of drug is proportional to the
amount of drug in the body at any time. Elimination occurs
through renal and biliary pathways, biotransformation and
to a lesser extent through excretion in expired air. Drug
levels in the peripheral tissues (muscle, lean tissue, fat

and tumor) will first increase, reach a maximum and then decline during the post-distributive phase (Fig. 3).

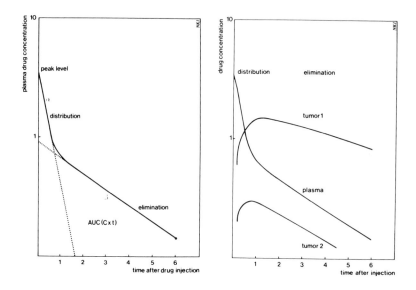

Fig. 2. Schematic representation of plasma levels of a
cytostatic agent after i.v.
administration. Concentration
and time in arbitrary units.

Fig. 3. Schematic representation of drug concentration
in peripheral tissues (including tumor)

The area under the plasma concentration curve (AUC) reflects the period during which the tumor cells are exposed to the concentration C of a drug (Cxt). Information on the impact of Cxt on tumor cell kill is of major importance for drug scheduling. In fact, experimental data suggest that peak plasma level is more important than AUC (Schabel 1982).

Another relevant pharmacokinetic parameter is the volume of distribution (Vd), representing the extent to which a drug distributes through body-fluid compartments, which is in essence the uptake by the tissues. The clearance from the central compartment is calculated from the dose divided by the area under the plasma concentration curve (AUC). Lastly, excretion from the body (e.g. renal clearance) is also a major pharmacokinetic parameter.

CONDITIONS AFFECTING BIOLOGICAL ACTIVITY

As mentioned above several conditions may greatly influence serum and tissue concentrations and subsequently the biological effect of a cytotoxic agent. These include the rate of metabolism of the parent drug to inactive or active metabolites, and the fraction of active compound which is bound to plasma proteins and blood cells. Concomitant drug therapy may alter protein binding and metabolism and lead to unexpected host toxicity. During combination chemotherapy, the anti-tumor effect of one drug may be altered by a second agent. Few clinical studies have investigated this phenomenon, in contrast to several animal studies. Likewise, changes in the effect of one anti-tumor agent may be seen following an effect on cellular kinetics caused by another drug of a combination regimen.

Dose dependent pharmacokinetics is reflected by an increase in the biological half-life and a greater than proportional increase in plasma concentration of the drug with increase in dose. An important cause for this is saturation of the capacity of an enzyme as carrier system for drug metabolism or excretion. It is obvious that more information on this phenomenon is essential since high dose chemotherapy is being applied at increasing frequency. Phase 1 clinical trials offer the possibility to study dose-dependent pharmacokinetics as in these studies the new drugs are administered over a wide range of doses. Dose-dependent pharmacokinetics may be of particular importance when high doses of drugs are being infused into the hepatic artery. Direct or indirect effects of the tumor on pharmacokinetics may have to be considered. Cancer patients usually have a decreased physical condition with malfunctioning of one or more organs, e.g. kidney or liver. Also compounds formed directly by or in response to a tumor may give rise to decreased organ functioning and hence affect the pharmacokinetics of a drug.

ROUTINE MONITORING OF ANTI-NEOPLASTIC AGENTS

Future routine use of drug level measurements in
clinical oncology will be necessary in case a correlation is
established between one or more pharmacokinetic parameters
of a drug and either anti-tumor activity or toxicity. Obviously, the availability of reliable and easy analytical
methods for drug assay is a prerequisite. In this respect
it is encouraging that for the majority of clinically used
anti-neoplastic agents a strong correlation has been
established between dose and toxicity in experimental
animals, regarding both host and tumor tissues (Schabel
1982). This dose-relationship is steep for homogeneous and
sensitive animal tumors. Obviously, tumor heterogeneity
and the presence of resistant cells may alter the steepness
of this correlation. It is the general experience in
clinical oncology that the dose-response curve for normal
tissues in man is also steep, i.e. small increments in the
dose of the cytostatic drug may lead to an unproportionally
increase in toxicity (Frei, Canellos 1980). For a limited
number of drugs such as methotrexate and carminomycin a
correlation has been established between one or more pharmacokinetic parameters and toxicity.

Moreover, standard clinical trials do not offer the option
to increase doses in case of limited toxicity, as this would
hamper the evaluation of treatment results. Also the
majority of clinical oncologists routinely tend to adhear
to standard dosages aiming not to be faced with serious
toxicity. While it has been even suggested that lower
dosages of cytotoxic drugs might be equally effective and
safer (Tattersall, Tobias 1976), there is now some evidence
from clinical investigations that dose-escalation does result
in better tumor response. Such studies include randomised
trials in Hodgkins- and non-Hodgkins lymphoma, lymphocytic
leukaemia and small cell bronchogenic carcinoma (Frei,
Canellos 1980). These tumors are generally sensitive and
may therefore respond in a first-order kinetics (Skipper
1975). However, exciting data also exist for less sensitive
tumors including melanoma, colo-rectal carcinoma, breast
cancer and osteogenic sarcoma (Frei and Canellos 1980).
Most likely these favourable findings are a reflection of
increased tissue levels of the drug and related pharmacokinetic parameters. The wide variation in response seen

after standard-dose treatment of human malignancies in apparently comparable patients may be explained by the administration of suboptimal drug doses to some patients.

One should bear in mind that pharmacokinetic studies of several drugs used in the general medical practice have learned that the administration of standard dosages results in a wide variation of serum concentrations and consequently in tissue response (Koch-Weser 1975). Indeed, the recent pharmacokinetic studies of anti-neoplastic agents have also shown great variations in the various parameters, but many data are from patients receiving combination chemotherapy which makes it impossible to study the relationship of the parameters with biological effects. Thus, there is almost a complete lack of clinical data with respect to the correlation between pharmacokinetic parameters and tumor response. The only possible exception is a report showing a correlation between plasma concentration of cytosine arabinoside and response of acute myeloid leukemia (van Prooyen 1977).

In this respect the enhanced anti-tumor effect observed following intra-arterial infusion as compared to intravenous drug administration is encouraging. Higher local drug concentrations with this method of administration most likely provide the basis for the improved responses.

Hopefully novel approaches of pharmacokinetic studies such as intrapleural and intraperitoneal drug administration may render more information on the relationship between drug concentration and anti-tumor effect in-vivo. Interestingly, in-vitro clonogenic cell experiments have shown that human tumor stem cell kill is dose-related.

It is encouraging that several recent treatment protocols which are now being used, give room for dose-escalation in case of minimal toxicity. It may be expected that correlations of pharmacokinetic parameters and anti-tumor effect will be difficult to establish in particular for solid tumors. Studies may require a great number of patients, since many other factors also play a role in the ultimate effect on the tumor cells (Table 1). It is nonetheless urgent to test the hypothesis of a relationship between pharmacokinetic parameters of anti-cancer agents and tumor response, both in animals and in humans. Hopefully the relative impact of peak levels versus AUC will be established.

> Table 1. Reasons that make interpretation
> of dose-response relationship more
> difficult
>
> - drugs are usually given in combination
> - AUC-plasma may not be proportional
>   to AUC-tumor tissue
> - varying blood supply (drug uptake)/
>   cytokinetics etc.
> - varying uptake into/excretion from
>   the cells
> - intrinsic mechanism leading to
>   decreased drug sensitivity

The sensitive and easy methods to measure drug concentration,
such as high pressure liquid chromatography and radio-immuno
assays, which have recently become available to many
laboratories will be of great help. The available evidence
does give hope that these pharmacokinetic data, in a
framework with other biochemical and cytokinetic data, may
ultimately lead not only to a safe but also a more effective
cytostatic treatment of the individual patient.

Frei E, Canellos GP (1980). Dose: A critical factor in
  cancer chemotherapy. Am J Med 69:585.
Koch-Weser J (1975). The serum level approach to individualization of drug dosage. Eur J Clin Pharmacol 9:1.
Prooyen van R, van der Kleyn E, Haanen C (1977). Pharmacokinetics of cytosine arabinoside in acute myeloid
  leukemia. Clin Pharmacol Ther 21:744.
Schabel FM Jr, Griswold DP Jr, Corbett TH, Laster WR Jr
  (1982). Increasing therapeutic response rates to anti-
  cancer drugs by applying the basis principles of pharmacology. Proceedings of a meeting entitled "Cancer 1981/
  Cancer 2001 - An International Colloquium", sponsored
  by the University of Texas System Cancer Center,
  M.D. Anderson Hospital and Tumor Institute, Houston,
  Texas, November 11, 1981.
Skipper HE (1975). Pharmacological basis of cancer chemo-
  therapy: closing remarks. In "Pharmacological basis of
  cancer chemotherapy," Baltimore: The Williams and Wilkins
  Company, p 713.
Tattersall MHM, Tobias JS (1976). How strong is the case
  for intensive cancer chemotherapy? Lancet 2:1071.
Wagner JG (1975). Fundamentals of clinical pharmacokinetics.
  Drug Intelligence Publications, Inc., Hamilton, Illinois.

13th International Cancer Congress, Part E
Cancer Management, pages 129–143
© 1983 Alan R. Liss, Inc., 150 Fifth Avenue, New York, NY 10011

CELL BIOLOGICAL SYSTEMS FOR PREDICTION OF INDIVIDUAL HUMAN TUMOR DRUG SENSITIVITY

Stephan Tanneberger, M.D., Ph.D. and
Eberhard Nissen, Ph.D.
Central Institute of Cancer Research,
Academy of Sciences, Berlin,
German Democratic Republic

For more than 15 years, along with some other groups, we have emphasized that the biological individuality of human tumors has been proven in clinical and cell biological levels and demands individualized, biology-adapted cancer treatment (Tanneberger et al. 1967). The prediction of individual human tumor drug sensitivity is one of the key problems within the conception of individualized cancer chemotherapy.

Cell biological systems for prediction of individual human tumor drug sensitivity have been elaborated and recommended for more than 20 years. The long history of predictive tests has repeatedly been reviewed (Tanneberger 1968; Dendy et al. 1973; Nissen et al. 1980; Hamburger 1981). An up to date summary is given in Table 1 in which the most important predictive tests are listed and classified by the principles of the technique used. The conclusions of the authors on the clinical value of the assays are added.

Approach	Method	Conclusion	Authors, Year
long-term tissue cultures	cell cultures/morphology	(+)	Lickiss et al. 1974
		(+)	Cobb et al. 1964
		+	Limburg 1973
		(+)	Tanneberger et al. 1967
		+	Terentieva et al. 1976
		+	Izsak et al. 1971
	cell cultures/trans-membrane potential	+	Walliser et al. 1981
	cell cultures/cell counting	+	Holmes et al. 1974
	cell cultures/auto-radiography	+	Murphy et al. 1975
		+	Zittoun et al. 1975
		+	Livingstone et al. 1980
	lymphocyte cultures tryphan blue dye exclusion	+	Durkin et al. 1979
	cell cultures/DNA or RNA synthesis	(+)	Mitchel et al. 1972
		+	Wheeler et al. 1974
		+	Shristav et al. 1980
	organ cultures/DNA synthesis	(+)	Tschao et al. 1962
		(+)	Tanneberger et al. 1973
		(+)	Nissen et al. 1978
	organ cultures/histo-chemistry	+	Hecker et al. 1976
	tumor slices/DNA, RNA, Proteinsyntesis, respiration glycolysis	+	Dickson 1976
	in-vitro-soft agar human tumor stem cell assay	(+)	Salmon et al. 1978
		+	v. Hoff 1979
		+	Tveit et al. 1980
		+	Alberts et al. 1980

Ap-proach	Method	Con-clu-sion	Authors, Year
short-term tissue incuba-tion + drug	cell suspen-sion/mor-phology biopsy/ autoradi-ography	+ + –	Dendy et al. 1973 Wright et al. 1973 Wolberg 1971
	cell suspen-sion/auto-radiography	+	Thirlwell et al. 1976
	cell suspen-sion/DNA or RNA	+ (+) + + + + + (+)	Andrysek 1973 Hirschmann 1973 Possinger et al. 1976 Mattern et al. 1976 Bastert et al. 1975 Volm 1975 Volm 1980 Schlag 1979
	biopsy/ DNA syn-thesis	(+)	Kaufmann et al. 1971
	cell suspen-sion/enzyme assay	+ (+) +	Kondo 1971 Di Paolo 1971 Knock et al. 1974

Tab. 1. Historical survey on in vitro prediction of human tumor drug sensitivity (modified from Tanneberger et al. 1982).

As shown in Table 1 most authors have evaluated their assays enthusiastically; the fact that no assay has achieved general clinical application is evidence enough that such evaluations have general-ly been overoptimistic. The in vitro soft-agar hu-man tumor stem cell assay strongly advocated over the last few years (Sikic et al. 1981) has also received 1980 a sober and more realistic evalu-ation by Rubniak and Hill and in 1981, during the First UICC Conference on Clinical Oncology by Steel.

Our own experiences concerning the use of in vitro methods to predict tumor response to anti-neoplastic chemotherapy fit this pattern. In 1964

we started very optimistically with a cell culture
technique, evaluating drug effects by morphological
criteria. Having cultivated several hundred tumor
specimens we recognized the limitations of this
assay and in light of our experience we developed
a second type of assay in 1969/70 using the organ
culture technique and evaluating the drug effects
by DNA-synthesis measurement (Tanneberger et al.
1973). Without doubt this organ culture assay was
a real advance in comparison to the former technique of in vitro prediction. As can be seen in
Figure 1 for example, the rate of in vitro maintenance for breast cancer specimen rose to 88,7%
in organ culture compared with only 32,8 % in
monolayer cell culture. Furthermore, the detection
of cell viability with the aid of DNA-synthesis
measurement is much more precise than with morphological methods.

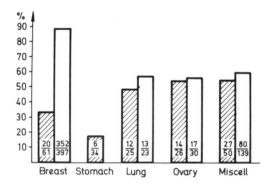

Fig. 1. Percentage of growing cultures of
different tumortypes cultivated in vitro
▨ cell culture technique (196 biopsies)
▢ organ culture technique (589 biopsies)

In our clinical studies as described earlier, the
survival rate of patients with ovarian cancer receiving predicted surgical adjuvant chemotherapy
had a tendency to be higher but the difference
to non-predicted adjuvant treatment was sta-

tistically not significant different. For lung
cancer no difference in outcome was found between
non-individualized and individualized surgical
adjuvant chemotherapy (Tanneberger et al. 1979).

A very promising result we obtained incor-
porating principles of individualized treatment in
a surgical adjuvant chemotherapy protocol for the
treatment of breast cancer stage III (UICC registered trial No 77-051). From January 1974 to
February 1981, 200 patients entered this study.
For the first 110 patients the control/treatment
ratio was 1 to 1, thereafter 1 to 2. 193 patients
are evaluable now. According to the protocol all

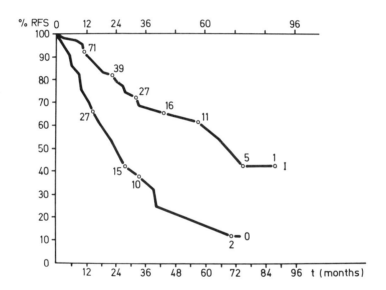

Fig. 2. Results of individualized surgical adjuvant chemotherapy in breast cancer stage III; drug
sensitive, ER$^{\pm}$ patients; treatment (I) 77 patients,
control (0) 36 patients; ( ) patients at risk;
$x^2 = 14,167$, p o,001; evaluation by Peek III/82

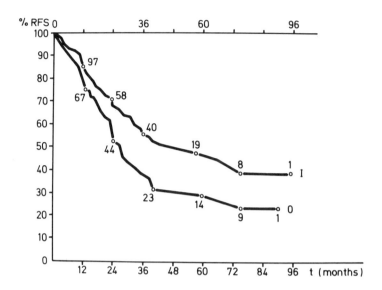

Fig. 3. Results of individualized surgical adjuvant chemotherapy in breast cancer stage III;drug
sensitive and non-sensitive, $ER^{\pm}$ patients;treat-
ment(I) 115 patients, control (0) 85 patients;
( ) patients at risk $x^2 = 5,812$, p 0,02;
evaluation by Peek III/82

patients (control and treatment arm) are investigated in vitro for drug sensitivity and estrogen
receptor content of the tumor. The control group
is treated by radical mastectomy only, the treatment group receives the predicted hormone-chemotherapy in the case of sensitivity and ER^+, and
no hormone or chemotherapy in case of drug resistance and ER^-. In case of insufficient in vitro
data for technical reasons, patients in the treatment arm receive surgical adjuvant treatment with
Cyclophosphamide alone. As shown in Figure 2
(statistically significant) longer relapse free
survival has been achieved if drug sensitive,
$ER^{\pm}$ patients are treated with the predicted
hormone-chemotherapy (77 patients) in comparison

to the relapse free survival of drug sensitive,
$ER^{\pm}$ patients, getting no surgical adjuvant treatment as control (36 patients). This difference
could not be observed (Figure 3) comparing the
total control (85 patients) with the total treatment arm (115 patients). Of course, the relevance
of this trial to the problem of correlation between
in vitro drug prediction and clinical response is
limited due to the combination of hormone- and
chemotherapy. Moreover, from our present viewpoint,
premenopausal controls should get a standard CMF
surgical adjuvant chemotherapy instead of no chemotherapy. Nevertheless this trial which addressed
the general problem of individualized chemotherapy
was confirming our present standpoint to the role
of drug prediction in antineoplastic therapy.

Considering the 20 year history of international experience concerning in vitro drug predictive
tests, including our own results, the following
conclusions seem to be justified: There are some
biologically and pharmacologically acceptable
approaches of proven predictive value for anti-
neoplastic drug efficacy in experimental systems
and also in man. But these approaches are complicated, time-consuming and need special laboratory
facilities. In contrast to some overoptimistic
evaluations in the past, there is no assay for
prediction of antineoplastic drug efficacy available at present which could be recommended for
general use in clinical practice. This criticism
applies also to the "tumor stem cell assays" which
have received wide publicity during the last few
years. Accordingly, human tumor drug sensitivity
prediction and individualized cancer chemotherapy
remains a top problem for applied cancer research.
Surgical adjuvant chemotherapy is a field of increasing activity currently; the importance of
drug sensitivity prediction is as a result, that
much the greater.

There are some crucial obstacles in the way
of elaboration an effective predictive test. Technical problems still exist in the in vitro methodology, but more fundamental problems result from

the heterogeneity of tumors in space and time
and of the variability of human tumor drug sensitivity.

Concerning the main problems there is the
following situation: Isolated cells for short-term
studies, monolayer cultures or soft-agar cloning
frequently cannot be obtained in sufficient a-
mounts, particularly in such clinically important
tumor types as breast and stomach cancer (18).
Furthermore, as emphasized by Dendy, the identification of isolated cells as neoplastic, essential
for a successful assay, is still an unsolved problem. The risk of selection from mixed cell populations must never be overlooked. Selection of subpopulations able to grow in vitro may automatically
introduce a false positive bias in the test procedure since tumor cells unable to grow under those
conditions may also be insensitive to any given
drug. Thus it was to be expected that assays such
as those described by us (Tanneberger et al. 1967)
or by Salmon (Salmon et al. 1978) would be much
better at predicting drug insensitivity than drug
sensitivity. Finally, the kinetics of isolated
single cells are very different from that of the
cells in tissue, a fact which can influence interpretation of drug sensitivity.

For tumor types, suitable for single cell
preparation, the measurement of the cloning ability of tumor cells in soft agar seemed to be the
most promising approach to determine the cell
viability. Cloning is a very precise test for cell
viability. Moreover cloning increases the chance
that from a mixed single cell population neoplastic cells are considered since neoplastic
cells have a selectively higher potential for
cloning in soft agar (Sikic et al. 1981; Tveit
et al. 1982).

Nevertheless there are increasing doubts as
to whether the optimism of some groups working
with the so-called human tumor stem cell assays
is justified. There are theoretical and practical
doubts concerning this approach. First of all,
the hypothesis that clonogenic cells are repre-

sentative human tumor stem cells needs further
support. Neither is there at present evidence
enough that the cells isolated from human tumors
which do clone are representative of the entire
in vivo stem cell population. For this reason
terms like colony forming assay or clonogenic tumor cell assay for this approach seem to be more
realistic than the term "human tumor stem cell
assay" often used by Salmon. In general the clonogenic tumor cell assay is restricted with respect
to the prediction "sensitive" by the tumor heterogeneity and, with respect to the prediction
"resistant" by cell cloning artefacts which possibly exist (Steel 1981). Finally the long duration of clonogenic tumor cell assay (10 days on
the average) limits clinical application.

Approaches as organ cultures or short-term
incubation techniques which avoid the disadvantages
of isolated cell-assays by working with tumor biopsies have other disadvantages resulting from the
human tumor heterogeneity. Heterogeneity of human
tumors refers to the balance between tumor and
normal cells in each tumor and each part of a tumor. Due to the heterogeneity of human tumors
there is a high risk of biopsying connective tissue
instead of neoplastic tissue. Knowledge of what
is in the test tube is essential for a succesful
in vitro assay but this is difficult to aquire
when working with biopsies. Furthermore many tumors are composed of mixed populations of tumor
cells with different growth properties and different drug sensitivities. Taking into account
tumor heterogeneity it seems clear that only those
predictive techniques will have a chance which
insure representative sampling of the entire tumor.

An additionally disadvantage of the short-
term incubation techniques is the risk to work
with "dying tissue" which is not representative
of a proliferating tumor. In organ culture by
contrast vital tumor tissue is under investigation.
The tumor cells metabolize in the normal biological
environment, the original biological architecture,
cellular interrelationships and function are largely retained. There are only minimal deviations of

the cell behaviour from the in vivo situation. To
this extent organ cultures have remarkable advantages in comparison to the short-term incubation
techniques and to other in vitro approaches.

To measure cell damage and cell death in
predictive tests often radioactive precursor incorporation has been used (Tchao et al. 1962;
Volm et al. 1980; Sanfillipo et al. 1981). The
measurement of DNA-, RNA- or protein synthesis
after 1 - 2 days of drug influence on metabolizing
cells no doubt adequately reflects cellular defects.
Nevertheless, since not all antineoplastic compounds act directly against DNA-, RNA- or protein
synthesis, precursor incorporation inhibition has
inherent limitations if used in short-term incubation assays. A realistic picture of ultimate drug
effects cannot be expected to be apparent within
few hours. Only in cases where the mechanism of
drug action in known, is short-term radioactive
precursor incorporation justified. Furthermore
the precursor to be incorporeated has to be chosen
according to the known mechanism of drug action.
Another limitation of short-term-precursor incorporation assays result from, the failure of DNA
precursors to be incorporated in cells with a long
cycle time. After explantation in an in vitro system the cell cycle time is commonly prolonged.
This phenomenon increases the risk of failure of
a short-term precursor incorporation assay.
A very basic obstacle for the prediction of
the tumor drug response is the great variability
of human tumor drug sensitivity depending on the
in vivo or in vitro biological environment of the
tumor and of the stage of tumor cell development
when testing occurs. In an experimental man-in
vitro-nude mice heterotransplantation system we
have demonstrated that human tumor cells change
such fundamental properties as growth rate and
karyotype as well as the drug sensitivity pattern
in a very dynamic way when growing under different
conditions (Nissen et al. 1980). The pharmacologic
heterogeneity among different metastases, as well
as between the metastasis and the primery tumor
are probably related to this phenomenon.

In our institute a new predictive test has been developed in 1979/80.

Our goals in developing this new test were to based on our positive experiences with organ cultures but to overcome the very critical problem of insufficient characterization of the tumor samples when using the conventional organ culture technique.

Organ cultures in our view are the most promising approach for sampling and maintainance of human tumors for in vitro drug prediction. Already Foley, 1964, and particularly Ambrose, 1968, have underlined that organ cultures meet the essential requirement of an in vitro predictive test much better than other approaches. As mentioned above, organ culture preserves the cellular interrelationships and, in contrast to single cell culture, there is no risk of selecting a small and unrepresentative proportion of the stem or total cell population. More than 10 years work with human tumor organ cultures have fully confirmed our expectations and the organ culture approach has since been reproduced by some groups, for example Dickson, 1976 and Masters, 1980 with success.

There are some alternative means to overcome the problem of insufficient characterization of tumor samples investigated in organ culture. Theoretically autoradiographic assessment of the drug effects appears to be such an alternative but this approach is not acceptable for practical reasons (long exposure time). Therefore we looked in an other direction, seeking a way to combine morphological control of the cultures and quantitative biochemical assessment of drug effects.

Based on our earlier efforts (Tanneberger 1969) using tissue slices instead of human tumor biopsies for organ culture, a new technique has been developed based on Krumdieck's approach (1980) to cut uniform vital slices of human tumors which can be characterized morphologically and to cultivate these slices in organ culture (Nissen et al. 1982).

The technique guarantees, in contrast to the conventional organ culture technique, strict morphological control of all cultures. Furthermore the metabolic activity of the tissue slices maintained in vitro is much higher than in maintained biopsies due to an improved cell-medium interaction and an improved oxygenation. We had already an optimal assessment technique for cell viability with the ^{3}H-thymidin incorporation measurement after 48 hours drug exposure and this technique has been succesfully incorporated in our new assay. As shown in Table 2 und 3 the new assay predicted very well the drug sensitivity of Lewis lung carcinoma in mice and of a transplantable rectal carcinoma of rats.

	in vitro		in vivo			
drug	ug/ ml	% inhibition of ^{3}H-thymidin uptake	day post implant.	inoculation ml cell susp.	dosage mg/kg	% tumor inhib.
CTX	12	87,0	7	2x0,1	120 i.p.	52
FU	10	88,4	2	2x0,05	100 i.p.	73
Dbl	1,0	25,8	2	2x0,05	5 i.v.	29
Crm	0,5	5,2	7	2x0,1	3 i.v.	35

Table 2. Antineoplastic effectivity of Cyclophosphamide (CTX), Fluorouracil (FU), Carminomycin (Crm) and Daunoblastin (Dbl) on Lewis lung carcinoma of the mouse (C 57 B^{0}l 6 - 12 animals/ group)

drug	in vitro dosage ug/ml	% inhibition of ^{3}H-thymidin uptake	day post implant.	in vivo inoculation ml cell susp.	dosage mg/kg	% ILS
CTX	20	65,0	14	0,5 i.p.	120 i.v.	100
	10	50,0	14	0,5 i.p.	60 i.v.	86
Crm	0,5	0	17	0,5 i.p.	3 i.v.	-17

Table 3. Antineoplastic effectivity of Cyclophosphamid (CTX), and Carminomycin (Crm) on rectal carcinoma MV 760 DMes of the rat (Wistar 12 animals/group).

In so far our first experience with the new assay suggest that this approach is a realistic route to individualized cancer chemotherapy. Nevertheless our knowledge of the previous history of such tests tempers our optimism. Here as everywhere in drug prediction, (and science in general), what A.Hamburger 1981 emphasized in an excellent review of predictive cancer chemotherapy holds true, namely "that a system must be utilized by many investigators before it can be effectively used as a clinical tool."

Dendy PP, Dawson MPA, Honess DJ (1973). Studies on the drug sensitivity of human tumor cells in short term culture. In Wüst G (ed): "Aktuelle Probleme der Therapie maligner Tumoren", Stuttgart: Georg Thieme, p 34.

Dickson JA, Suzangar M (1976). In vitro sensitivity testing of human tumor slices to chemotherapeutic agents. In Dendy PP (ed): "Human tumors in short-term culture", New York: Academic Press, p 107.

Hamburger AW (1981). Use of in vitro tests in predictive cancer chemotherapy. J Natl Cancer Inst 66:981.

Krumdieck CL, Dos Santos JE, Ho KJ (1980). A new instrument for the rapid preparation of tissue slices. Anal Biochem 104:118.

Masters JRW, Krishnaswamy A, Rigby CC, O'Donoghue EPN (1980). Quantitative organ culture: An approach to prediction of tumour response. Br J Cancer 41, Suppl IV:199.

Nissen E, Arnold W, Weiss H, Tanneberger St (1980). Some further characteristics of human mesothelioma cells. In De Brabander M (ed): "Cell movement and neoplasia", Oxford, New York: Pergamon Press, p 171.

Nissen E, Projan A, Tanneberger St (1980). In vitro-Vorhersage der Wirkung von Zytostatika im Konzept der individualisierten antineoplastischen Chemotherapie beim Menschen. In Tanneberger St (ed): "Experimentelle und klinische Tumorchemotherapie" Berlin: Akademie-Verlag, p 103.

Nissen E, Tanneberger St, Weiss H (1982). Zur in vitro Kultivierung vitaler Gewebeschnitte als eine neue Variation der Organkulturtechnik. Acta biol med germ, in press.

Rupniak T, Hill BT (1980). The poor cloning ability in agar of human tumour cells from biopsies of primary tumours. Cell Biol Int Rep 4: 479.

Salmon SE, Hamburger AW, Soehnlen BJ, Durie, BGM, Alberts DS, Moon TE (1978). Quantitation of differential sensitivity of human tumour cells to anticancer drugs. N Engl J Med 298:1321.

Sanfillippo O, Daidone MG, Costa A, Canetta R, Silvestrini R (1981). Estimation of differential in vitro sensitivity of non-Hodgkin lymphomas to anticancer drugs. Eur J Cancer 17:217

Sikic IS, Taber RL (1981). Human tumor clonogenic assays. Cancer Chemother Pharmacol 6:201.

Steel G (1981). Human tumour kinetics, in vitro sensitivity. 1. Conference Clinical Oncology UICC, Lausanne, October.

Tanneberger St, Bacigalupo G (1967). Die Benutzung von Zellkulturen zur Ermittlung der Sensibilität menschlicher Tumoren gegenüber Zytostatika. Dtsch Gesundh Wes 22:11.

Tanneberger St (1968). Gewebekultur und Krebschemotherapie. Arch Geschwulstforsch 31:387.

Tanneberger St (1969). Versuche zur Erweiterung der Möglichkeiten für in vitro-Studien an menschlichen Tumoren. Experientia 25:334.

Tanneberger St, Mohr A (1973). Biological cha-
    racterization of human tumours by means of organ
    culture and individualized cytostatic cancer
    treatment. Arch Geschwulstforsch 42:307.
Tanneberger St, Nissen E, Schälike W (1979). Pre-
    diction of drug efficacy potentialities and lim-
    itations. In Fox BW (ed): "Advances in medical
    oncology, research and education, Vol. 5, Basis
    for cancer therapy 1" New York/Oxford: Pergamon
    Press, p 107.
Tanneberger St, Nissen E (1982). The role of in
    vitro techniques in assessing antineoplastic
    therapeutic activities. In Tanneberger St,
    Davis W (eds): "The control of tumour growth
    and its biological bases" Berlin: Academic Press.
Tchao R, Easty GC, Ambrose EJ, Raven RW, Bloom HJG
    (1968). Effect of chemotherapeutic agents and
    hormones in organ cultures of human tumours.
    Europ J Cancer 4:39.
Tveit KM, Fodstad O, Lotsberg I, Vaage, Piehl A
    (1982). Colony growth and chemosensitivity in
    vitro of human melanoma biobsies. Relationship
    of clinical parameters. Int J Cancer 29: in
    press.
Volm M (1980). Sensibilitätstestung menschlicher
    Tumoren gegenüber Zytostatika mit einem In-
    vitro-Kurzzeittest. Dtsch med Wschr 105:1493.

13th International Cancer Congress, Part E
Cancer Management, pages 145–149
© 1983 Alan R. Liss, Inc., 150 Fifth Avenue, New York, NY 10011

CLINICAL APPLICATION AND LIMITATION

Sándor Eckhardt, M.D.

Department of Chemotherapy
National Institute of Oncology
Budapest, Hungary 1525

Despite the availability of approximately 120 cytostatic drugs currently used in clinical cancer therapy only a limited amount of patients with malignancies could be cured by cytostatic agents alone /1,5-2,0 %/ while in a considerable propor- tion of cases chemotherapy became an important component of the multimodality treatment approach /25-30 %/. Cytostatic therapy resulted in pallia- tive effects in 25-30 % of all cancer patients, while the remaining part of patients treated by cytostatic agents did not show any response. /Table 1/.

RESULTS OF CHEMOTHERAPY
/1982/

Response	% of all patients
Cure	1.5 - 2.0
Increased lifespan	25.0 - 30.0
Improved quality of life	25.0 - 30.0
No effect	38.0 - 48.5

Malignant diseases which can be considered as curable by chemotherapy are: acute lymphocytic and acute myelogenous leukemia of children and young adults, Burkitt-tumour, trophoblastic disease, Wilms-tumour and certain pediatric malignancies. More recently, Hodgkin's disease and non-Hodgkin lymphoma, testicular cancer are main targets for curability by chemotherapy /Table 2/.

MALIGNANT DISEASES CURABLE BY CHEMOTHERAPY

Childhood ALL, AML
Burkitt lymphoma
Trophoblastic disease
Wilms tumour, rhabdomyosarcoma
Hodgkin's disease
Non-Hodgkin lymphoma
Testicular cancer /non-seminoma/

1.5-2.0 % of all cancer patients

Diseases in which cytostatic drugs play a decisive role in a form of a multimodality approach are some acute and chronic leukemia and lymphomas, breast cancer, ovarian cancer, prostatic cancer and microcellular cancer of the lung /Table 3/.

MALIGNANT DISEASES WITH INCREASED
LIFESPAN DUE TO CHEMOTHERAPY

Acute leukemias in adults
Chronic leukemias
Multiple myeloma
Breast cancer
Ovarian cancer
Prostate cancer
Small cell lung cancer

25-30 % of all cancer patients

Palliation is the only result of chemotherapy in about a third of all malignancies, such as head and neck, colorectal and other GI-tract carcinomas. Nevertheless, some patients gain not only relief of severe symptoms but also have a prolongation of their lifespan and are able to maintain a reasonable quality of life /Table 4/.

MALIGNANT DISEASES IN WHICH IMPROVED QUALITY OF
LIFE OF PATIENTS CAN BE ACHIEVED BY CHEMOTHERAPY

Head and neck cancer
GI-tract cancer
Non-small cell lung cancer
Uterine cancer
Bone and soft tissue sarcoma

25-30 % of all cancer patients

There are, however, neoplastic diseases in
which chemotherapy did not yield any benefit to
the patients /e.g. renal cancer, gall bladder
cancer, glioblastomas etc./ /Table 5/.

MALIGNANT DISEASES REFRACTORY TO
CHEMOTHERAPY

Stomach cancer
Pancreas, gall bladder cancer
Liver cancer
Kidney cancer
Brain tumours
Melanoma

38.0-48.5 % of all cancer patients

A special application of chemotherapy, while
still under debate regarding its usefulness, is
the adjuvant prophylactic chemotherapy which is
certainly modifying the fate of a number of breast
and testicular cancer patients as well as that
of patients with osteogenic sarcoma /Table 6/.

MALIGNANT DISEASES TREATED BY ADJUVANT
CHEMOTHERAPY

Results +	+	−
Breast	Lung	Stomach
Non-seminoma	/small cell/	Lung
Osteogenic sc.	Colorectal	/non-small
Chorionepithelioma	Ovary	cell/
Wilms tumour		Melanoma
Rhabdomyosc.		

Since results of cancer chemotherapy are far
from being satisfactory it is of paramount importance to analyze the series of limitations encountered in this field.

One major limitation is the inadequacy of
preclinical testing systems for predictability of
drug effect in man. So far transplantable and chemically induced experimental tumours served as a
basis for selecting cytostatic agents for clinical
testing in the majority of cases. More recently,
however, there are also other approaches such as
the human tumour xenograft systems or the clonogenic assays which are models more close to human
malignancies. Nevertheless, their value still has
to be assessed. It is also of particular importance to learn more about testing the biological response modifiers and that of hormone active substances.

Another difficulty for having greater success
with chemotherapy is the lack of proper knowledge
on mechanism of action of new agents. The rational
design of drug schedules and combinations is an
immense field of research in which so far only few
results were achieved. As a result of this incapa-
bility of designing rational drug schedules in human malignancies,many drugs which were earlier rejected as too toxic or ineffective compounds have
to be revisited. As an example, Cisplatin has to
be mentioned which although known for many decades
was not used in clinics before its proper mode
of administration was elaborated. Nowadays it is

considered as a powerful cytostatic agent with acceptable toxicity.

Drug interactions play an important role in the success or failure of cancer chemotherapy. Metabolic or catabolic enzyme inducers may decisively influence cytostatic effect. Nevertheless, very few data are available in this respect. Data on tissue distribution of drugs, especially those of the elimination, are also not always available, thus, limiting the rational design of clinical chemotherapy.

Heterogenecity of human tumours and difficulties in tumour sampling are also limitations of major importance. Results reached in this field by application of various cell separation techniques seem to be encouraging, however, they are hardly applicable in clinical conditions.

Insufficiently conclusive results obtained in the study of human neoplastic cells and the still openly discussed interpretation of the immunogenecity of malignant tumours are major limitations to the success of cytostatic treatment. We have to learn more about the immune modulatory effect of cytostatic agents in order to be able to protect the host against the deleterious effect of anticancer drugs.

CONGRESS SYMPOSIA

CHILDHOOD TUMORS Massimo, L., Italy,
Chairman; Evans, A., USA, Co-Chairman; Rainier
Room

Recent Advances in the Management of Children
with Wilms' Tumor. *National Wilms' Tumor
Study Group, Philadelphia, PA USA.

Prognostic Factors in the Treatment of
Neuroblastoma. *Green, A. A., Hayes, F. A.,
George, S., Look, A. T. and Mauer, A. M.,
Memphis, TN USA. (By Title Only)

Chemotherapy as Initial Treatment in
Rhabdomyosarcoma. *Voute, P. A. and
Kindertumoren, W., Amsterdam, The Netherlands.
(By Title Only)

Medulloblastoma. *Wilson, C. B., San Francisco,
CA USA. (By Title Only)

Histopathology as a Prognostic Indicator in
Tumors of Childhood. *Beckwith, J. B.,
Seattle, WA USA.

Please note: Papers that are listed as "By Title
Only" were presented at the 13th International
Cancer Congress, but are not included in these
volumes.

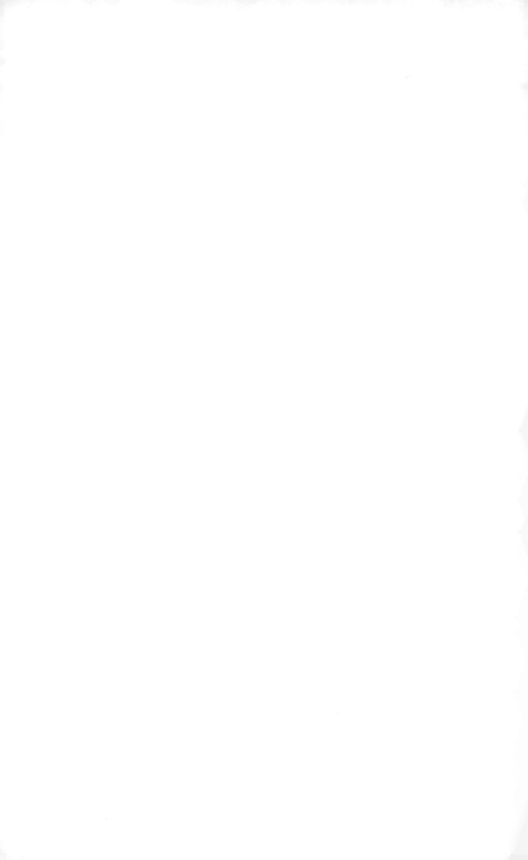

13th International Cancer Congress, Part E
Cancer Management, pages 153–158
© 1983 Alan R. Liss, Inc., 150 Fifth Avenue, New York, NY 10011

RECENT ADVANCES IN THE MANAGEMENT OF CHILDREN WITH WILMS'
TUMOR

National Wilms' Tumor Study Group

The management of patients with Wilms' tumor reflects
the progress made in the treatment of children with solid
tumors of childhood. There have been three major goals in
pediatric oncology: (1) To cure more children with cancer, (2) To lessen treatment-associated morbidity, and (3)
To identify genetic and other etiologic factors. The advances made against Wilms' tumor are a heartening reflection of the progress being made along all three lines.*

Nine out of every 10 children with Wilms' tumor died
in the early years of this century. The first advances
were made by pioneering surgeons who lessened the mortality rate, and devised now-standard transabdominal
approaches to these huge tumors. The lesion was found to
be radio responsive; postoperative radiation therapy was
therefore added as a routine measure. By the 1940's and
50's, 2-year survival rates of close to 50% were being
reported by leading institutions. The multi-modal team,
thus first given impetus, was enlarged when actinomycin-D
was found to be an effective drug against the nephroblas-
toma. The team approach to the child with Wilms' tumor,
coupled with the routine administration of postoperative
radio- and chemotherapy led to over-all survival rates in
the 80% range. Meanwhile, cooperative groups had been
formed, and addressed certain of the salient questions
concerning Wilms' tumor. Cancer and Acute Leukemia Group B

---

* References to the Wilms' tumor work to be cited are to
be found in article by D'Angio, et al. included in the
list of additional reading appended.

investigators demonstrated that adjuvant actinomycin-D (AMD) had a role in the management of Wilms' tumor patients. Children's Cancer Study Group research established that multiple courses of AMD gave better results than a single para-operative course. Southwest Oncology Group members, meanwhile, expanded an observation made by physicians at the M.D. Anderson Hospital, and demonstrated that vincristine (VCR) also was strongly active against the Wilms' tumor. It was not known whether AMD or VCR was the better agent; meanwhile, there were several other outstanding questions regarding staging, the role of radiation therapy, and epidemiologic factors. Accordingly, the American cooperative groups dealing with childhood cancer banded together to form the National Wilms' Tumor Study (NWTS) in 1969. A series of investigations undertaken by the NWTS used a clinical-pathologic grouping system shown in Table 1. The results of these studies have established the following:

1. There are important tumor sub-types that affect the kidneys of children, one set being associated with a generally favorable outlook (Favorable Histology or FH), and the other having ominous overtones (Unfavorable Histology or UH).

2. Routine postoperative radiation therapy need not be given to children with Group I FH tumors who also receive AMD and VCR.

3. Group I FH patients fare no worse when given AMD and VCR for six rather than 15 months.

4. A combination of AMD plus VCR is better than either agent alone, and the addition of adriamycin (ADR) provides even better protection for Groups II-IV.

Meanwhile, cooperative groups in Europe and in the U.K. addressed other questions. The International Society of Pediatric Oncology demonstrated that preoperative irradiation or chemotherapy lessened the likelihood of tumor rupture at surgery even though survival was not adversely affected by tumor spillage. Children with this complication require total abdominal irradiation, with obvious connotations for both the male and female gonad, so that it clearly is better avoided. Members of the U.K. Medical Research Council Study Group established that more

intensive courses of VCR gave results that were superior
to the three-monthly schedule employed by the NWTS.

Table 1
NATIONAL WILMS' TUMOR STUDY
Grouping System

I   Tumor limited to the kidney and completely excised.

The surface of the renal capsule is intact. The
tumor was not ruptured before or during removal.
There is no residual tumor apparent beyond the margins of resection.

II Tumor extends beyond the kidney, but is completely
excised.

There is local extension of the tumor, i.e., pene-
tration beyond the pseudocapsule into the perirenal
soft tissues, or periaortic lymph node involvement.
The renal vessel outside the kidney substance is in-
filtrated or contains tumor thrombus. There is no
residual tumor apparent beyond the margins of resection.

III Residual nonhematogenous tumor confined to the abdo-
men.

Any of the following may occur:

a. The tumor has ruptured before or during surgery,
    or a biopsy has been performed.
b. Implants are found on peritoneal surfaces.
c. Lymph nodes are involved beyond the abdominal
    periaortic chains.
d. The tumor is not completely resectable, because
    of local infiltration into vital structures.

IV Hematogenous metastases.

Deposits beyond Group III, e.g., lung, liver, bone,
and brain.

V   Bilateral renal involvement either initially or
subsequently.

Ancillary information also was gathered concerning the frequency of incorrect preoperative diagnosis (about 5%), the frequency of bilateral tumors (about 5%) and similar data of clinical importance. Epidemiologic studies identified the frequency of hemihypertrophy (3%), aniridia (1%) and genito-urinary anomalies (4%). Familial features were also studied. There were, for example, 3 families with more than one member having had Wilms' tumor among the 547 registered patients in the first NWTS. That study also demonstrated that there were 6 sets of twins encountered (no co-twins both with Wilms' tumors, however.)

These and other data have been utilized in fashioning the third NWTS. A new staging system has been adopted, and promises to provide better discriminants among patients with regional spread. The salient differences from the grouping method are shown in Table 2. NWTS-3 seeks in favorable histology patients to determine (a) whether a short course (10 weeks) of AMD plus VCR suffices for children with stage I lesions of favorable histologic type, (b) whether a more intensive course of AMD plus VCR will produce results in stages II and III that are consonant with those produced by triple agent chemotherapy (AMD + VCR + ADR), (c) whether postoperative irradiation is needed in stage II children, (d) and whether 1000 rather than 2000 rad flank irradiation suffices for stage III patients. Thus, the questions for these patients at relatively low risk are whether therapy can be reduced even further, and therefore lessen the short- and long-term toxicities. The problem is different for those at high risk; namely, those with tumors of unfavorable histologic types, or those with metastases at diagnosis. Here, better therapies are needed.

NWTS-3 has therefore added cyclophosphamide to AMD, VCR, and ADR to see whether that four drug regimen gives better results than the last-named three drugs alone. NWTS-3 also is producing data on the health status of children followed for five or more years after cure. The effects of therapy on various organ systems is being studied so that adversities can be identified with precision and means of mitigating them can be devised.

Table 2
NATIONAL WILMS' TUMOR STUDY
Staging: Differences From Grouping System

I   Same as Group I

II Same as Group II except:

   a. Biopsy or local spillage of tumor may have oc-
       curred *

   b. Lymph nodes may not be involved *

III Same as Group III except:

   a. Lymph nodes at any level are involved *

   b. There has been massive tumor spillage (local
       spills or biopsies do not qualify) *

IV Same as Group IV

V   Bilateral renal involvement at diagnosis *

   An attempt should be made to stage each side at
diagnosis *

Staging criteria are the same for tumors of favorable or
unfavorable histology. Both staging and histologic type
should be specified for all patients. *

* Indicates points of difference from Grouping System
shown in Table I.

Finally, etiologic factors are being investigated
through questionnaires gathering information on environmental and genetic factors in order to seek clues as to
the causes of Wilms' tumor.

The goals of pediatric oncology remain the same, and
the advances made against Wilms' tumor are a heartening
demonstration of how far medicine has progressed towards
achieving those goals.

ACKNOWLEDGEMENT

The authors acknowledge the contribution made by the many surgeons, pediatricians, and radiation therapists who treated these children and without whom the study would have been impossible.

Supported in part by U.S.P.H.S. Grant No. CA-11722.

ADDITIONAL READING

D'Angio, G.J., Beckwith, J.B., Breslow, N.E., Bishop, H.C., Evans, A.E., Farewell, V., Fernbach, D., Goodwin, W.E., Jones, B., Leape, L.L., Palmer, N.F., Tefft, M., and Wolff, J.A.: Wilms' Tumor: An Update. Cancer 45: 1791-1798, 1980.

van Eys, J. and Sullivan, M.P. (eds) Status of the Curability of Childhood Cancers, New York, Raven Press, 1980.

13th International Cancer Congress, Part E
Cancer Management, pages 159–164
© 1983 Alan R. Liss, Inc., 150 Fifth Avenue, New York, NY 10011

HISTOPATHOLOGY AS A PROGNOSTIC INDICATOR IN TUMORS OF
CHILDHOOD

J. Bruce Beckwith, M.D.

Director of Laboratories
Children's Orthopedic Hospital and Medical Center
Seattle, Washington USA 98105

One of the primary missions of the tumor histopathologist
is to identify structural characteristics of neoplasms that
have prognostic importance. Moderate success has been achieved with certain tumors of adults, for which grading systems
have been developed that correlate reasonably well with
prognosis. Recently, admirable efforts have been made to
develop sound morphometric criteria of such grading systems
(Baak 1982), and with the advent of widely available, simple,
computer-assisted graphic analyzers this approach should
soon become widespread.

The tumors of childhood, however, present some formidable obstacles to the development of adequate grading systems.
We have discussed these problems in detail elsewhere
(Beckwith 1979) and will review them more briefly at this
time.

PROBLEMS IN DEVELOPING GRADING SYSTEMS FOR CHILDHOOD TUMORS

1. Tumors of children are uncommon.

The solid tumors of children occur so rarely that even the most
frequent types occur only a few hundred times per year in the
USA (Young, Miller 1975). Therefore, no single institution
can hope to assemble a sizeable series of comparable cases
of any one tumor type. Without a large number of cases uni-
formly staged and treated, only the most obvious of morphological prognostic criteria can be recognized and validated.
In recent years this problem has been overcome for several
tumor types by the development of several large collaborative

therapeutic trials for childhood tumors, in which the
systematic acquisition of histopathological materials
has been a part of the study design.

2. Childhood tumors may present as multicentric primary neoplasms.

    This problem arises in relation to Wilms' tumor, where
multicentric and bilateral origin of this neoplasm is well
recognized. It is also likely that some neuroblastomas,
especially of the IV-S variety, may arise as multicentric
tumors. When the various primary tumors present differing
appearances, considerable difficulty may arise in developing
staging criteria, as it may not be obvious which pattern
was responsible for an observed metastasis, and it may not
be clear if some secondary sites represent metastasis, or
a metachronous new primary lesion.

3. Many pediatric tumors are complex, mixed embryonal neoplasms.

    Teratomas, osteosarcomas, and Wilms' tumors are examples
of tumors in which an immense spectrum of cell and tissue
types, with widely differing degrees of differentiation, may
occur within a single tumor. Such neoplasms present a
formidable problem in terms of developing a rational grading
system, because of the large number of variables which must
be considered.

WILMS' TUMOR - AN APPROACH TO THE GRADING OF MIXED TUMORS

    In 1969, the USA National Wilms' Tumor Study (NWTS)
was inaugurated. This afforded, for the first time, the
opportunity to study histopathological material from a
population of many hundreds of cases that had been clinically
managed in uniform and standardized fashion. From the outset,
one of the primary objectives of the NWTS was to determine
whether there were histopathological criteria that could be
correlated with therapeutic responsiveness.

    In designing an approach to this problem, we were
challenged by the extraordinary structural diversity of
Wilms' tumors. A wide variety of cell and tissue types may

be seen in these tumors. Some Wilms' tumors, for example, are composed almost exclusively of sheets of primitive blastemal cells, while others may consist of a monomorphous population of highly differentiated tubular cells, and in still others the picture may be dominated by differentiated or undifferentiated stromal tissues. Among tissue types that may be seen in Wilms' tumors are those of nephrogenic type, such as glomeruloid and tubular formations, as well as a wide variety of heterotopic tissues such as skeletal muscle, cartilage, mucinous epithelium, squamous epithelium, argentaffin cells, ganglion cells, etc.

We considered the following possible factors that might be of prognostic importance:

1. Prognosis might be related to the presence or absence or specific histological elements.

We developed a "catalog" of 30 definable cell types or patterns of tissue aggregations, each of which was tabulated as present or absent for every tumor studied.

2. The relative proportion of differentiated or undifferentiated tissues might be an important variable.

After developing criteria for degrees of differentiation in epithelial and stromal cells (all blastemal cells were by definition considered undifferentiated) we estimated the total proportion of the sampled regions of each tumor that was "undifferentiated" or "differentiated".

3. Cell turnover rate might be an important variable.

This possibility was considered, but because of the problems inherent in counting mitotic figures (Silverberg 1976), plus the observation that mitotic figures often seemed to differ in number in the various cell types of a given Wilms' tumor, we have deferred the evaluation of this possibility.

4. Cell atypia might be an important prognostic factor.

Since in most tumor grading systems extreme cellular pleomorphism (anaplasia) is a negative prognostic indicator, we evaluated this possibility. Arbitrarily we chose a defini-

tion of anaplasia as being present when all three of the
following criteria were met for any cell type within the
tumor:
- a) Enlargement of nuclei to at least three times the
     diameter of adjacent nuclei of the same cell type.
- b) Marked, easily recognized hyperchromasia of the en-
     larged nuclei.
- c) Multipolar mitotic figures.

The results of our analysis for the first NWTS (NWTS-1)
have been published elsewhere (Beckwith, Palmer 1978) and for
NWTS-2 in summary form (Beckwith 1980). The earlier analysis
suggested that, using the therapeutic protocols of NWTS-1,
neither the presence of any one cell type, the relative proportions of differentiated stromal or tubular cells, the proportion of blastema, nor the proportion of undifferentiated
cellular elements were prognostically significant. However,
anaplasia as defined above was a major indicator of adverse
prognosis. The summary results for NWTS-1 and 2 are presented
in Table 1.

	ANAPLASIA PRESENT	ANAPLASIA ABSENT
Total Cases	49	720
Relapses	27 (55.1%)	101 (14.0%)
Tumor Deaths	23 (46.9%)	39 (5.4%)

Table 1. Significance of anaplasia in NWTS-1 and NWTS-2.
This table presents only cases presenting without metastases
(Clinical Groups I-III), excluding cases with sarcomatous
renal tumors, and those dying without evidence of residual
or recurrent tumor.

Clearly the presence of even a single microscopic focus
of anaplsia seriously increases the chance of tumor relapse
and death due to tumor. Fortunately, anaplasia is relatively
uncommon, occurring in only 6.8% of tumors in this series.
Therefore, the great majority of Wilms' tumors, presenting
with metastases or anaplasia, can be expected to have a very
high survival rate, when the NWTS therapeutic protocols have
been utilized.

Two distinctive sarcomatous tumors were also encountered
during our review of NWTS-1 (Beckwith, Palmer 1978). These,

which we now refer to as the Malignant Rhabdoid Tumor of
Kidney (MRTK) (Haas et al 1981) and the Clear Cell Sarcoma
of Kidney (CCSK) are now recognized to be distinct neoplastic
entities not closely related to kidney. The MRTK is thought
possibly to be of neuroectodermal origin (Haas et al 1981),
though certain mesenchymal cells of origin have not yet
been excluded. CCSK, also known as Bone Metastasizing Renal
Tumor of Childhood by Marsden and Lawler (1980), is of uncertain origin and is characterized by a rather high incidence
of osseous metastases, in sharp contrast to Wilms' tumor,
which rarely metastasizes to bony sites.

DISCUSSION

The results with Wilms' tumor, presented above, illustrate
some of the potential difficulties, as well as the potential
rewards, of evaluating histopathology as a prognostic indicator of childhood tumors. Results from collaborator studies
of other childhood solid tumors, including rhabdomyosarcoma,
gliomas, and neuroblastomas, are currently in progress in
other centers.

It is clear that without the existence of major multi-
center cooperative studies of these rare tumors of childhood,
further progress toward histopathological grading of pediatric
tumors will be limited.

SUMMARY

Because of their relative rarity and structural complexities, many of the solid tumors of children present
formadible obstacles to the development of histopathological
grading systems. However, the cooperative clinical trials
now in progress in many nations provide a unique opportunity
to overcome these difficulties. The results of the NWTS are
briefly summarized as an illustration of the potential value
of this approach.

Baak JPA. Kurver PHJ, DeSnoo-Niewlaat AJE, et al (1982).
   Prognostic indicators in breast cancer-morphometric methods.
   Histopathology 6:327-340.
Beckwith JB, Palmer NF (1978). Histopathology and prognosis
   of Wilms' Tumor. Cancer 41:1937-1948.
Beckwith JB (1979). Grading of pediatric tumors. pp 39-44

in: Care of the Child with Cancer. American Cancer Society.

Beckwith JB (1980). The pathology of renal tumor in children. pp 73-78 in: Recent Advances in Management of Children with Cancer. The Children's Cancer Association of Japan, Tokyo.

Haas JE, Palmer NF, Weinberg AG, et al (1981). Ultrastructure of malignant rhabdoid tumor of the kidney: a distinctive renal tumor of children. Hum Pathol 12:646-657.

Marsden HB, Lawler W (1980). Bone metastasizing renal tumour of childhood. Histopathological and clinical review of 38 cases. Virchows Archiv A Path Anat and Histol 387:341-351.

Silverberg SG (1976). Reproducibility of the mitosis count in the histologic diagnosis of smooth muscle tumors of the uterus. Hum Pathol 7:451-454.

Young JL Jr, Miller RW (1975). Incidence of malignant tumors in United States children. J Pediatr 86:254-258.

Supported by Grant CA 11722 from the National Institute of Health (National Wilms' Tumor Study).

CONGRESS SYMPOSIA

BASIC AND CLINICAL STUDIES ON HORMONE RECEPTORS
Bresciani, F., Italy, Chairman; Rosen, F., USA,
Co-Chairman; Playhouse

Criteria of Hormone-Responsiveness in Cancer
Biopsies. *Jungblut, P. W., Hannover, W. Germany.
(By Title Only)

The Use of Monoclonal Antibodies in Estrogen Receptor Assays. *Greene, G. L. and Jensen, E. V.,
Chicago, IL USA. (By Title Only)

Steroid Hormone Receptors in Breast Cancer.
*McGuire, W. L., San Antonio, TX USA. (By
Title Only)

A Rationale for Combined Antiestrogen Plus
Progestin Administration in Breast Cancer.
*Baulieu, E-E., Bicette, France.

Steroid Receptors in Prostate Neoplasms.
*Robel, P. and Hechter, O., Bicetre, France and
Chicago, IL USA.

The Importance of Estrogen and Progesterone Re-
ceptor in Primary Breast Cancer. *Clark, G. M.,
McGuire, W. L., Hubay, C. A., Pearson, O. H. and
Carter, A. C., San Antonio, TX USA and
Cleveland, Ohio USA and Brooklyn, NY USA.

Please note: Papers that are listed as "By Title
Only" were presented at the 13th International
Cancer Congress, but are not included in these
volumes.

13th International Cancer Congress, Part E
Cancer Management, pages 167–173
© 1983 Alan R. Liss, Inc., 150 Fifth Avenue, New York, NY 10011

A RATIONALE FOR COMBINED ANTIESTROGEN PLUS PROGESTIN
ADMINISTRATION IN BREAST CANCER

Etienne-Emile Baulieu

INSERM U 33, Lab Hormones, 94270 Bicêtre, France

In more than two-thirds of breast cancers (unselected
cases), estradiol receptor (ER) is found in concentration
believed to be sufficient for mediating estrogen action.
These cases are "ER+". It is known that most tumors are
heterogeneous in terms of receptor containing cells, and
that estradiol receptor is a necessary but not sufficient
cellular component for obtaining a response to estrogens or
antiestrogens. In fact, $\sim$ 50 % of patients whose tumors are
ER+ (> 20 fmol/mg cytosol protein) respond to hormonal
manipulation (Jensen et al 1967; McGuire et al 1975). By far
these ER+ responsive cancers are those which contain, in
addition, progesterone receptor (PR+ > 20 fmol/mg cytosol
protein) (Horwitz et al 1975; McGuire et al 1977), a
marker of estrogen action (Milgrom et al 1973) ($\sim$ 30 % of
cancers are ER+, PR+, and 80 % of those cases are responsive
to hormonal therapy). However not only some ER+, PR+ cases
do not respond to endocrine treatments, but more interestingly $\sim$ 30-40 % of ER+ PR- tumors are responsive. We have proposed a "hormonal challenge test" (Namer et al 1980) which
may be able to detect early such patients likely to benefit
from appropriate adjunctive hormonal therapy. The test is
based on the ER-dependent PR increase provoked by the antiestrogen tamoxifen.

Hormonal challenge test with tamoxifen

Tamoxifen is an antiestrogen showing insignificant
effect on the division and growth of estrogen target cells,

not only in avian (Sutherland et al 1977) but also in
mammalian species (Jordan et al 1978). It binds to ER,
occupying estradiol binding sites. Wherever the receptor is
localized in the cytoplasmic or in the nuclear compartment
of estradiol target cells, there is formation of antiestro-
gen-receptor complexes in as much as the concentration of
the antiestrogen and its relative affinity for the receptor
are appropriate to compete with estradiol. These antiestro-
gen-receptor complexes do not promote the division of
target cells, like estrogen-receptor complexes. However, in
several instances, they are responsible for the synthesis
of specific proteins, in particular that of PR. Such "disso-
ciated" effect, with absence of estrogen-like action on
cell multiplication and estrogen like positive effect on
specific protein synthesis, in particular PR, make tamoxifen
an interesting drug for challenging the estrogen responsive
machinery of cancer cells, without risk of stimulation of
tumor growth. The hormonal challenge test with tamoxifen
consists in measuring PR in tumors samples before and after
administration of the drug. The increase in PR concentration
indicates a potential for these patients to benefit from
hormonal therapy.

In a small number of breast cancer patients with
cutaneous metastases (Namer et al, 1980), tamoxifen (30 mg x
7 d) displayed properties predictable from laboratory
animal and in vitro experiments. No ER- tumors showed a
response. Approximately 50 % of the ER+ cases did not
respond, including some cases originally with PR+. As
expected (Horwitz et al 1975), most ER+, PR- cancers did
not respond, but there was a definitive increase of PR in
one case. Like in endometrial cancer (Robel et al 1978;
Mortel et al 1981), it appears that a dynamic test may be
more valuable than a single set of receptor measurements in
assessing hormone sensitivity of breast carcinoma.

In animal experiments, tamoxifen binds to ER in the
cytoplasm, and the tamoxifen-ER complexes migrate to the
nucleus, resulting in a decrease of the cytoplasmic receptor
concentration. The latter finding was observed in all ER+
breast cancer samples after tamoxifen administration,
indicating that tamoxifen had reached its target cells.
Whether this decrease is only due to transfer of the tamoxifen ER complexes to the nucleus, or also to the diminution
of the total ER concentration following a week of antiestrogen
treatment is not known, since ER had not been measured in
the nuclear fraction. In any event our preliminary results

have been confirmed (Pouillart et al 1981). The use of
needle biopsies (drill), combined with appropriate miniaturi-
zation of the technique of receptor determination (Magdelénat
1979; Magdelénat et al 1981) should make possible the use
of the hormonal challenge test in other metastases and in
the primary tumor itself, even at an early stage of the
disease.

Combined administration of antiestrogen and progestin

We have suggested that, in addition to the predictive
value of the challenge test, and besides the proper antiestrogen effect of tamoxifen (Mouridsen et al 1978, Manni
et al 1979), the utilization of this agent may also be
viewed as a potential primer for progestin action.

Progestin treatment of breast cancer is not new. Many
authors have reported on the anti estrogenic properties of
progesterone especially on estrogen stimulated growth (Stoll
1967; Segaloff et al 1967; Rubens et al 1976; Muggia et al
1968). However the administration of "low" doses of progestin, in the order of $< \sim 100$ mg/d, appears to be the least
efficient hormonal treatment of breast cancer. Recently
Pannuti and several others (Panutti et al 1980, Role of
Medroxyprogesterone in Endocrine Related Tumors, 1983) have
successively used much larger doses of medroxyprogesterone
acetate (MPA), and obtained results comparable to other
active hormonal therapy, i.e. tamoxifen and aminogluthetimid
(a suppressor of steroid biosynthesis). Even if only
minimal side effects have yet been reported, administration
of 1 g/d and of even larger doses (Role of Medroxyprogesterone in Endrocine Related Tumors, 1983) of a steroid for
several weeks may not be justified. Unforeseen difficulties
may occur, related in particular to the known effects of
large doses of progesterone in the CNS (Phillipps 1974).

The determination of progesterone action is rather
complex. Besides a direct effect on breast cancer cells,
negative feed-back mechanism on pituitary function and
general anabolic activity may be important. These effects
are either totally or partly mediated by receptor mechanisms,
i.e. the progesterone receptor (for breast, hypothalamic
and pituitary cells) and possibly by the androgen and the
glucocorticosteroid receptors for the poorly defined anabolic activity. However we wonder what could be the consequences of the several hundreds ng/ml concentration of progestin
established in the plasma during high dose administration.

Are there unknown beneficial specific mechanisms ? or is it
only a manner to compensate the low PR concentration,
decreased by the treatment by progestin itself as in the
uterus (Milgrom et al 1973), according to the law of mass
action :

size of progestin effect : f (progestin) (PR).

This "equation" indicates that, for a given hormone
concentration, within certain limits, the receptor concentration is critical. Likewise, for a given receptor concentration,
within certain limits, the concentration of hormone is
critical.

It is therefore more promising, in our opinion, to
try to rescue the PR concentration, therefore rendering the
cells potentially more responsive to progestin. Hopefully
it then would be sufficient to establish progestin concentrations nearer to physiological levels, in contrast to the
presently proposed administration of very high doses of
MPA.

Efficient schedule and dose of antiestrogen and progestin administrations are yet to be established. Some investigators (Robustelli Della Cuna 1983) are even still proposing
the use of an estrogen (ethinylestradiol) rather than
antiestrogen as a primer for progesterone action, in order
to increase the number of cells entering cell division
cycle and promote progesterone action (Periti et al 1983).
In view of mitogenic effect of estrogens, we prefer antiestrogen, since it appears as active as estrogen in the rescue
of PR. It remains to be established however whether simultaneous is preferable to the sequential administration of
antiestrogen and progestin. We favor the discontinuous
schedule, since the aim is to overcome the negative progesterone effect on its receptor concentration (Milgrom et al 1973).
Among the possibilities, one can consider either alternate
administration of tamoxifen and progestin for each 4 to
15 day period, or continuous administration of tamoxifen
with progestin given every 4-15 days.

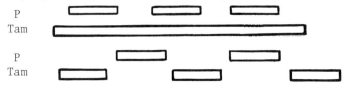

Figure 1 : Rectangles indicate a period of treatment. Small
rectangles may be 4-15 days long.

Interrupting both hormonal treatments for a few days from time to time, can also be proposed, to use possible rebound phenomenon prior to further courses of treatment. In any case, the pharmacokinetic particularities of antiestrogen and progestin should always be considered, and in particular the prolonged action of tamoxifen and of intramuscularly administered progestin.

REFERENCES

Horwitz KB, McGuire WL, Pearson OH, Segaloff A (1975). Predicting response to endocrine therapy in human breast cancer : a hypothesis. Science 189:726.
Jensen EV, DeSombre ER, Jungblut PW (1967). Estrogen receptors in hormone-response tissues and tumors. In Wissler RW, Dao TL, Wood S (eds): "Endogenous Factors influencing Host Tumor Balance", University of Chicago Press, pp. 15-30.
Jordan VC, Dix CJ, Naylor KE, Prestwich G, Roswby L (1978). Nonsteroidal antiestrogens : their biological effects and potential mechanisms of action. J. Toxicol. Environ. Health. 4:363.
Magdelénat H (1979). Simultaneous determination of estrogen receptor and progesterone receptor on small amounts of breast tumors cytosol. Cancer Treat. Rep. 63:1146.
Magdelénat II, Toubeau M, Picco C, Bidron C (1981). Détermination des récepteurs d'oestrogènes et de progestérone sur forages biopsies des tumeurs mammaires. In Martin PM (eds): "Récepteurs Hormonaux et Pathologie Mammaire", Medsi, Paris, pp. 107-119.
Manni A, Trujillo JE, Marshall JS, Brodkey J, Pearson OH (1979). Antihormone treatment of stage IV breast cancer. Cancer 43:444.
McGuire WL, Carbone PP, Vollmer EP (eds) (1975): "Estrogen Receptors in Human Breast Cancer", Raven Press, New York.
McGuire WL, Raynaud JP, Baulieu EE (eds) (1977): "Progesterone receptors in Normal and Neoplastic Tissues", Raven Press, New York.
Milgrom E, Luu Thi M, Atger M, Baulieu EE (1973). Mechanisms regulating the concentration and the conformation of progesterone receptor(s) in the uterus. J Biol Chem 248:6366.
Mortel R, Levy C, Wolff JP, Nicolas JC, Robel P, Baulieu EE (1981). Female sex steroid receptors in postmenopausal

endometrial carcinoma and biochemical response to an antiestrogen. Cancer Res 41:1140.

Mouridsen H, Palshof T, Patterson J, Battersby L (1978). Tamoxifen in advanced breast cancer. Cancer Treat Rev 5:131.

Muggia FM, Cassileth PA, Ochoa M Jr, Flatw FA, Gellhorn A, Human GA (1968). Treatment of breast cancer with medroxyprogesterone acetate. Ann Inter Med 68:328.

Namer M, Lalanne C, Baulieu EE (1980). Increase of progesterone receptor by tamoxifen as a hormonal challenge test in breast cancer. Cancer Res 40:1750.

Pannuti F, DiMarco AR, Martoni A, Fruet F, Stocchi E, Burroni P, Rossi AP, Cricca A (1980). Medroxyprogesterone acetate in treatment of metastatic breast cancer : seven years of experiences. In Iacobelli S, Di Marco A (eds): "Role of Medroxyprogesterone in Endocrine-Related Tumors, Progress in Cancer Research and Therapy", vol 15, pp.73-92.

Periti et al (1983) In Campio L, Robustelli Della Cuna G, Taylor RW (eds): "Role of Medroxyprogesterone in Endocrine-Related Tumors" vol 3, Raven Press, New York. (in press).

Philipps GH (1974). Structure-activity relationships in steroidal anaesthetics. In Massley MJ, Millar RA, Sutton JA (eds): "Molecular Mechanisms in General Anaesthesia" Churchill Livingstone, London pp. 32-47.

Pouillart P, Palangié T, Jouve M, Garcia-Giralt E, Magdelénat H (1982). Hormono-thérapie des cancers mammaires : administration séquentielle de tamoxifen et d'acétate de médroxyprogestérone. Bulletin du Cancer 69:176.

Robel P, Levy C, Wolff JP, Nicolas JC, Baulieu EE (1978). Réponse à un antiestrogen comme critère d'hormonosensibilité du cancer de l'endomètre. CR Acad Sci Paris 287:1353.

Robustelli Della Cuna et al (1983) In Campio L, Robustelli Della Cuna G, Taylor RW (eds): "Role of Medroxyprogesterone in Endocrine-Related Tumors" vol 3, Raven Press, New York. (in press).

Rubens RD, Knight RK, Hayward JL (1976). Norethisterone acetate in the treatment of advanced breast cancer. Eur J Cancer 12:563.

Segaloff A, Cuningham M, Rice BF, Weeth JB (1967). Hormonal therapy in cancer of breast XXIV - effects of corticosterone or medroxy progesterone on the clinical cause and hormonal excetion. Cancer 20:1673.

Stoll A (1967). Progestin therapy of breast cancer : comparison of agents. Br Med J 3:338.

Sutherland RL, Mester J, Baulieu EE (1977). Tamoxifen is a potent "pure" antiestrogen in chick oviduct. Nature 267:434.

13th International Cancer Congress, Part E
Cancer Management, pages 175–182
© 1983 Alan R. Liss, Inc., 150 Fifth Avenue, New York, NY 10011

STEROID RECEPTORS IN PROSTATE NEOPLASMS

Paul   Robel, M.D.[1] and Oscar HECHTER, Ph.D.[2]

[1]Lab. Hormones 94270 Bicêtre, France and [2]Northwestern Medical School, Chicago, Ill 60611, USA.

Benign prostatic hyperplasia (BPH) has a distinctive periurethral origin and does represent hyperplasia of generally mixed epithelial-stromal elements. In marked contrast, prostatic cancer primarily involves epithelial elements in the peripheral regions of the "prostate proper". Both diseases occur in ageing males with considerable frequency (review in Hechter 1976).

The prostatic gland is strictly dependent on androgens for its function and normal development. After castration, the gland rapidly atrophies. It regains its normal function after androgen administration. Interestingly both the formation of dihydrotestosterone (DHT) (the active metabolite of testosterone in the prostate), and the level of androgen receptor (AR) are under the control of testosterone (Moore, Wilson 1973; Blondeau et al 1982). Androgens are of importance also for abnormal development of the human prostate since neither prostatic cancer nor hyperplasia ever occur in males castrated before the age of 40. Approximately 75 to 80 percent of prostatic cancer patients treated by bilateral orchiectomy or with estrogens respond objectively (regression of tumor) or subjectively (relief of symptoms). Prompted by these observations many investigators began to explore the prostate to determine whether or not any correlation with the response to hormonal therapy existed. However, the simplifying assumption that androgen action in all cell types of an androgen target tissue is essentially similar is now open to debate. The possibility has been raised that interaction between stromal and epithelial cells may play a role in the coordinated growth of the prostate gland, and that certain cell types in the prostate may be dependent upon other steroid hormones (eg estrogen, progesterone, etc...).

METHODS

Despite considerable efforts to improve the specificity and accuracy of sex steroid receptor assays in human pros- tate, a survey of the literature shows that no agreement has been reached on the quantitative and even qualitative features of those receptors (review in Robel 1980).

Androgen Receptor

It is generally agreed that most androgen receptor sites are occupied by endogenous dihydrotestosterone and are located in the nuclear compartment. Moreover, the prostate contains systems which readily inactivate steroid receptors (proteases, phosphatases) and natural receptor ligands (steroid metabolizing enzymes). Therefore, the exchange assays, required for the measurement of occupied receptor sites, must be performed at the optimal temperature of 0-4°C. At this temperature, the half-time of dissociation of DHT-AR complexes, corrected for AR inactivation, is appro- ximately 60 h, and the time required for > 90 % exchange is > 200 h. Human prostate extracts also contain other andro- gen-binding components [Sex hormone binding plasma protein

Table 1. Exchange Assay of AR in Prostatic Homogenate.

Ligand : ^{3}H-R-1881 (+ Trimacinolone Acetonide).
Protective measures : Washout of secretory proteases, Molybdate (20 mM), PMSF (0.5 mM).
Incubation : Temperature, 0-4°C ; Duration 96 h.
Separation of bound ligand : Hydroxylapatite batch procedure ; Scatchard plot with Rosenthal correction. Results expressed in pmol/mg DNA.

In spite of the protective measures used, some inactivation of receptor sites still occurs, such that maximal exchange obtains after 72 to 96 h and represents about 60 percent of preexisting AR sites.

(Bordin, Petra 1980; Mercier-Bodard et al 1982) and progesterone receptor (Asselin et al 1976)]. Based on the above
summarized observations, we have described an exchange assay
for AR in human prostate, that can be applied with minor
modifications to estrogen (ER) and progestin (PR) receptors
(Table 1).

SEX STEROID RECEPTORS IN NORMAL AND HYPERPLASTIC HUMAN
PROSTATE

Since the original work of Siiteri and Wilson (1970),
several reports have confirmed that BPH contains significantly larger concentrations of DHT than normal human prostate (NHP). Such difference may well be explained by an
increased concentration of AR in the BPH cells. Ekman et al
(1979) have reported a tendency for larger number of specific R-1881 binding sites in the central (cranial) than in
peripheral (caudal) parts of normal human prostate, and a
larger concentration of such sites in BPH than in NHP, but
their experimental conditions did not provide a specific
assay for AR. Our own results (Eychenne et al, unpublished)
do not show any significant difference in AR levels between
NHP and BPH (Table 2).

Table 2. Sex Steroid Receptors in Human Prostate (pmol/mg
DNA, mean $\pm$ sem).

		AR	ER	PR
Normal	Cranial	1.4 $\pm$ 0.4 (7/7)	0.5 $\pm$ 0.4 (3/6)	2.3 $\pm$ 0.6 (6/6)
	Caudal	1.8 $\pm$ 0.5 (8/8)	0.1 $\pm$ 0.1 (4/7)	1.8 $\pm$ 0.7 (6/8)
Hyperplastic		1.6 $\pm$ 0.2 (14/14)	< 0.1[+] (4/14)	0.8 $\pm$ 0.2° (12/14)

() Proportion of R + cases ; [+]$p < 0.05$ vs normal cranial and
caudal ; °$p < 0.01$ vs normal cranial.

Several publications have reported a specific progestin receptor in human prostate cytosol (Gustaffson et al 1978). It was claimed that its concentration was much larger in BPH than in NHP. The present results, on the contrary, show a significantly larger level of PR in normal cranial prostate than in BPH. This discrepancy is likewise due to the labile character of PR, which does not survive either to post-mortem conditions or to initial freezing and thawing of surgical samples.

Finally, we can confirm the presence of an estradiol receptor-like component in the human prostate. The frequency of its occurrence is open to debate. Our results are in excellent agreement with those of Murphy et al (1980), in that ER is often found in NHP, contrary to BPH (Table 3).

Table 3. Frequency of Estrogen Receptor in Human Prostate.

Normal : Cranial : 8/16 ; Caudal : 14/23
Hyperplastic : 16/123
Malignant : 25/62

(Pooled data from Concolino et al 1980, Ekman et al 1979, Hawkins et al 1976, Murphy et al 1980, Raynaud et al 1980, Tilley et al 1980, Wagner 1980, Robel, Hechter, present work).

Several publications have reported that PR and ER were mainly located in the stromal cells of human prostate. However, we have observed that the mechanical disruption procedures used for the fractionation of prostate samples into epithelial and stromal elements result in gross damage of epithelial cells, which preferentially lose soluble cytoplasmic components such as arginase or steroid receptors. For example, we have found 1.6 ± 0.2 pmol of AR/mg DNA (mean $\pm$ sem n = 14) in unfractionated BPH, but only 0.5 ± 0.2 pmol in BPH epithelium (n = 5), and 0.7 ± 0.2 pmol in BPH stroma (n = 4). Moreover, we have used linear regressions to relate the activities of acid phosphatase (AP), a very specific marker of epithelial cells, with PR and AR concentrations in 10 BPH surgical samples. Significant positive correlations were obtained between [PR] and [AP] (slope 0.02, intercept 0.06, $r = 0.81$, $p < 0.05$) and between [AR] and [AP] (slope 0.03, intercept 0.28, $r = 0.80$, $p < 0.05$). The latter results constitute strong indirect evidences for a predominant localization of AR and PR in the epithelial compartment of unfractionated BPH.

PREDICTIVE VALUE OF AR AND OF DHT IN PROSTATIC CANCER

Clinical correlations between androgen receptors and the response of prostate cancer are few. Most of them are based on assays of cytosolic receptors the reliability of which remains questionable. It is also unfortunate that positive responses to hormone therapy have been evaluated in terms of objective remissions, without consideration of the duration of remission and of the duration of survival. Some authors have reported a positive correlation between the presence of cytoplasmic AR and the frequency of objective remissions (Ekman et al 1979; Martelli et al 1980; Pertschuk et al 1982), whereas others have found no correlation at all (De Voogt, Dingjan 1978; Wagner, Schulze 1978; Trachtenberg, Walsh 1982). It is not surprising that measurements performed on small numbers of tumors, with methods that greatly underestimate the actual concentration of AR, have led to divergent conclusions.

Therefore the recent findings of Ghanadian et al (1981) and of Trachtenberg and Walsh (1982) deserve mention. Both groups have reported a clearcut correlation between nuclear AR and the response to endocrine therapy. In particular, the latter authors have observed that in patients with nuclear AR levels superior to 110 fmol/mg DNA, both the durations of response (17.3 vs 7.1 months) and of survival (24.7 vs 14.4 months) were largely increased.

Another approach to the prediction of androgen responsiveness of prostatic cancer is the one proposed by Geller et al (1979). In previously untreated patients with stage D carcinoma, DHT tissue concentrations were correlated with objective responses of patients to anti-androgen treatment. Tissue DHT levels greater than 2.0 ng/g were considered as indicative of tumour "differentiation" and response to treatment was noted in 9 of 10 patients.

More specific measurements of prostatic DHT in the nuclear compartment or as receptor-DHT complexes (Blondeau et al 1982) may still improve its predictive value.

PREDICTIVE VALUE OF ER IN PROSTATIC CANCER

Diethylstilbestrol has been widely used for the conservative treatment of prostatic carcinoma ; 75-80 percent of all prostatic carcinomas respond to estrogen therapy (Ferguson 1972). The current opinion is that estrogens effectively suppress circulating testosterone levels. However a direct inhibitory action of estrogens on tumor growth should be discussed. In this connection, two groups have reported some relationship between response and ER. Sidh et al (1979) found that 9 of the 15 patients who responded favourably to endocrine therapy showed higher estradiol binding compared with DHT binding, a situation found in only 1 of 18 non responders. De Voogt and Dingjan (1978) also stated that in 12 out 19 patients who showed a good response or remained stationary the cytosol ER values exceeded 100 fmol/mg protein, whereas only 3 out of 15 patients with lower ER values responded well to endocrine therapy. These results should be considered as preliminary.

CONCLUSION

Adequate methodology is now available for the accurate measurement of androgen, progestin, and estrogen receptors in human prostate, whenever relatively large surgical specimen are provided to the Biochemist. Although encouraging results have already been recorded, it seems unlikely that we shall come to any useful conclusions about the predictive value of receptor measurements in the treatment of prostate carcinoma, until a much larger body of cases is accumulated.

REFERENCES

Asselin J, Labrie F, Gourdeau Y, Bonne C, Raynaud JP (1976). Binding of ^{3}H-methyl trienolone (R-1881) in rat prostate and human benign prostatic hypertrophy (BPH). Steroids 28:449.
Blondeau JP, Baulieu EE, Robel P (1982). Androgen-dependent regulation of androgen nuclear receptor in the rat ventral

prostate. Endocrinology 110:1926.

Bordin S, Petra PH (1980). Immunocytochemical localization of the sex steroid-binding protein of plasma in tissues of the adult monkey Macaca Nemestrina. Proc Natl Acad Sci USA 11:5678.

Concolino G, Marocchi A, Ricci G, Liberti M, Di Silverio F, Bracci U (1980). Steroid receptors and endocrine therapy of prostatic carcinoma. In Schröder FH, De Voogt HJ (eds): "Steroid Receptors, Metabolism, and Prostatic Cancer", Amsterdam: Excerpta Medica, p 202.

De Voogt HJ, Dingjan P (1978). Steroid receptors in human prostatic cancer. A preliminary evaluation. Urol Res 6: 151.

Ekman P, Snochowski M, Dahlberg E, Bression D, Högberg B, Gustaffson JA (1979). Steroid receptor content in cytosol from normal and hyperplastic human prostates. J Clin Endocrinol Metab 49:205.

Ferguson JD (1972). Secondary endocrine therapy. In Stolt BA (ed): "Endocrine Therapy in Malignant Disease", London: Saunders Co Ltd, p 263.

Geller J, Albert J, Loza D (1979). Steroid levels in cancer of the prostate. Markers of tumour differentiation and adequacy of anti-androgen therapy. J Ster Biochem 11:631.

Ghanadian R, Auf G, Williams G, Davis A, Richards B (1981). Predicting the response of prostatic carcinoma to endocrine therapy. Lancet 2:1418.

Gustaffsson JA, Ekman P, Poussette A, Snochowski M, Högberg B (1978). Demonstration of a progestin receptor in human benign prostatic hyperplasia and prostatic carcinoma. Invest Urol 15:361.

Hawkins EF, Nijs M, Brassinne C (1976). Steroid receptors in the human prostate. 2. Some properties of the estrophilic molecule of benign prostatic hypertrophy. Biochem Biophys Res Commun 70:854.

Hechter O (1976). Reflection on the NIH Workshop on BPH. In Grayhack JT, Wilson JD, Scherbenske MJ (eds): "Benign Prostatic Hyperplasia", Washington DC: DHEW Publication N°(NIH)76-1113, p 269.

Martelli A, Soli M, Bercovich E, Prodi G, Grilli S, De Giovianni C, Galli MC (1980). Correlation between clinical response to antiandrogenic therapy and occurrence of receptors in human prostatic cancer. Urology 16:245.

Mercier-Bodard C, Roux C, Groyer MT, Devin J, Dadoune JP, Robel P (1982). SBP-like immunoreactive protein in human prostate epithelial cells. Biology of the Cell 45:186.

Moore RJ, Wilson JD (1973). The effect of androgenic hormones on the reduced nicotinamide adenine dinucleotide phosphate : Δ4-3-ketosteroid-5α-oxidoreductase of rat ventral prostate. Endocrinology 93:581.

Murphy JB, Emmott RC, Hicks L, Walsh PC (1980). J Clin Endocrinol Metab 50:938.

Pertschuk LP, Rosenthal HE, Macchia RJ, Eisenberg KB, Feldman JG, Wax SH, Kim DS, Whitmore WF, Abrahams JI, Gaetjens E, Wise GJ, Herr HW, Karr JR, Murphy GP, Sandberg AA (1982). Correlation of histochemical and biochemical analyses of androgen binding in prostatic cancer. Cancer 49:984.

Raynaud JP, Bouton MM, Martin PM (1980). Human prostate hyperplasia and adenocarcinoma : steroid hormone receptor assays and therapy. In Schröder FH, De Voogt HJ (eds): "Steroid Receptors, Metabolism, and Prostatic Cancer", Amsterdam: Excerpta Medica, p 165.

Robel P (1980). Sex-steroid hormone receptors and human prostatic hyperplasia and carcinoma. Ann Clin Res 12:216.

Sidh SM, Young JD, Karmi SA, Powder JR, Bashirelahi N (1979). Adenocarcinoma of prostate : role of 17β-estradiol and 5α-dihydrotestosterone binding proteins. Urology 13:597.

Siiteri PK, Wilson JD (1970). Dihydrotestosterone in prostatic hypertrophy. J Clin Invest 49:1737.

Tilley WD, Keightley DD, Marshall VR (1980). Oestrogen and progesterone receptors in benign prostatic hyperplasia in humans. J Ster Biochem 13:395.

Wagner RK (1980). Lack of correlation between androgen receptor content and clinical response to treatment with diethylstilboestrol (DES) in human prostate carcinoma. In Schröder FH, De Voogt HJ (eds): "Steroid Receptors, Metabolism, and Prostatic Cancer", Amsterdam: Excerpta Medica, p 190.

13th International Cancer Congress, Part E
Cancer Management, pages 183–190
© 1983 Alan R. Liss, Inc., 150 Fifth Avenue, New York, NY 10011

THE IMPORTANCE OF ESTROGEN AND PROGESTERONE RE-
CEPTOR IN PRIMARY BREAST CANCER

GM Clark, Ph.D., WL McGuire, M.D., CA Hubay, M.D.,
OH Pearson, M.D., AC Carter, M.D.
UT Health Science Center, San Antonio, TX 78284,
Case Western Reserve University, Cleveland, Ohio
44106, Downstate Medical Center, Brooklyn N.Y.
11203

Estrogen receptor (ER) has been well documented as an important predictor of long disease-free intervals and survival for patients with primary breast cancer (Knight et al 1977). In advanced breast cancer it has been hypothesized that the presence of progesterone receptor (PgR) might be a sensitive marker for predicting response to endocrine therapy (Horwitz et al.1975; McGuire 1978). We have recently found that PgR was more important than ER in predicting disease-free survival for a group of patients with Stage II breast disease that was treated according to a randomized protocol[1].

This report examines the generality of that result by extending our analysis to include patients from another clinical research institution. The additional patients were not treated according to a rigid clinical protocol, but rather received treatments in much the same way as the majority of breast cancer patients in a community practice. Of interest was whether the relationships between steroid receptors and disease-free survival that we have previously reported would hold with this new group of patients with different demographic and treatment profiles. The relationship between steroid receptor levels and both disease-free and overall survival were examined in detail.

[1]Clark et al. submitted for publication.

MATERIALS AND METHODS

The patients included in these analyses were located in two separate geographical locations: Ohio -- (Case Western Reserve University Headquarters in Cleveland) or New York -- (Downstate Medical Center Headquarters in Brooklyn).

Patients from Ohio have been described in previous publications (Hubay et al. 1980; Hubay et al. 1981). They were randomized to receive one of three treatment modalities: 1) cytoxan, methotrexate, 5-fluorouracil (CMF); 2) CMF plus tamoxifen (CMFT); 3) CMFT plus bacillus Calmette-Guerrin vaccination. Patients from New York were treated on an individual basis including: 1) neither chemotherapy nor endocrine therapy, 2) chemotherapy alone, 3) endocrine therapy alone, 4) combined chemotherapy and endocrine therapy. All patients had a radical or modified radical mastectomy with the biopsy specimen from the primary tumor sent to San Antonio for ER and PgR assays.

Steroid Receptors

The methodologies for the steroid receptor assays performed in San Antonio have been previously described (McGuire et al. 1977; Powell et al. 1979). Specimens were considered ER+ if they contained at least 3 femtomoles of specific binding sites per mg protein and PgR+ if they contained at least 5 femtomoles/mg protein.

Statistical Methods

Survival and disease-free survival curves were calculated by the method of Kaplan and Meier (Kaplan, Meier 1958). Tests of differences between curves were made using the log-rank test for censored survival data (Mantel 1966). Cox's partially non-parametric regression model was used to evaluate the predictive power of various combinations of prognostic factors in a multivariate manner (Cox 1972; Breslow 1975). This model is as follows:

$$\lambda(t) = \exp \left(\beta_1 (X_1 - \bar{x}_1) + \cdots \beta_k (X_k - \bar{x}_k) \right) \lambda_o(t)$$

Where λ (t) is the hazard function at time t; the β's are regression parameters estimated by the data; the X's are patient characteristics possibly related to prognosis; the $\bar{x}$'s are average values of patient characteristics; and λ_o(t) is an arbitrary hazard function when no patient characteristics are included in the model. The hazard function gives the risk of death for an individual known to be alive at time t, so that components that tend to increase the hazard function tend to decrease the survival time. The patient characteristics included in the models were ER and PgR status, the number of positive nodes, size of primary tumor, menstrual status, age, treatment modalities, and institution.

RESULTS

A total of 418 patients were included in these analyses, 189 from Ohio and 229 from New York. Table 1 presents a comparison of the demographic characteristics of the patients from Ohio and New York.

TABLE 1

Patient Characteristics

	Ohio Hospitals (N = 189)	New York Hospitals (N = 229)	P-Value
MENOPAUSAL STATUS			.05
Pre	61 (32%)	53 (24%)	
Peri + Post	128 (68%)	172 (76%)	
AGE			.04
<50	65 (35%)	53 (24%)	
>50	123 (65%)	171 (76%)	
POSITIVE NODES			.77
1-3	90 (48%)	108 (49%)	
>3	99 (52%)	112 (51%)	
SIZE OF PRIMARY			.003
<2 cm	72 (38%)	53 (24%)	
>2 cm	116 (62%)	165 (76%)	

TREATMENT					<.001
No Chemo, No Endocrine	0		102	(44%)	
Chemotherapy alone	64	(34%)	85	(37%)	
Endocrine therapy alone	0		13	(6%)	
Both Chemo and Endocrine	125	(66%)	29	(13%)	

ER STATUS					.30
ER-	45	(24%)	66	(29%)	
ER+	144	(76%)	163	(71%)	

PgR STATUS					.30
PgR-	79	(42%)	109	(48%)	
PgR+	109	(58%)	120	(52%)	

MEDIAN FOLLOWUP	43 Months	19 Months	<.001

New York patients tended to be older and have larger primary tumors. The treatment modalities were more diverse as would be expected for non-protocol patients. The median followup times were significantly longer for Ohio patients than for New York patients (43 months and 19 months, respectively, $p<.001$). There were no significant differences in the distribution of either of the steroid receptors or the number of positive nodes.

Table 2 presents the results of the survival and disease-free survival analyses when the potential prognostic factors were considered one at a time.

TABLE 2

UNIVARIATE SURVIVAL ANALYSES

	Disease-Free Survival	Overall Survival
PROGNOSTIC FACTOR		
Menopausal status	.76	.93
Age	.12	.70
Number of positive nodes	<.0001	.0005
Size of primary tumor	.10	.035
Chemotherapy	.25	.012

Endocrine therapy	.18	.045
ER status	<.0001	<.0001
PgR status	<.0001	<.0001
Institution	.09	.014

The number of positive nodes and both of the steroid receptors were significantly correlated with disease-free survival. The differences between institutions was of marginal significance. In addition to these factors, the treatment modalities and the size of the primary tumor were also related to overall survival. Patients who received chemotherapy or endocrine therapy had longer survival than those who did not.

We examined several subsets of the potential prognostic factors using Cox's multiple regression technique. This procedure can incorporate several prognostic factors simultaneously. If a particular variable is deemed statistically significant, the implication is that if all other factors in the model are held constant, then a change in the value of the variable in question will significantly affect the survival.

For disease-free survival, only three prognostic factors were significant when analyzed simultaneously: the number of positive nodes, PgR, and ER. The following model was obtained for predicting disease-free survival based on these factors:

$$\log_e\left(\frac{\lambda(t)}{\lambda_o(t)}\right) = .761 \ (\text{Nodes} - .518) - .476 \ (\text{PgR} - .545)$$
$$- .480 \ (\text{ER} - .737)$$

For overall survival, the significant prognostic factors were: the number of positive nodes, ER, Chemotherapy, PgR. Using these variables, the following prediction equation was obtained:

$$\log_e\left(\frac{\lambda(t)}{\lambda_o(t)}\right) = .858 \ (\text{Nodes} - .518) - .851 \ (\text{ER} - .737)$$
$$- .827 \ (\text{Chemo} - .742) - .723 \ (\text{PgR} - .545)$$

Patients who did not receive chemotherapy and who had ER- and PgR- tumors with more than 3 positive nodes comprised a particularly poor prognostic group. It was of interest that once other variables were taken into account, the differences between institutions disappeared. Table 3 presents the p-values for the prognostic factors in these models as well as p-values for the variables not in the model.

TABLE 3

MULTIVARIATE SURVIVAL ANALYSES

Disease-Free Survival		Overall Survival	
FACTORS IN THE MODEL	P-VALUE	FACTORS IN THE MODEL	P-VALUE
Positive Nodes	<.0001	Positive Nodes	.0002
PgR Status	.012	ER Status	.001
ER Status	.017	Chemotherapy	.002
		PgR Status	.007
FACTORS NOT IN THE MODEL	P-VALUE	FACTORS NOT IN THE MODEL	P-VALUE
Chemotherapy	.10	Menopausal Status	.44
Institution	.15	Endocrine Therapy	.53
Size of Primary Tumor	.19	Size of Primary Tumor	.59
Age	.27	Institution	.68
Endocrine Therapy	.38	Age	.74
Menopausal Status	.93		

The number of positive nodes was the single most important factor in each of these models. Both steroid receptors were also significant factors in each model. PgR was slightly more important than ER for predicting long disease-free survival, but ER was more important than PgR for predicting overall survival. Patients who received chemotherapy tended to have longer survival, but this variable did not help to predict time of recurrence.

We next examined the relationship between ER and PgR more closely by considering four groups of patients: 1) ER+/PgR+, 2) ER+/PgR-, 3) ER-/PgR+, 4) ER-/PgR-. (The third group comprised only 13 patients and was not further analyzed). There was a significant improvement in both disease-free survival and overall survival corresponding to the presence of the steroid receptors. ER+/PgR- patients fared better than ER-/PgR- patients, and ER+/PgR+ patients had significantly better prognosis than ER+/PgR- patients.

DISCUSSION

We have recently found that PgR was more important than ER in predicting disease-free survival. But these conclusions were based on a controlled clinical trial. It was of interest to know whether patients who were treated according to a strict protocol in a clinical trial might constitute a prognostically different population than patients who received individualized therapies. When the potential prognostic factors were examined one at a time, there appeared to be significant differences between the two institutions. Patients on the clinical trials were younger, had smaller tumors, and all received chemotherapy. However, when examined from a multivariate point of view, the only institutional difference which impacted on survival was whether or not the patient received chemotherapy. None of the factors which differed between institutions were related to time to recurrence. The number of positive nodes and the steroid receptor levels dominated all other patient characteristics in predicting disease-free and overall survival.

PgR status enhanced the predictive power of ER as evidenced by the significant differences observed between the ER/PgR groups. This underscores the importance of our previous suggestion that PgR be routinely measured and incorporated into future adjuvant therapy trials.

Breslow NE (1975). Analysis of survival data under the proportional hazards model. Int Stat Rev 43:45.
Cox DR (1972). Regression models and life tables (with discussion). J Royal Stat Soc (B) 34:187.
Horwitz KB, McGuire WL (1975). Predicting response to endocrine therapy in human breast cancer: a hypothesis. Science 29:726.
Hubay CA, Pearson OH, Marshall JS, et al. (1980). Antiestrogen, cytotoxic chemotherapy and Bacillus Calmette-Guerin vaccination in Stage II breast cancer: a preliminary report. Surgery 87:494.

Hubay CA, Pearson OH, Marshall JS, et al. (1981). Adjuvant therapy of Stage II breast cancer: 48 month follow-up of a prospective randomized clinical trial. Breast Cancer Res and Treatment 1:77.

Kaplan EL, Meier P (1958). Nonparametric estimation from incomplete observations. J Am Stat Assoc 53:457.

Knight WA III, Livingston RB, Gregory EJ, McGuire WL (1977). Estrogen receptor as an independent prognostic factor for early recurrence in breast cancer. Cancer Res 37:4669.

Mantel N (1966). Evaluation of survival data and two rank order statistics arising in its consideration. Cancer Chemoth Rep 50:163.

McGuire WL, De La Garza M, Chamness GC (1977). Evaluation of estrogen receptor assays in human breast cancer tissue. Cancer Res 37:737.

McGuire WL (1978). Hormone receptors: their role in predicting prognosis and response to endocrine therapy. Seminars in Oncology 5:428.

Powell B, Garola RE, Chamness GC, McGuire WL (1979). Measurement of progesterone receptor in human breast cancer biopsies. Cancer Res 39:1678.

CONGRESS SYMPOSIA

CELLULAR AND HUMORAL MARKERS OF CANCER CELL
ACTIVITY Wahren, B., Sweden, Chairman;
Chu, T. M., USA, Co-Chairman; Flag Pavilion A

Expression of Organ-Specific Neoantigens by
Human Cancer. *Thomson, D. M. P., Montreal,
Quebec, Canada.

Multiparameter Studies in Malignant Lymphoma
Based on Studies in 1192 Cases. *Lukes, R. J.,
Taylor, C. R. and Parker, J. W., Los Angeles, CA
USA.

Membrane and Other Phenotypes of Leukemia Cells.
*Minowada, J., Buffalo, NY USA.

Human Tumor Nucleolar Antigens. *Busch, H.,
Busch, R. K., Chan, P. K., Kelsey, D. and
Spohn, W. H., Houston, TX USA.

Protein Hormone-Like Materials from Normal and
Cancer Cells -- "Ectopic" Hormone Production.
*Odell, W. D. and Saito, E., Salt Lake City,
Utah USA.

Please note: Papers that are listed as "By Title
Only" were presented at the 13th International
Cancer Congress, but are not included in these
volumes.

13th International Cancer Congress, Part E
Cancer Management, pages 193–202
© 1983 Alan R. Liss, Inc., 150 Fifth Avenue, New York, NY 10011

EXPRESSION OF ORGAN-SPECIFIC NEOANTIGENS BY HUMAN CANCER

D.M.P. THOMSON

MONTREAL GENERAL HOSPITAL RESEARCH INSTITUTE

1650 Cedar Avenue, Montreal, Quebec, Canada

INTRODUCTION

During the past decade, enthusiasm for human immunity to cancer neoantigens has been seriously challenged. Even when antitumor immunity has been detected, the importance is summarily dismissed as of either little relevance to in vivo events or as artifactual. This negative view comes from the failure of transplantation tests to reveal any immunogenicity in a series of spontaneous mouse tumors, from the finding that athymic mice do not have a high incidence of spontaneous tumors, from the lack of in vitro assays to detect antitumor immunity reproducibility, from the inability to identify the elusive neoantigens, and from the failure of immunotherapy to make major advances in dealing with clinical cancer. Despite the serious challenge, investigators who are working with the tumor antigen-induced leukocyte adherence inhibition (LAI) phenomenon (Halliday and Miller, 1972) have provided much evidence for specific antitumor immunity in animal and human cancers (See Review, Cancer Research, 1979; Thomson, 1982).

Research in my laboratory with a modified version of the assay called tube LAI (Grosser and Thomson, 1975) has shown that the assay can be divided into three parts: immunologic recognition of antigen, generation of leukotriene mediators from monocytes, and leukotriene-induced inhibition of the adherence of leukocytes to glass (Grosser et al., 1976; Marti et al., 1976; Thomson et al., 1982a,b). The nature of the organ-specific tumor neoantigen (OSN) to which the human immune response is directed continues to be defined (Thomson et al., 1982a), but disappointingly to us the OSN has not yet been purified. In this paper, we will present evidence using two different in vitro assays that suggests that human immunity to OSN is probably the most important component of resistance to human cancer.

The epitope on the OSN, to which the human antitumor response is directed, is identical for cancers of the same organ and histogenesis. OSNs of different organs do not share the same epitope (Thomson, 1982a). However, the epitopes are similar enough in breast and lung cancers that cross-reactivity can be detected, although leukocytes from patients with breast cancer have a stronger response to breast cancer extracts than lung cancer and vice versa for leukocytes from patients with lung cancer.

TUMOR ANTIGEN-INDUCED LEUKOCYTE MOBILITY (ADHERENCE INHIBITION)

The adherence of leukocytes to glass is often regarded as an active event; thus, nonadherence is viewed as negation of an active process. Our results indicate that the adherence of leukocytes to glass is a comparatively passive event since neither oxidative metabolism, an intact cytoskeletal microtubular system nor calcium movement are required, whereas tumor antigen-induced LAI requires all these cellular events. Since tumor antigen induced LAI depends upon active physiologic events and the generation of chemoattractants, we think that the locomotion from glass should be named more appropriately; we have therefore chosen the term "mobility" in place of "adherence inhibition".

Tumor Antigen-Induced Release of Leukotrienes

Human monocytes armed with cytophilic IgG antitumor antibody are responsible for recognizing and binding allogeneic OSN (Grosser et al., 1976; Marti et al., 1976). When the cytophilic antibody on the monocyte binds tumor antigen, cross-linking of the antibody and bridging of the Fc receptors triggers the second messenger function of cyclic AMP and calcium, generating a mediator that excites the mobility of leukocytes. Synthesis of the mediator is dependent upon the 5-lipoxygenase pathway but not the cyclooxygenase pathway of arachidonic acid metabolism (Thomson et al., 1982a,b). The mediator has been identified pharmacologically as a leukotriene (LT) (Thomson 1982a,b). We determined the amount of FPL 55712, a competitive antagonist of SRS-A, that was required to block authentic LT and tumor antigen from inducing leukocyte mobility. From this we estimated that the equivalent of 2×10^{-11}M LTD_4 generated by monocytes during the LAI assay was sufficient to mediate the phenomenon (Thomson et al. 1982a). Macrophage/monocytes represent a major source of LT. The specific LT generated by the armed monocytes challenged with tumor antigen has not been identified; however, authentic LT - $B_4 > D_4 > C_4$ - induce mobility of leukocytes at concentrations as low as 10^{-11}M (Thomson et al., 1982a).

Chemoattractant-Induced Leukocyte Mobility

When we realized that leukocyte mobility (non-adherence) was mediated by LT of which LTB can cause leukocytes to aggregate, to move (chemokinesis), to degranulate to a limited extent and to show chemotaxis (Goetzl, 1980), we examined the direct effects of other chemoattractants on leukocyte mobility. Compared to the effects in chemotaxis assays, chemoattractants often excited leukocyte mobility at lower concentrations in the LAI assay. At high concentrations, LTB_4, FMLP, C_5a and PAF caused leukocytes to be less mobile. Maximum mobility was induced by about 2×10^{-11}M LTB_4, 2×10^{-9}M LTD_4, 2×10^{-8}M LTC, 2×10^{-9}M PAF, 2×10^{-8}M FMLP and 2×10^{-10}M C_5a.

T-LYMPHOCYTES RECOGNIZE AUTOLOGOUS TUMOR ANTIGEN (ASSAYED BY TRANSMEMBRANE POTENTIAL ASSAY)

Membrane potential ($\Delta\Psi$) of cells can be measured by the distribution of a lipophilic cation, ^{3}H-tetraphenyl-phosphonium (Shenouda et al., 1982). Moreover, when a signal is transduced from a membrane stimulus, a series of changes take place in the membrane which results in $\Delta\Psi$ changes. Stimuli from immune complexes or chemoattractants induce $\Delta\Psi$ changes. Consequently, we developed a transmembrane potential assay to measure any early signalling event after leukocytes bound tumor antigen.

With the $\Delta\Psi$ assay, the findings of the LAI assay were confirmed. OSN induced $\Delta\Psi$ changes of sensitized leukocytes. $\Delta\Psi$ changes and leukocyte mobility were closely correlated, suggesting that $\Delta\Psi$ change was part of the signalling event that triggered the mobility of leukocytes. When monocytes armed with cytophilic anti-tumor antibody bound OSN, a signal was tranduced. The LT generated from the monocytes transduced a second signal in mononuclear cells and PMN cells. Thus two separate signals are transmitted when leukocytes interact with OSN. Leukocytes from patients with advanced cancer transmit neither the first nor second signal when they bind tumor antigen.

T cells from cancer patients do not transmit a signal when they are incubated with allogeneic tumor extracts of the same organ. But T cells do show $\Delta\Psi$ changes when incubated with autologous cancer extracts. The results suggest that the T cell response to human tumor antigens might be retricted by the Major Histo-compatibility Complex (MHC) similar to the findings for animal and human T cell responses to viral antigens. Initial experiments in which class I MHC proteins are sterically hindered by monoclonal anti-HLA antibody blocked transduction of the $\Delta\Psi$ change signal, suggesting that T cell recognition of class I MHC proteins and tumor antigens must occur concomitantly. When all appropriate controls are completed, we will know whether the pre-liminary results are valid.

FEATURES OF FETAL-CANCER ORGAN-SPECIFIC NEOANTIGEN

The OSN is an integral membrane protein that is made water-soluble by papain digestion. In KBr gradients OSN is found in the upper fraction with HLA and β_2 micro-globulin (β_2m). It co-isolates with β_2m on anti-β_2m affinity chromatography. The papain soluble molecule on molecular-sieve chromatography is found at mol. wts. from 150,000 to 25,000, suggesting that it forms aggregates and is cleaved by papain at different points

(Thomson, 1982).

The physicochemical properties of OSN from different organs are remarkably similar, indicating that they probably have a common framework structure with the OSN epitope for cancers of different organs residing in the same domain. T cells may recognize the same OSN molecule; but because T cells are MHC restricted, they may respond only if OSN is recognized concomitantly with autologous class I MHC antigens. There are, of course, other possibilities: T cells and cytophilic antitumor antibody may recognize different epitopes on the OSN or the T cell response may be directed to molecules unique for each tumor that may or may not be MHC restricted.

Recent studies in our laboratory show that fetal organs express the OSN as early as 13 weeks till about 19 weeks. Moreover, multiparous women show an immune response to the OSN of fetal organs or cancer from about 4 to 7 months gestation. Thus the OSN is a product of genes expressed in the fetus and may play an important role in cell-to-cell recognition in fetal development. Cancers are associated with phenotypic characteristics of embryonic tissues because neoplastic cells, unlike normal, have a block in their differentiation. Expression of OSN by cancer cells seems to be a stable property since the OSN is expressed by cancer cells grown in tissue culture or in nude mice (Thomson, 1982). As a product of a fetal gene, the OSN is unusual in the sense that it elicits an immune response in the host.

When cells become dysplastic or cancerous, they express once again the OSN; differentiation is blocked before the point where OSNs stop being expressed. Leukocytes from patients with cancer show no response to extracts of the equivalent normal tissue. However, leukocytes from patients with severe dysplatic changes in the epithelium of an organ often react to cancer extracts of the same organ. Positive assays are observed with leukocytes from about 6 to 12 percent of patients with severe benign breast disease, 30 percent with colon adenomas, ⩾50 percent with bladder dysplasia and ⩾50 percent with atrophic gastritis and polyps. Besides, leukocytes from most patients with in situ cancer respond positively. These results indicate that the OSN is expressed before the cell acquires its invasive properties.

EVIDENCE FOR THE IMPORTANCE OF ANTITUMOR IMMUNITY IN VIVO

Excited Mobility of Leukocytes from Patients with Advanced Cancer

Leukocytes from control subjects are equally mobile to two different cancer extracts (Fig. 1). Leukocytes from patients with early breast cancer, Stage I and Stage II, show mobility with the breast cancer extract but not with the control cancer extract (p <0.001) (Fig. 1). Conversely, leukocytes from patients with advanced breast cancer Stage II ⩾4 LN, III, or IV, show equal mobility to both the breast and control cancer extracts (p> 0.05).

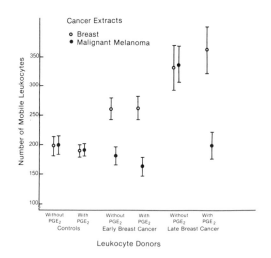

Figure 1 shows the number of mobile leukocytes excited by breast cancer and control cancer extracts without and with 5 min preincubation of leukocytes with PGE_2 before the assay.

Consequently, the difference in mobility is nearly zero. The most important observation in Figure 1, however, is that the cells of patients with advanced cancer have had mobility excited in vivo which explains the high mobility with the control cancer extract.

PGE$_2$, by elevating intracellular cyclic AMP, stops the mobility and returns the cells to a resting state and, if properly titrated, allows the cells to show mobility when incubated with the sensitizing OSN (Fig. 1). Thus in advanced cancer the mobility of leukocytes has been activated in vivo because monocytes have

Table 1

Effect of PGE$_2$ on the Mobility (Nonadherence Property) of Normal Leukocytes Exposed to LTD$_4$†

Treatment of Leukocytes	Mean ± SE of Mobile Cells Extract Containing LTD$_4$	Extract Not Containing LTD$_4$	Difference in Mobile Cells (LMI)
Initial exposure to 2×10^{-11}M LTD$_4$	403 ± 58	267 ± 53	50
Initial exposure, then washed and re-exposed to 2×10^{-11}M	351 ± 61	324 ± 45	8*
Initial exposure and incubated with 3×10^{-6}M PGE$_2$ and re-exposed to 2×10^{-11}M LTD$_4$	337 ± 46	250 ± 47	34*

†Adapted from Thomson et al., 1982a;
*The difference in mean mobile cells is statistically significant by Student's paired t test (p <0.001).

generated LT after binding free circulating OSN (Grosser and Thomson, 1976; Thomson et al., 1982a, b). And cells already in the midst of their programmed response to OSN or LT cannot respond to repeat stimuli (Table 1).

We also tested the response of leukocytes to LT, C_5a, and FMLP. Leukocytes from patients without cancer and patients with early cancer are mobilized by the chemoattractants with or without elevating intracellular cyclic AMP. Leukocytes from patients with advanced cancer are mobile, and the chemoattractants induce no additional cells to become mobile. However, if the mobility is stopped by raising intracellular cyclic AMP, the cells can then be induced to become mobile again by either the sensitizing OSN or chemoattractants (Fig. 2). In advanced cancer, leukocytes are able to recognize

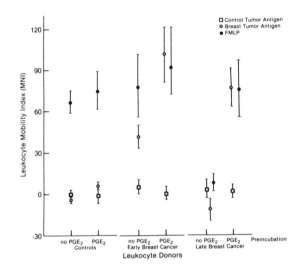

Figure 2 shows the LMIs of leukocytes from subjects with-out cancer, early cancer and late cancer to OSN or to the chemoattractant FMLP. Leukocytes from controls and patients with early cancer are mobilized by FMLP, whereas leukocytes from patients with advanced cancer are not. Elevating intracellular cyclic AMP stops the mobility of the leukocytes from patients with advanced cancer and allows them to respond to OSN and FMLP.

and bind circulating tumor antigen; however, they are already expressing the appropriate physiologic response after contacting OSN and are refractory to transmitting a signal or generating LT. Moreover, once the physiologic response of mobility is triggered, it continues for at least 2 hr, the duration of the LAI assay. Accordingly, the lack of immune response of patients with advanced cancer to different stimuli is engendered by the intensity of the antitumor response and its resultant inflammatory products. The response to chemoattractants such as FMLP, LT or C_5a can be used therefore to predict the tumor burden of the patient.

CONCLUSION

The tube assay measures locomotion of leukocytes, depending upon the generation of immunopharmacologic substances similar to leukotrienes by monocytes when they bind tumor antigen. The mobility requires oxidative metabolism, electron transport, microfilaments, microtubules and transmembrane signalling, many of the same physiologic events that are essential for chemokinesis and chemotaxis. Moreover, tumor antigen-induced leukocyte mobility is more than an interesting in vitro phenomenon, for about 50 percent of leukocytes from patients with advanced cancer are activated in vivo in a manner identical to that observed by tumor antigen in vitro. Leukotrienes and prostaglandins may be critical to a fully developed local host inflammatory response (Lewis and Austen, 1981). Results of our recent studies imply that armed human monocytes reacting with tumor cells in vivo will release leukotrienes that manifest vasoactive, permeability-augmenting and chemotactic activities which can modulate the microenvironment to recruit protective proteins and cells to the inflammatory site (Lewis and Austin, 1981). Free tumor antigen shed from the tumor, however, by triggering leukocyte mobility at a distance from the tumor cell may prevent leukocyte-tumor cell contact that is essential for killing of tumor cells. Having shown this in vivo effect of the inflammatory response to cancer, we believe that added emphasis needs to be given to the importance of the immune response to tumor antigens of human cancer.

REFERENCES

Goetzl EJ (1980). Mediators of immediate hypersensitivity derived from arachidonic acid. N Engl J Med 303:822.

Grosser N, Marti JH, Proctor JW, Thomson DMP (1976).
Tube leukocyte adherence inhibition assay for the detection of anti-tumour immunity.: I. Monocyte is the
reactive cell. Int J Cancer 18:39.

Grosser N, Thomson DMP (1975). Cell-mediated antitumour
immunity in breast cancer patients evaluated by antigen-
induced leukocyte adherence inhibition in test tubes.
Cancer Res 35:2571.

Grosser N, Thomson DMP (1976). Tube leukocyte (monocyte)
adherence inhibition assay for the detection of anti-
tumour immunity.: III. "Blockade" of monocyte reactivity
by excess free antigen and immune complexes in advanced
cancer patients. Int J Cancer 18:58.

Halliday WJ, Miller S (1972). Leukocyte adherence inhibition: a simple test for cell-mediated tumor immunity
and serum blocking factors. Int J Cancer 9:477.

Lewis RA, Austen KF (1981). Mediation of local homeo-
stasis and inflammation by leukotrienes and other mast
cell-dependent compounds. Nature (Lond) 293:103.

Marti JH, Grosser N, Thomson DMP (1976). Tube leukocyte
adherence inhibition assay for the detection of anti-
tumour immunity.: II. Monocyte reacts with tumour antigen
via cytophilic anti-tumour antibody. Int J Cancer 18:48.

Review (1979). Cancer Res 39:551-662.

Shenouda G, Thomson DMP, Bach MK (1982). Tumor antigen
induced changes in transmembrane potential of leukocytes
of cancer patients and modulation by leukotrienes and
prostaglandins. In Bockman R (ed): "Prostaglandins and
Cancer: First International Conference," New York: Alan
R. Liss, p 679.

Thomson DMP (1982). "Assessment of Immune Status by the
Leukocyte Adherence Inhibition Test." New York, Academic
Press, p 1.

Thomson DMP, Phelan K, Morton DG, Bach MK (1982a). Armed
human monocytes challenged with a sensitizing cancer
extract release substances pharmacologically similar to
leukotrienes. Int J Cancer 30: (in press).

Thomson DMP, Phelan K, Scanzano R, Fink A (1982b).
Modulation of antigen-induced leukocyte adherence
inhibition by metabolites of arachidonic acid and intracellular nucleotides. Int J Cancer 30: (in press).

13th International Cancer Congress, Part E
Cancer Management, pages 203–213
© 1983 Alan R. Liss, Inc., 150 Fifth Avenue, New York, NY 10011

MULTIPARAMETER STUDIES IN MALIGNANT LYMPHOMA
BASED ON STUDIES in 1186 CASES

R.J.Lukes, M.D., C.R. Taylor, M.D., D.Phil. and
J.W. Parker, M.D.
Department of Pathology
University of Southern California
School of Medicine
2025 Zonal Avenue, Los Angeles, California 90033

For decades the malignant lymphomas have been the subject of debate and controversy as a result of the limited understanding of lymphopoiesis and the lack of technical precision in cell characterization and identification. In 1972, at an international lymphoma conference in West Germany, we proposed a functional approach for these disorders in an attempt to relate the lymphomas to the remarkable developments in immunology of the 1960's (Lukes, 1974a). A multiparameter technical approach was outlined for the redefinition of the malignant lymphomas and an immunological classification including T and B cell subtypes was proposed (Lukes, 1974b). This approach was based upon the description of T and B cell systems in experimental animals, the observation of congenital immune defects in the T and B cell systems in man, the availability of techniques for characterizing T and B cells and our morphologic studies of the lymphocyte transformation phenomenon with mitogens. It was predicted that the (1) non-Hodgkin's lymphomas principally involved T and B cell types; (2) nodular lymphomas of Rappaport (Rappaport,1966) are lymphomatous follicles composed of follicular center cells and therefore are B cells; and (3) large cell lymphomas designated as the histiocytic type by Rappaport (Rappaport,1966) primarily are transformed lymphocytes of T and B cell types and rarely of genuine histiocytic type.

In the intervening years numerous investigators, including ourselves, using an ever expanding array of techniques have established the malignant lymphomas as neoplasms of the immune system composed principally of T and B cell types and rarely of genuine histiocytes (Aisenberg 1975, Braylan 1975, Gajl-Peczalska 1975, Green 1975, Leech 1975, Lennert 1978, Lukes 1977, Lukes,

1978a, Lukes 1978a, Lukes 1978b, Lukes 1979, Lukes 1982, Parker 1979, Taylor 1979, Van Heerde 1980). Nodular lymphomas are accepted as lymphomatous follicles (Jaffe 1974, Lennert 1978, Lukes 1978a, Lukes 1978b, Lukes 1982) and the large cell lymphomas as a heterogeneous group principally of T and B cell subtypes (Stein 1980, Strauchen 1978).

Acute lymphocyte leukemia of childhood is also acknowledged to be a heterogeneous group of disorders with T and B cell subtypes and even the so-called "null" cell type of recent years seems likely to be established as a special B cell possibly involving the precursor cell of the bone marrow. The recently developed monoclonal antibodies (MOAb) techniques brings a superior level of precision to cell characterization. In a brief period of two years it has had a major impact on the clarification of acute lymphocytic leukemia variants. Currently the rapid expansion of the available types of MOAb employed in cytofluorographic studies of cell suspensions and in immunoperoxidase labelled form on frozen sections is changing dramatically our knowledge of the non-Hodgkin's lymphomas.

The purpose of this report will be to summarize briefly (1) the current effectiveness of the various technical parameters employed in cytological characterization and diagnosis of malignant lymphomas; (2) the results of the multiparameter studies in relationshp to our immunologic classification; and (3) the potential future value of these techniques both in the diagnosis of malignant lymphoma and the investigation of the biology of these disorders. The views presented will be based on our experience with multiparameter studies on over 6000 specimens including those from over 1186 cases of non-Hodgkin's lymphomas.

MULTIPARAMETER APPROACH

In our approach fresh specimens of lymph nodes, spleen, peripheral blood, bone marrow and extranodal lymphoid tumors from such sites as the conjunctiva and adnexal structures, skin and lung are collected through our Southern California Lymphoma Group of 30 cooperating hospitals and evaluated in a central laboratory with a battery of techniques. Through the years over 6000 specimens, including over 1186 cases cases of non-Hodgkin's lymphoma, many with multiple specimens plus Hodgkin's disease and a variety of other abnormal lymphoid processes have been studied. A wide variety of techniques have been eveluted continually for their potential usefulness in the definition of the cytologic types of malignant lymphoma. The technical components of the multiparameter approach are listed in Table 1.

Table 1

MULTIPARAMETER APPROACH

1. Special morphology - paraffin and plastic sections
2. Cytochemistry - imprints, smears and frozen sections
3. Electron microscopy
4. Immunoperoxidase labelled Ab on paraffin sections for CIg and phagocytic enzymes
5. Phenotyping
   a) manual techniques; also cytospin on E-rosettes
   b) cytofluorography; MOAb and Ab for SIg
   c) Frozen sections; immunoperoxidase labelled MOAb and Ab for CIg and SIg
6. Cell kinetics
7. Cytogenetics
8. HLA-studies
   Ab-antibodies   MOAb-Monoclonal Antibodies
   CIg-cytoplasmic immunoglobulin   SIg-surface immunoglobulin

Table 2

DISTRIBUTION OF NON-HODGKIN'S CASES
MULTIPARAMETER STUDIES (6/30/82)

CYTOLOGIC TYPES

B-CELL	Cases	Percent
Small lymphocyte-B	124	10.5
Plasmacytoid lymphocyte	85	7.1
Follicular Center Cell	(667)	(56.2)
Small cleaved	347	29.3
Large cleaved	52	4.4
Small noncleaved	104	8.8
Large noncleaved	82	6.9
Immunoblastic sarcoma-B	54	4.6
(Hairy cell luekemia)	28	2.4
B-CELL total	876	73.9

T-CELL		
Small lymphocyte	36	3.0
Convoluted T-cell	98	8.3
Cerebriform	37	3.1
(Sezary's & MF)		
Immunoblastic sarcoma-T	50	4.2
Lymphoepithelioid cell	17	1.4
T-CELL total	238	20.1

HISTIOCYTE	4	0.3
U-CELL	68	5.7
	1186	

Of critical importance is the care and attention given to the preparation of cell suspensions and to the collection of tissue for fixation and preparation of histiological sections for special morphological and immunohistological studies. Multiple tissue imprints are prepared for cytologic evaluation and cytochemistry. Tissue blocks are frozen in isopentane to prepare frozen sections for cytochemistry and immunoperoxidase labelled monoclonal antibodies and antibodies for surface and cytoplasmic immunoglobulins. Our approach from the onset has been to establish initially the morphological diagnosis according to the immunologic classification of Lukes and Collins shown in Table 2 and then critically relate the results of the multiparameter studies to the morpholoical diagnosis. The morphologic findings of the cytologic types have been an effective predictor of these results.

In the following sections, the value of individual components will only be highlighted since they have been presented in detail previously (Lukes, 1978a; Lukes, 1978b; Lukes 1982).

SPECIAL MORPHOLOGY

Effective cytologic evalution and accurate morphologic diagnosis are dependent upon careful attention to the important initial step of tissue collection and fixation which is commonly disregarded. Thin (2 mm.) tissue blocks of fresh tissue are cut cross-section to the long axis of the lymph node and fixed in B-5 or Zenker's solutions for not longer than 2 hours to avoid excessive hardening. Histologic sections are cut at 4 micons, stained routinely with hematoxylin and eosin, periodic acid Sciff (PAS), methyl green pyronine (MGP) and Giemsa methods and compared to the findings in Wright's stained tissue imprints. This interpretation is related to the results of the multiparameter studies.

CYTOCHEMISTRY

A battery of cytochemical techniques has been used in the study of tissue imprints, smears of peripheral blood and bone marrow and at times on cytocentrifuge preparations of cell suspensions. In addition to Wright's stain for morphology they include a wide variety of procedures including peroxidase, sudan black and chloracetate esterase stains all of which have been extremely helpful in the diagnosis of poorly differentiated granulocytic leukemia. Acid phosphatase activity in the form of a single punctate globule in the Golgi area has been demonstrated in a high proportion of cases with convoluted T cell lymphoma-leukemia in our experience. Its effectiveness, however, is dependent upon the time interval between preparations of tissue imprints or smears and fixation with the optimum interval being 24-48 hours. In small T cell lymphoma-leukemias variable acid phosphatase activity is found in diffuse granular form. Tartrate resistant acid phosphatase activity is demonstrated usually, but not always, in hairy cell leukemia.

Demonstration of alpha naphthyl butyrate activity is currently the most reliable method of establishing the identity of histiocytes and monocytes although immunohistologic methods for phagocytic enzymes on paraffin sections have recently come into prominence.

Other staining techniques are helpful but less specific. Oil red O staining of lipid cytoplasmic vacuoles in small non-cleaved FCC (Burkitt and non-Burkitt varients) has been variably demonstrated.

IMMUNOHISTOLOGY

A vast literature describing the value of this approach has accumulated in a brief period and is summarized in a number of reports (Lukes 1982, Taylor 1979).

The value of the application of fluorescent labelled antibodies to tissue imprints, smears, frozen sections and even paraffin sections for the localization of antigens has long been acknowledged. The substitution of immunoperoxidase as the label for the antibody recognition has two advantages; (1) improved morphology for cytologic identification; and (2) permanently stained specimens. If the antigen is present in quantity and can survive fixation and histologic preparatory techniques, the antigen can be demonstrated in paraffin sections with excellent morphology (Burns 1974, Taylor 1974). In the brief period since the technique was originally published the successful demonstration of over 100 antigens in tissue has been reported. Identification of cytoplasmic immunoglobulin, both heavy and light chains, in monoclonal form in B cell lymphomas of various cytologic types (Taylor 1979)) and tissue sites has been of great value in the study of these disorders. Its effectiveness at times is limited in our experience by faulty fixation and tissue processing in referral case material. Similar labelled antibodies for phagocytic enzymes, muramidase (lysozyme), alpha-1 antitrypsin and alpha-1 antichymotrypsin have proven to be effective in our hands and have expanded our armamentarium for the identification of histiocytic lymphoma and monocytic leukemia in paraffin sections.

ELECTRON MICROSCOPY

The ultrastructural features of the cytologic types of lymphoma cells in general confirm the light microscopy impressions. Certain subtle nuclear and cytoplasmic features not always apparent in paraffin sections, may be evident ultrastructurally. These included limited nuclear irregularities at times in the small cleaved FCC or convoluted T cells. Cytoplasmic features, such as rough endoplasmic reticulum indicating plasmacytoid differentiation may be found in plasmacytoid lymphocytic lymphoma and B immunoblastic sarcoma when not definite in paraffin sections. Similarly microvilli of hairy cell leukemia may be better appreciated with the electron microscope. The technique also enables the study of cellular interrelations of lymphoma cells, e.g., stromal cells and is of special value in differentiating poorly differentiated tumors from malignant lymphomas through the identification of specific cytoplasmic granules, melanosomes, desmosomes and other organelles.

IMMUNOLOGIC PHENOTYPING

In a brief period of less than a decade voluminous literature has developed on the use of a variety of manual techniques in the study of lymphomas and related leukemias which we have summarized and evaluated at intervals (Lukes 1977, Lukes 1978a, Lukes 1978b, Lukes 1979, Lukes 1982). However, they are already threatened with extinction by the recently developed monoclonal antibodies (MOAb) produced in the mouse hibridoma system with their application in cytofluorographs or on specially frozen sections.

Manual techniques

A variety of erythrocyte rosette techniques combined with the study of surface immunoglobulin (SIg) have provided the basic evidence of the immunologic nature of lymphomas and related leukemias even though numerous complexities and pitfalls have been uncovered. The demonstration of monoclonality of SIg, a single light immunoglobulin (Ig) chain and usually one heavy Ig chain, has been accepted as support for the B cell nature of lymphomas, although in a small proprotion of cases little or no SIg is detectable. Non-specific absorption of Ig to the cell surface or by Fc bending of Ig also have resulted in frequent problems in false polyclonality obscuring the monoclonality of B cell neoplasms. Incubation at 37oC for 45 minutes and the use of F(ab')2 antibody reagents has largely eliminated this problem in our experience. Rosette techniques, though informative, are less specific in cell identification with the exception of E rosettes for T cells. Spontaneous sheep erythrocytes (E) rosettes have been an effective marker of T cells. It is essential in T cell lymphomas and leukemia to demonstrate rosette formation about the critical cells in cytocentrifuge preparations since residual normal cells are usually present and may account for misleading high percentages of T cells in lymphomas and leukemias of B cells. Detection of complement receptors (EAC) and Fc receptors (EA) have yielded important information, but both have proven to be present on T and B cells as well as monocytes. Using the EAC technique on frozen sections, Jaffe showed the follicular nature of nodular lymphomas (Jaffe 1974).

Cytofluorography

This automated fluorescent laser beam flow system using MOAb plus heteroantibodies for SIg seems likely to replace the above traditional manual methods. The greater objectivity and accuracy of the technique, the large number of cells evaluated together with the enormous potential of the MOAb approach are bringing a new level of sophistication and accuracy to surface marker studies in lymphomas and leukemias. The impact of this approach seems only limited by the number and specificity of the MOAb which are expanding at a rapid rate. At the moment we are employing routinely the MOAb on all lymphomas and related leukemias shown in Table 3.

Table 3

MONOCLONAL ANTIBODIES

PAN T
E-rosette receptor
Helper or inducer T cell
Suppressor or cytotoxic T cell
Cortical thymocyte
Prothymocyte   (These antibodies are for the
CALLA   most part available from more than
Monocyte   one commercial source.)

Frozen Sections

Immunoperoxidase labelling of heteroantibodies for immunoglobulin and MOAb for a wide variety of antigens in numerous cell types, permits the demonstration of the topographic distribution of various cell types in lymphomas and leukemia (Stein 1980, Taylor 1974). This approach focuses attention on the important interrelationships of T cells in B cell lymphomatous processes particularly FCC lymphomas with a follicular pattern and T cell subtypes. Of greatest importance, there is minimal antigen loss, the cells are accurately labelled, morphologic detail is good and permanent sections are available for subsequent study. This capability on frozen sections overcomes numerous problems of the past such as the sampling errors or small sample sizes encountered in the study of cell suspensions. It has overcome situations where cell suspensions were difficult to acquire because of dense stroma such as in dermal lymphomas and sclerosing lymphomas since the cells may be investigated in a sense in situ . Both cytoplasmic Ig (CIg) and SIg are identified thus eliminating the problem in which SIg may be low or absent in plasmacytoid processes where little SIg may be present. Finally, it is possible to search for the labelling of antigens on the fragile high proliferative rate cell types particularly the large cell types that are vulnerable to the trauma of cell preparation techniques where often few if any cells have survived for study in our experience in the past.

RESULTS OF MULTIPARAMETER STUDIES

The results of our studies since 1974 on 1186 cases of non-Hodgkin's lymphomas and over 6000 specimens only can be summarized and commented upon briefly because of space limitations. For further information refer to the detailed reports . A wide variety of specimens have been studied including lymph nodes, spleen, peripheral blood, bone marrow, and numerous extra nodal sites as well as pleural, ascitic and spinal fluids. The techniques employed have evolved over the years both in number and diversity. The effectiveness of the techniques have gradually improved as well and the use of MOAb and heteroantibodies in the cytofluorograph and in immunoperoxidase labelled form on frozen sections from our recent experience unquestionably will lead to a much greater level of precision , objectivity and accuracy.

T-Cell Lymphomas

Of the 1186 cases of non-Hodgkin's lymphomas (Table 2) 238 (20.1 %) are of T cell types with convoluted lymphocyte being the most common with 98 cases (8.3%) and immunoblastic sarcoma of T cells the second most common with 54 cases (4.8%). Until recently these have been confirmed only by E rosette determinations with morphologic demonstration of the lymphoma forming E rosettes in cytocentrifuge preparations. For over a year, essentially all cases have been studies in parallel with manual, cytofluorography and frozen section techniques. The use of MOAb have dramatically improved the precision in T cell lymphoma characterization.

B-Cell Lymphomas

Of the 1186 cases of non-Hodgkin's lymphomas evaluated, 876 (74.1%) have been of B-cell types with 667 cases (56.2%) being of follicular center cell types (FCC). The small cleaved FCC with 347 cases (29.3%) is the most common cytologic type. In the early years, using manual techniques, monoclonality with SIg was in the range of 60% with considerable problem with polyclonality resulting from absorption or binding of Ig to the surface membrane. Incubation at 37^oC for 45 minutes plus the use of $F(ab')_2$ reagents has largely eliminated polyclonality. In the past year approximately 90% of B cell types mark in a monoclonal manner. Cytofluorographic studies using the same approach yield similar results. Application of similar immunoperoxidase labelled antibodies to special frozen sections appears to provide superior results because it also identifies CIg and overcomes the loss of cells in dense stroma or in the preparation of fragile high proliferative rate cell types. Thus monoclonality may approach 100%. Most importantly this approach allows the study of the interrelationship of B cell lymphoma types with stromal cells and T cell subtypes and a valid comparison with the permanent paraffin sections.

Monocyte-Macrophage Proliferations

Only four cases (0.3%) of the population (Table 2) have been demonstrated to be of this type. This diagnosis was confirmed by alpha napthyl buterate esterase stains on imprints and immunoperoxidase stains for muramidase (lysozyme) on paraffin section. Expansion of our capability by the addition of immunoperoxidase stains for alpha-1 antitrypsin and alpha-1 antichymotrypsin plus MOAb for monocytes is likely to improve the effectiveness of our studies.

Future Studies

Over the next few years the expansion of the number and type of MOAb undoubtedly will greatly improve the capability of the multiparameter approach for the characterizaiton of lymphomas and leukemias. Cancer Centers will be the ideal locations for evaluating their capability and role in future use and also serve as regional resources for communities. Once the value of certain MOAb is established, selected MOAb will be applied in local hospitals by pathologists especially on frozen sections of initial biopsy material. Unquestionably, the ideal therapy in the future will be more biological and even immunological and precise cell characterization will be the essential basis for therapy.

Aisenberg AC, Long JC (1975). Lymphocyte surface characteristics in malignant lymphoma. Am J Med 58:300.

Braylan RC, Jaffe ES, Berard CW (1975). Malignant lymphomas: Current classification and new observations. In Somers SC (ed): "Hematologic and Lymphoid Pathology Decennial 1966-1975". New York:Appleton-Century-Crofts.

Burns J, Hambridge M, Taylor CR (1974). Intracellular Immunoglobulin: A study of three standard tissue processing methods using horseradish peroxidase and fluorochrome conjugates. J Clin Path 27:548.

Gajl-Peczalska KJ, Bloomfield CD, Coccia PF, Sosin H, Brunning R Kersey, JH (1975). B and T cell lymphomas. Am J Med 59:674.

Green I, Jaffe E, Shevach EM, Ederson RL, Frank MM, Berard CW (1975). Determination of the origin of malignant reticular cells by the use of surface membrane markers. In Rebeck JW, Berard CW, Abell MR (eds): "The Reticuloendothelial System". International Academy of Pathology Monograph No. 16. Baltimore: Williams & Wilkins, p 282.

Jaffee ES, Shevach, EM, Frank MM, Berard CW, Green I (1974).Nodular lymphoma: Evidence for origin from follicular B lymphocytes. N Engl J Med 290:813.

Leech JH, Glick AD, Waldron JA, Flexner JM, Horn RG, Collins RD (1975). Immunologic, histochemical and ultrastructural studies of malignant lymphomas presumed to be of follicular center cell origin. J Natl Cancer Inst 54:11.

Lennert K (1978). "Malignant Lymphomas other than Hodgkin's Disease". Berlin: Springer, part 6, p 529.

Lukes RJ, Collins RD (1974a). A functional approach to the classification of malignant lymphomas. Recent Results Cancer Res 46:18.

Lukes RJ, Collins RD (1974b). Immunologic characterization of human malignant lymphomas. Cancer 34:1488.

Lukes RJ, Collins RD (1977). The Lukes-Collins classification and its significance. Cancer Treat Rep 61:971.

Lukes RJ, Taylor CR, Parker JW, Lincoln TL, Pattengale PK, Tindle BH (1978a). A morphologic and immunologic surface marker study of 299 cases of non-Hodgkin's lymphomas and related leukemias. Am J Pathol 90:461.

Lukes RJ, Parker JW, Taylor CR, Tindle BH, Cramer AD, Lincoln TL (1978b). Immunologic Approach to non-Hodgkin's lymphomas and related leukemias: Analysis of the results of multiparameter studies 425 cases. Semin Hematol 15:322.

Lukes RJ (1979). The immunologic approach to the pathology of malignant lymphomas. Am J Clin Path 72:657.

Lukes RJ, Taylor CR, Parker JW (1982). Immunological surface marker studies in the histopathological diagnosis of non-Hodgkin's lymphomas based on multiparameter studies of 790 cases. In Rosenberg S, Kapan H. eds: "Malignant Lymphomas", New York: Academic Press, p 309.

Parker, JW (1979). Immunologic Basis for the Redefinition of Malignant Lymphomas. Am J Clin Path 72:670.

Rappaport, H (1966). Tumors of the Hematopoietic System. Atlas of Tumor Pathology, Section III, Fascicle 8. Washington, D.C.: Armed Forces Institute of Pathology.

Stein H, Bond A, Tolksdorf G, Lennert K, Rodt H, Gerdes J (1980). Immunohistological analysis of the organization of normal lymphoid tissue and non-Hodgkin's lymphomas. J Histochem Cytochem 28:746

Strauchen JA, Young RC, DeVita VT (1978). Clinical relevance of the histopathological subclassification of diffuse "histiocytic" lymphoma. N Engl J. Med 299:1382.

Taylor CR, Mason DY (1974). Immunohistological detection of intracellular immunoglobulin in formalin-paraffin sections from multiple myeloma using the immunoperoxidase technique. Clin Exp Immunol 18:417.

Taylor CR (1979). Results of multiparameter studies of B-cell lymphomas. Am J Clin Path 72:687.

Tubbs RR, Sheibani K, Sebek BA, Weiss RA, Sebek BA (1980). Immunohistochemistry of fresh frozen tissue with indirect immunoperoxidase technique. Am J Clin Path 75:172.

Van Heerde P, Feltkamp C., Feltkamp-Vroom T, Koudstaal J. Van Unnik J (1980). Non-Hodgkin's lymphoma. Immunohistochemical and electron microscopical findings in relations to light microscopy. A study of 74 cases. Cancer 46:2210.

Warnke R, Pederson M, Christopher W, Levy R (1978). A study of lymphoproliferative diseases comparing immunofluorescence and immunohistochemistry. Am J Clin Path 70:867.

13th International Cancer Congress, Part E
Cancer Management, pages 215–227
© 1983 Alan R. Liss, Inc., 150 Fifth Avenue, New York, NY 10011

MEMBRANE AND OTHER PHENOTYPES OF LEUKEMIA CELLS

Jun Minowada, M.D., D.M.S.

Roswell Park Memorial Institute
Buffalo, N.Y. 14263, U.S.A.

INTRODUCTION

The study of immunological and other phenotypes of
leukemia-lymphoma cells has provided much knowledge in
insight into hematopoietic malignancy and normal
differentiation. It has also provided diagnostic and
prognostic correlates in leukemia-lymphomas (Knapp 1981;
Greaves et al 1981; Minowada 1982). Recent advances in
cell technology such as hybridoma technique, gene
cloning, lymphokines, and in vitro growth-differentiation
factors have further enhanced progress in the study of
hematopoietic cells (Kohler and Milstein 1975; Korsmeyer
et al. 1981; Morgan et al. 1976; Collins et al. 1978).

Pulvertaft in 1964 (Pulvertaft 1964), for the first
time, established a permanent hematopoietic cell line
from an African Burkitt lymphoma. Until we established
and characterized a set of sheep
erythrocyte-rosette-forming acute lymphoblastic leukemia
(ALL) cell lines (MOLT 1-4) (Minowada et al. 1972),
however, immunological studies on human leukemia-lymphoma
cells were rather unremarkable. During the past decade,
increasing numbers of proven leukemia-lymphoma cell lines
have been established and characterized (Minowada 1978;
Minowada et al. 1982a). Nearly 100 of such
leukemia-lymphoma cell lines now available together with
studies of fresh leukemia-lymphoma cases were in part
responsible for the progress of leukemia research.
Reasons for this are based on their individual
monoclonality, arrested differentiation characteristics

and stability of these chararacteristics during long-term culture (Minowada et al. 1982a).

A total of 73 leukemia-lymphoma cell lines which represent lymphoid leukemia (non-T, non-B common ALL, T-, Pre-B- and B-ALL), myelomonocytic leukemias, erythriod precursor, lymphomas and myelomas were studied by the multiple markers. A total of 595 patients with four major subtypes of leukemia (ALL, AML, CLL and CML in blastic phase) were similarly studied by the multiple markers. The results thus obtained indicated that the human leukemia exhibits monoclonality, arrested differentiation marker profile, and the marker profiles of leukemia reflecting normal counterparts of hematopoietic differentiation.

MATERIALS AND METHODS

Fresh Uncultured Leukemia and Leukemia Cell Lines.

Leukemic samples (blood and bone marrow) were obtained from patients in the area hospitals as part of a routine immunological diagnosis. All samples were isolated on Ficoll-Hypaque gradient, 30 minutes at 400 g at 22°C. A panel of 73 proven leukemia-lymphoma cell lines as shown in Table 1 were maintained in the laboratory as described previously (Minowada et al. 1982b). The 22 T-cell, 38 B-cell and 4 myeloid leukemia-lymphoma cell lines are grouped by the presence of definitive marker; T-antigen (T-Ag), immunoglobulin (SmIg or CyIg) and myeloid-antigen (MAg), respectively. Remaining 9 non-T, non-B-cell leukemia-lymphoma lines were lacking all these antigens.

Multiple Marker Assay.

As previously reported (Minowada et al. 1982), a number of immunologic, enzymatic and functional analyses (the conventional markers) were used to obtain a particular marker profile to respective immunological subtypes of leukemia relative to the scheme of hematopoietic cell differentiation (Minowada 1982; Minowada et al. 1982b). In addition, relevant murine

HUMAN LEUKEMIA LYMPHOMA CELL LINES (JANUARY '82)

T CELL	ORIGIN	B-CELL	ORIGIN	B-CELL	ORIGIN	MYELOID-CELL	ORIGIN
1 CCRF-CEM	ALL	1 NALM 1*	CML	20 OGUN	BL	1 HL-80	APL
2 CCRF HSB 2	ALL			21 B35M	BL	2 ML 1-3	AML
3 MOLT 1-4	ALL	2 BALL 1	ALL	22 AL 1	BL	3 KG-1	AML
4 RPMI 8402	ALL	3 BALM 1-2	ALL	23 SL 1	BL	4 THP 1	AMOL
5 HPB ALL	ALL	4 NALM 6-15*	ALL	24 NK 9	BL		
6 JM	ALL	5 NALM 17-18*	ALL	25 DAUDI	BL		
7 PEER	ALL	6 KOPN 1-8*	ALL	26 B46M	BL	NON-T, NON-B CELL	
8 P12/Ichi	ALL	7 HPB Null*	ALL	27 NAMALVA	BL		
9 DND 41	ALL	8 LAZ 221*	ALL	28 RAMOS	BL	1 K-562	CML
10 KE 37	ALL			29 BJAB	BL		
11 P30/OKUBO	ALL			30 DG 75	BL	2 REH	ALL
12 MOLT 10	ALL	9 U-698-M	LS	31 CHEVALLIER	BL	3 KM 3	ALL
13 HD Mar 2	HD (?)	10 BALM 3-5	LB	32 DND 39	BL	4 NALL 1	ALL
		11 TANAKA	LB	33 KOBK 101	BL	5 NALM 16	ALL
14 HPB-MLT	ATL	12 MANACA 2	LB			6 KOPN-K	ALL
15 TALL 1	ATL	13 SKW-4	LB	34 RPMI 8226	MM		
16 MT 1	ATL	14 RIVA	LB	35 U 266	MM	7 KLM 2 (+)	AMOL
17 HUT 78	SS	15 SCOTT	LB	36 ARH 77	MM		
18 CTCL 2	SS	16 SU-DHL 4	LY			8 U-937	LY
19 HUT 102	MF	17 EB3	BL	37 JOK 1	HCL	9 SU-DHL 1	LY
		18 RAJI	BL	38 KHT-M	HCL		
20 SKW 3	CLL	19 HR1K	BL				
21 A3/KAWAKAMI	LY						
22 KOPT KI	LS						

ALL · ACUTE LYMPHOBLASTIC LEUKEMIA
HD · HODGKIN'S DISEASE
ATL · "ADULT T-CELL LEUKEMIA"
SS · SEZARY SYNDROME
MF · MYCOSIS FUNGOIDES
CLL · CHRONIC LYMPHOCYTIC LEUKEMIA
CML · CHRONIC MYELOCYTIC LEUKEMIA
LS · LYMPHOSARCOMA

LB · B-CELL LYMPHOMA
LY · LYMPHOMA
BL · BURKITT LYMPHOMA
MM · MULTIPLE MYELOMA
HCL · HAIRY CELL LEUKEMIA
APL · ACUTE PROMYELOCYTIC LEUKEMIA
AML · ACUTE MYELOBLASTIC LEUKEMIA
AMOL · ACUTE MONOCYTIC LEUKEMIA
* · PRE-B-CELL LEUKEMIA

monoclonal hybridoma antibodies from the panel of 64
preparations were used on some samples in indirect
immunofluorescence test. By the conventional multiple
markers, immunologic subtypes of leukemia are identified
as shown in Table 2.

RESULTS AND DISCUSSION

Leukemia–Lymphoma Cell Lines.

From 22 T-cell leukemia-lymphoma cell lines in Table
1, further immunologic subtypes of T-cell malignancy were
defined by particular combination of 4 markers (Ia, T-Ag,
cALL and TdT), i.e., types I, II, III, IV and V,
respectively. Of 38 B-cell leukemia-lymphoma cell lines,
immunologic subtypes were further defined by particular
combination of 5 markers (CyIgM, SmIgM, SmIgG, cALL, and
TdT). Six of those B cell lines were identified as Pre-B
ALL line on the basis of cytoplasmic μ-chain without
detectable SmIg. Some of them, if not all, were found to

MARKER PROFILE OF LEUKEMIA

DX	IMMUNOLOGIC SUBTYPE		E	EA	EAC	SmIg	CyIg	T-Ag	Ia	cALL	M-Ag	TdT	MLC-S
ALL	T	I	-	-	-	-	-	+	+	+	-	+	+/-
		II	+	-	+	-	-	+	-	+	-	+	-
		III	+	-	+/-	-	-	+	-	-	-	+	-
		IV	+	-	+/-	-	-	+	-	-	-	-	-
		V	+	-	+/-	-	-	+	+	-	-	-	+/-
	Pre B		-	-	-	-	+	-	+	+/-	-	+/-	+
	B	I	-	+/-	+/-	+ (μ)	+	-	+	+	-	-	+
		II	-	+/-	+/-	+ (μ)	+	-	+	-	-	-	+
		III	-	+/-	+/-	+ (γ)	+	-	+	-	-	-	+
	Common		-	-	-	-	-	-	+	+	-	+	+
	Null		-	-	-	-	-	-	+/-	-	-	+/-	+/-
AML	AML	I	-	-	-	-	-	-	+	-	-	-/+	+
		II	-	-	-	-	-	-	+	-	+	+	+
		III	-	+	+/-	-	-	-	+/-	-	+	-	+
CLL	B		-	+	+	+	+	-	+	-	-	-	+
	T		+	-	-	-	-	+	-	-	-	-	-
CML-BP	"Lymphoid"		-	-	-	-	-/+	-	+	+	-	+	+
	"Mixed"		-	+/-	+/-	-	-	-	+	+/-	+	+/-	+
	"Myeloid"		-	+/-	+/-	-	-	-	+/-	-	+	-	+

Abbreviations used: Dx=diagnosis, E: sheep erythrocyte rosette; EA=rosette formed by bovine erythrocyte–IgG antibody complex; EAC=rosette formed by bovine erythrocyte–IgM antibody–complement complex; SmIg-CyIg=surface membrane or cytoplasmic immunoglobulins; T-Ag=T-antigens; Ia=Ia-like HLA-DR antigen; cALL=common ALL associated antigen; M-Ag=myelomonocyte antigen; TdT=deoxynucleotidyl transferase; MLC-S=stimulating capacity in "one–way" mixed leukocyte culture; ALL=acute lymphoblastic leukemia; AML=acute myeloblastic leukemia; CLL=chronic lymphocytic leukemia; CML-BP=blastic phase in chronic myelocytic leukemia.

be positive for TdT. Four myeloid leukemia lines included a promyelocyte leukemia (HL-60), 2 AML (KG-1 and ML 1~3) and a monoblastic leukemia (THP-1).

Of particular interest was that 3 T-cell lines (HUT-102, CTCL-2 and MT-1) were positive for C-type retrovirus known as HTLV (Human T-cell Leukemia Virus) or ATLV (Adult T-cell Leukemia Virus) (Gallo 1981; Poiesz et al. 1981; Hinuma et al. 1981; Miyoshi et al. 1980). Most of B-lymphoma lines derived from African Burkitt lymphoma had Epstein-Barr virus genome (Minowada et al. 1982b).

The cALL antigen which was thought originally as a non-T, non-B common ALL specific antigen (Greaves et al. 1975) was found to distribute not only in leukemias of much wider lineages (Minowada et al. 1978) but also in some normal lymphoid precursor cells (Greaves and Janossy 1978). Furthermore, it distributes in cells of non-hematological origins (Metzgar et al. 1981). Nevertheless, the cALL antigen is a most useful leukemia-associated antigen in operational sense (Greaves 1982).

Fresh, Uncultured Leukemias.

Table 3 summarizes the results of 595 leukemic patients for their immunologic membrane phenotypes as determined by the conventional multiple marker assay (Table 1).

IMMUNOLOGICAL SUBCLASSIFICATION OF LEUKEMIA
(595 Patients at RPMI: 1975-Aug. 1982)

DX	IMMUNOLOGIC TYPE	% INCIDENCE (NO./TOTAL)	REMARKS
ALL	T	15% (32/210)	E^+: 63% (20/32) E^+EAC^+: 25% (8/32) $cALL^+$: 47% (15/32) Ia^+: 13% (4/32)
	B	5% (10/210)	$cALL^+$: 30% (3/10)
	COMMON	74% (156/210)	$CyIgM$: 18% (16/87)
	NULL	6% (12/210)	Ia^+: 75% (9/12)
AML	I	10% (13/134)	Ia^+: 78% (105/134)
	II	46% (62/134)	MAg^+: 90% (121/134)
	III	44% (59/134)	
CLL	B	99% (166/167)	
	T	1% (1/167)	
CML-BP	LYMPHOID	21% (18/84)	
	MIXED	35% (29/84)	$cALL^+$: 56% (47/84)
	MYELOID	44% (37/84)	

Some of the recent cases were analyzed a battery of relevant monoclonal antibodies in addition to the conventional markers. As previously reported (Minowada et al. 1982a), in 22 cases of T-cell ALL studied an extremely heterogeneous marker profile was seen just as seen with those 22 T-cell leukemia-lymphoma lines. It was then clear that the observations between lines and fresh leukemia cells could be interpreted interchangeably. It is remarkable, therefore, that the stability of the marker profiles in the permanent leukemia-lymphoma cell lines is so consistent for years in vitro cultivation. Nonetheless, recent studies demonstrated clearly that the marker profile of such leukemic T cell lines can be modulated by treatment with various differentiation inducers (Collins et al. 1977; Collins et al. 1978; Koeffler and Golde 1978; Delia et al. 1982; LeBien et al. 1982).

Concerning the marker profiles of myeloid leukemia, it has become increasingly clear that these leukemias are as heterogeneous as lymphoid leukemias (Roberts and Greaves 1978; Sagawa et al. 1980; Greaves 1982; Minowada 1982; Griffin et al. 1981). Since it has been known the clonal stem cell involvement in the CML (Fialkow et al. 1967; Boggs 1974), the immunological study on this disease has shown further unequivocal evidence for such multiple lineage involvement of leukemic clones (Janossy et al. 1976; Lozzio and Lozzio 1980; Andersson et al. 1979; LeBien et al. 1979; Minowada et al. 1979). Furthermore, our recent observation with a set of monoclonal antibodies demonstrated that in substantial cases of the lymphoid crisis in CML the leukemic blasts exhibit a dual marker expression of both lymphoid (cALL) and myeloid (M-Ag) antigens (Minowada unpublished data) which is in contrast to the marker profile of all Ph' negative acute leukemias thus far studied. It might indicate that the cellular origin or leukemic expression between ALL/AML and CML in blast phase may be different.

Hematopoietic Differentiation Scheme Based on the Study of Leukemia-Lymphomas.

Data are accummulated, as described briefly in the preceeding sections, that the findings are reasonably consistent with our interpretation which has been provided a model scheme of normal hematopoietic differentiation in man (Minowada 1978; Minowada 1982;

Minowada et al. 1982a). Various model schemes by several
investigators have been put forward in the literature
(Greaves and Janossy 1978; Greaves 1982; Foon et al.
1982; Reinherz et al. 1980; Cooper 1981; Magrath 1981).

Figure 1 illustrates a scheme of hematopoietic
differentiation which is based on the leukemia-lymphoma
marker study. Figures 2 and 3 represent further details
of myeloid lineage and T-lymphoid lineage, respectively.

HEMATOPOIETIC CELL DIFFERENTIATION

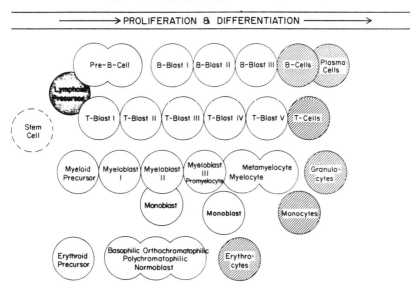

Fig. 1. Based on the description in this paper. See
Tables 1, 2, and 3.

SUMMARY

A total of 73 leukemia-lymphoma cell lines and 595
patients with leukemias were summarized for their marker

profiles. Neither specific leukemia antigen nor marker
profiles aberrant from those normal counterparts were
documented. Monoclonality and particular fixed profile
at varying points in differentiation pathway were
uniquely observed in all leukemia–lymphomas studied. An
extreme heterogeneity in the leukemia–lymphoma marker
profiles leads to a model scheme of normal hematopoietic
cell differentiation.

MYELOID CELL DIFFERENTIATION & LEUKEMIA

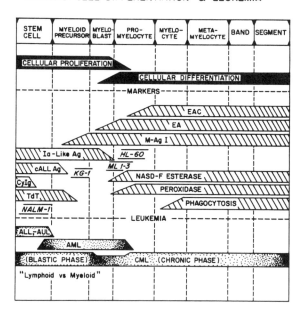

Fig. 2. Morphological, cytochemical, functional and
immunological parameters are illustrated, relative to
both leukemic and normal myeloid cells. Four leukemia
cell lines (NALM–1, KG–1, ML 1~3 and HL–60) are assigned
at appropriate position according to the data of their
marker profiles.

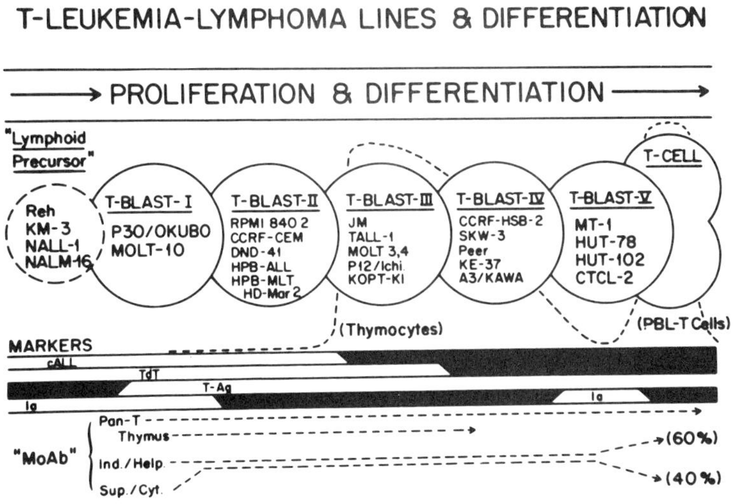

T-LEUKEMIA-LYMPHOMA LINES & DIFFERENTIATION

Fig. 3. Marker profiles of the stages of T-blast I, II, III, IV and V are shown in Table 2. The lymphoid precursor exhibits cALL, Ia and TdT. Four common ALL lines and 22 T-cell leukemia lines are assigned in respective compartments according to their marker profiles. Normal thymocytes and peripheral-mature T cells are shown in broken-line with relative quantity in the vertical axis. Data with relevant monoclonal antibodies (Minowada et al. 1982a) are illustrated in the lower part of the figure.

ACKNOWLEDGMENTS

This study was supported by grants CA-14413, AI-08899 and BRSG from the National Institutes of Health, U.S.P.H.S., from AAROC, and Institutional grant IN-54U from the American Cancer Society. The author gratefully acknowledges many colleagues who provided various essential contributions to this study.

REFERENCES

Anderson LC, Jokinen M, Gahmberg CG (1979). Induction of erythroid differentiation in the human leukaemia cell line K562. Nature 278:364.

Boggs DR (1974). Hematopoietic stem cell theory in relation to possible lymphoblastic conversion of chronic myeloid leukemia. Blood 44:449.

Collins SJ, Gallo RC, Gallagher RE (1977). Continuous growth and differentiation of human myeloid leukaemic cells in suspension culture. Nature 270:347.

Collins SJ, Ruscetti FW, Gallagher RE, Gallo RC (1978). Terminal differentiation of human promyelocytic leukemia cells induced by dimethyl sulfoxide and other polar compounds. Proc Natl Acad Sci USA 75:2458.

Cooper MD (1981). Pre-B cells: Normal and abnormal development. J Clin Immunol 1:81.

Delia D, Greaves MF, Newman RA, Sutherland DR, Minowada J, Kung P, Goldstein G (1982). Modulation of T leukaemic cell phenotype with phorbol ester. Int J Cancer 29:23.

Fialkow PJ, Gartler SM, Yoshida A (1967). Clonal origin of chronic myelocytic leukemia in man. Proc Natl Acad Sci USA 58: 1468.

Foon KA, Schroff RW, Gale RP (1982). Surface markers on leukemia and lymphoma cells: Recent advances. Blood 60:1.

Gallo RC (1981). Growth of human normal and leukemic T-cells: T-cells growth factor (TCGF) and the isolation of a new class of RNA tumor viruses (HTLV). Blood Cells 7:313.

Greaves MF (1982). "Target" cells, cellular phenotypes, and lineage fidelity in human leukaemia. J Cellular Phys Supplement 1:113.

Greaves MF, Brown G, Rapson NT, Lister TA (1975). Antisera to acute lymphoblastic leukemia cells. Clin Immunol Immunopath 4:67.

Greaves M, Janossy, G (1978). Patterns of gene expression and the cellular origins of human leukaemias. Biochem Biophys Acta 516:193.

Greaves MF, Janossy G, Peto J, Kay H (1981). Immunologically defined subclasses of acute lymphoblastic leukaemia in children: Their relationship to presentation features and prognosis.Brit J Haematol 48:179.

Griffin J, Ritz J, Nadler L, Scholssman S (1981).
Expression of myeloid differentiation antigens on
normal and malignant myeloid cells. J Clin Invest
68:932.
Hinuma Y, Nagata K, Hanaoka M, Nakai M, Matsumoto T,
Kinoshita K, Shirakawa S, Miyoshi I (1981). Adult
T-cell leukemia: Antigen in an ATL cell line and
detection of antibodies to the antigen in human sera.
Proc Natl Acad Sci 78:6476.
Janossy G, Greaves MF, Revesz T, Lister TA, Roberts M,
Durrant J, Kirk B, Catovski D, Beard MEJ (1976). Blast
crisis of chronic myeloid leukaemia (CML) II. Cell
surface marker analysis of 'lymphoid' and myeloid
cases. Brit J Haematol 34:179.
Knapp W (ed) (1981) "Leukemia Markers" Acad Press, London.
Koeffler HP, Golde DW (1978). Acute myelogenous leukemia:
A human cell line responsive to colony-stimulating
activity. Science 200:1153.
Kohler G, Milstein C (1975). Continuous cultures of
fused cells secreting antibody of predefined
specificity. Nature 256:495.
Korsmeyer SJ, Hieter PA, Ravetch JV, Poplack DG, Leder P,
Waldmann TA (1981). Patterns of immunoglobulin gene
arrangement in human lymphocytic leukemias. In Knapp W
(eds): "Leukemia Markers" London: Academic Press, p 85.
LeBien T, Bollum R, Yasmineh W, Kersey J (1982). Phorbol
ester-induced differentiation of a non-T, non-B
leukemic cell line: Model of human lymphoid progenitor
cell development. J Immunol 128:1316.
LeBien TW, Hozier J, Minowada J, Kersey JH (1979).
Origin of chronic myelocytic leukemia in a precursor of
pre-B lymphocytes. New Engl J Med 301:144.
Lozzio BB, Lozzio CB (1980). Review: Properties and
usefulness of the original K-562 human myelogenous
leukemia cell line. Leuk Res 3:363.
Magrath IT (1981). Lymphocyte differentiation: An
essential basis for the comprehension of lymphoid
neoplasia. J Nat Cancer Inst 67:501.
Metzgar R, Borowitz M, Jones N, Dowell B (1981).
Distribution of common acute lymphoblastic leukemia
antigen in nonhematopoietic tissues. J Exp Med
154:1249.

Minowada J (1978). Markers of human leukaemia-lymphoma cell lines reflect haematopoietic cell differentiation. In Serrou B, Rosenfeld C (eds): "Human Lymphocyte Differentiation: Its Application to Cancer", Elsevier/North Holland Biomedical Press, Amsterdam, pp.337.

Minowada J (1982). "Immunology of Leukemic Cells" in Gunz F and Henderson ES (eds.), "Leukemia", Grune and Stratton, New York, pp.119.

Minowada J, Janossy G, Greaves MF, Tsubota T, Srivastava BIS, Morikawa S, Tatsumi E (1978). Expression of an antigen associated with acute lymphoblastic leukemia in human leukemia-lymphoma cell lines. J Nat Cancer Inst 60:1269.

Minowada J, Koshiba H, Janossy G, Greaves MF, Bollum FJ (1979). A Philadelphia chromosome positive human leukaemia cell line (NALM-1) with pre-B characteristics. Leukemia Res 3:261.

Minowada J, Minato K, Srivastava BIS, Nakazawa S, Kubonishi I, Tatsumi E, Ohnuma T, Ozer H, Freeman AI, Henderson ES, Gallo RC (1982a). A model scheme of human hematopoietic cell differentiation as determined by leukemia-lymphoma study: T-cell lineages. In Serrou B and Rosenfeld C (eds.), "Current Concepts in Human Immunology and Cancer Immunomodulation ", Elsevier/North Holland Biomedical Press, Amsterdam, pp. 75.

Minowada J, Ohnuma T, Moore GE (1972). Rosette-forming human lymphoid cell lines. I. Establishment and evidence for origin of thymus-derived lymphocytes. J Nat Cancer Inst 49:891.

Minowada J, Sagawa K, Trowbridge IS, Kung PD, Goldstein G (1982b). Marker profiles of 55 human leukemia-lymphoma cell lines. In Rosenber SA and Kaplan HS (eds.), "Malignant Lymphomas: Etiology, Immunology, Pathology, Treatment", Acad Press, New York, pp.53.

Miyoshi I, Kubonishi I, Sumida M, Hiraki S, Tsubota T, Kimura I, Miyamoto K, Sato J (1980). A novel T-cell derived from adult T-cell leukemia. Gann 71:155.

Morgan DA, Ruscetti FW, Gallo R (1976). Selective in vitro growth of T lymphocytes from normal human bone marrows. Science 193:1007.

Poiesz BJ, Ruscetti FW, Mier JW, Woods AM, Gallo RC (1981). T-cell lines established from human T lymphocytic neoplasias by direct response to T-cell growth factor. Proc Natl Acad Sci USA 77: 6815.

Reinherz EL, Kung PC, Goldstein G, Levey RH, Schlossman SF (1980). Discrete stages of human intrathymic differentiation: Analysis of normal thymocytes and leukemic lymphoblasts of T-cell lineage. Proc Natl Acad Sci USA 77:1588.

Roberts MM, Greaves MF (1978). Maturation linked expression of a myeloid cell surface antigen. Brit J Haematol 38:439.

Sagawa K, Koshiba H, Lok MS, Freeman AI, Preisler HD, Henderson ES, Minowada J, Pressman D (1980). Membrane phenotypes of myeloid leukemia cells: An attempt at subgrouping AML and CML in man. Proc Amer Assoc Cancer Res 21:208.

Pulfertaft RJ (1964). Cytology of Burkitt's tumour (African lymphoma). Lancet i:238.

13th International Cancer Congress, Part E
Cancer Management, pages 229–246
© 1983 Alan R. Liss, Inc., 150 Fifth Avenue, New York, NY 10011

Human Tumor Nucleolar Antigens

H. Busch, R.K. Busch, P.K. Chan, D. Kelsey,
W.H. Spohn
Department of Pharmacology, Baylor College of
  Medicine
Houston, Texas 77030

Our initial experiments, (R.K. Busch et al., 1974), indicated that immunization of rabbits with nucleoli of normal rat liver and rat hepatomas resulted in formation of "nucleolus-specific" antibodies. In this original work, there was also the suggestion by complement fixation analysis that there might be some differences in the antigens in the tumors by comparison with nontumor tissues.

We found that by Ouchterlony analysis there were indeed antigens in the Novikoff rat hepatoma that were not present in normal rat liver and vice versa (Busch and Busch, 1977). Chemical characterization of these antigens was undertaken from both sources; one tumor antigen was isolated which had a molecular weight of approximately 60,000 and an isoelectric point of approximately 5.3. It was also found that the mRNA for the tumor antigens was not expressed in normal rat liver.

HUMAN TUMOR NUCLEOLAR ANTIGENS

The information base developed from the studies on the rodent antigens led us to search for the rodent tumor antigens in human specimens. With the aid of Dr. F. Gyorkey of the Veterans Administration Hospital of Houston, Texas, a series of human malignant tumors were analyzed. The antigen was not found, and, accordingly, the immunizations were done with nucleolar preparations from the readily available HeLa cells which resulted in antihuman tumor nucleolar antibodies that were used in subsequent studies.

Nucleolar Antigens in Human Tumors

Although the studies on the nucleolar antigens of the
rodent tumors and nontumor tissues indicated that there
might be important differences in these nucleolar proteins,
initial attempts to extend these studies to human neoplasms
met with the problem that human tumor nucleoli did not
exhibit bright fluorescence when treated with antibodies to
rat tumor nucleoli. After preliminary studies showed that
these antibodies did not produce corresponding immunoreact-
ivity with nucleolar antigens of human tumor specimens,
nucleolar preparations and nuclear Tris extracts (0.01 M
Tris HCl/pH8.0) of human HeLa cells were used as immunogens.
Happily, the immunized rabbits developed antihuman tumor
nucleolar antibodies (Davis et al., 1979; Busch et al., 1979).

A broad array of human and malignant tumors contains
nucleolar antigens recognizable by bright nucleolar fluores-
ence (Busch et al., 1979). These tumors include (Table 1)
carcinomas of many types, a variety of sarcomas, and many
hematological neoplasms. To discriminate the nucleolar
fluorescence of the tumors from that found in other tissues,
such as placenta, extensive absorption of nontumor antibodies
from the antisera, Ig or IgG fractions, was done. First,
because the HeLa cells initially used were grown in fetal
calf serum, fetal calf serum was an essential absorbent.
Second, since most human normal tissues were not widely
available for isolation, a source of nuclei or nuclear products was necessary. Inasmuch as placentas are ordinarily discarded and are a good source of nuclei, they were utilized as
a source of nuclear extracts for absorption (Davis et al.,
1979; Busch et al., 1979). In addition, normal human serum
contains some minor cross-reactive elements so that absorption
was done with serum proteins or whole serum.

Although it would be highly desirable to have a precipi-
tating antibody of the type found with the anti-Novikoff
hepatoma antibodies, such precipitins have not yet been found
with human tissues despite the use of multiple rabbits, sheep,
and goats. It appears that the antigenic determinants of
human nucleolar antigens differ from those of the rodent, but
as yet no specific information is available on either the
amino acid or other determinants in either of these types of
antigens.

Table 1. Bright Nucleolar Fluorescence in Human Malignant
Tumor Specimens

I. Carcinomas

   1. Lung
      adenocarcinoma(3)
       oat cell(4)
      squamous cell(22)
   2. Gastrointestinal
      oral cavity(8)
      pharynx(4)
      esophagus, squamous cell(5)
      stomach, adenocarcinoma(5)
        metastasis: liver
        metastasis: liver node
      colon, adenocarcinoma(9)
        metastasis: liver(2)
        transplantable carcinoma (GW-39)
      liver, primary carcinoma(3)
      pancreas(4)
   3. Genitourinary
      kidney(4)
      prostate, adenocarcinoma(22)
      bladder(4)
   4. CNS
      glioblastoma(1)
      astrocytoma(5)
   5. Endocrine
      breast(88)
      cervix(4)
      parathyroid(1)
      thyroid(5)
   6. Skin
      basal cell(8)
      eccrine gland(1)
      squamous cell(7)
        metastasis: lymph node
      melanoma, malignant(4)
        cerebral metastasis(1)
      sweat gland(3)

II. Sarcomas

    1. Chondrosarcoma(1)
    2. Fibrosarcoma(4)
    3. Giant cell tumor(1)
    4. Granulocytic myoblastoma(2)
    5. Leimyosarcoma(4)
    6. Lymphoma(10)
    7. Meningiosarcoma(1)
    8. Myoblastoma(2)
    9. Osteogenic(6)
    10. Pulmonary blastoma(1)
    11. Reticulum cell sarcoma(1)
    12. Synovial sarcoma(1)

III. Hematological Neoplasma

    1. Acute lymphoctyic leukemia(2)
    2. Acute myelocytic leukemia(7)
    3. Acute monocytic leukemia(2)
    4. Chronic myelocytic leukemia(5)
    5. Hodgkins disease(9)
    6. Leukemia: CLL(12), Hairy cell(1)
    7. Mycosis fungoides
    8. Plasmacytomas(7)

The numbers in parenthesis are numbers of samples in these
initial experiments. In subsequent studies, 94% of all
types of human cancers have exhibited bright nucleolar
fluorescence with these antibodies.

Antibodies to Other Tumors

    For comparative purposes, two malignant tumors other
than HeLa cells were used as sources of the antigen. The
Namalwa cell line is a derivative of a Burkitt tumor provided
to us by the National Cancer Institute and the Frederick Cancer Research Center through the generosity of Drs. V. DeVita,
J. Douros, and Fred Klein. A human prostate carcinoma grown
in tissue culture was used by Dr. F. Gyorkey and Mrs. P.
Gyorkey. Both of these tumors contain nucleolar antigens as
demonstrated by production of antinucleolar antibodies with
similar titers and specificities in rabbits. With the prostatic carcinoma, a nucleolar preparation was used for immunization and a Tris extract of nuclei of the Namalwa cells was

used as the immunogen. The similarity of the results obtained suggested that there were common antigens in these cells and the HeLa cells.

Are the Tumor Nucleolar Antigens Present in Nontumor Tissues?

It is logical to ask whether antigens of the type found reflect a neoplastic process or a normal process involved in growth cell division or other normal physiological effect. Our theory of carcinogenesis (Busch, 1976) pointed out that cancer is probably the result of misapplication of normal gene readouts as a dysplastic phenomenon involving fetal genes rather than a process which involves "totally new" events, such as integration of a viral genome or other gene aberration. Accordingly, a search has been made for the antigens in a variety of normal, growing, and fetal tissues. As noted in Table 2, the nucleolar antigens were absent from most of the nontumor tissues studies which presumably exhibited show growth or none at all.

An important question was whether the nucleolar antigens were present in normal growing nontumor tissues. In studies on bone marrow, skin Malpigian layers, and intestinal epithelium, the nucleolar antigens were not found. In studies on bone marrow of patients with leukemias, the neoplastic cells contained the antigens, but their nontumor counterparts in the same maturation series did not contain the antigens (Smetana et al., 1979). As controls for the nontumor tissues, studies were made on cells of patients with acute infectious mononucleosis and lymphoid hyperplasia, but neither exhibited bright nucleolar fluorescence under the circumstances of these studies. These results like those indicated above suggested that immunological analysis of whole cells, cell suspensions, or cell sections for the nucleolar antigen could be useful for immunodiagnosis of malignant disease.

In extending the studies to various types of tissues, fetal tissues were studied, partly because in earlier studies nucleolar fetal antigens were found to be expressed in the Novikoff hepatoma (Davis et al., 1978; Yeoman et al., 1976) and also because there may be important conclusions if the neoplastic cells contained functional fetal antigens (Busch, 1976). In more mature fetal tissues, such as 9-month fetal lung or 6-month fetal liver, no evidence was found for bright nucleolar fluorescence. However, examination of the IMR-90 and WI-38 diploid fetal fibroblast lines in tissue culture indicated that they exhibited brightly positive nucleolar

Table 2. Negative Nucleolar Fluorescence in Human Tissues

   I. Normal tissue

      1. Lung
      2. Gastrointestinal
         stomach
         intestine
            small, crypts of Lieberkuhn
            large
         liver
         pancreas
      3. Genital urinary
         kidney
         bladder
         prostate
      4. Endocrine
         thyroid
         breast
         placenta
      5. Skin

  II. Hematologic

      1. Bone marrow
      2. Lymph nodes
         lymphocytes
         hyperplastic lymph nodes
      3. Benign growing tissues
         thyroid, goiter
         prostate, hyperplastic

 III. Inflammatory diseases

      1. Chronic ulcerative colitis
      2. Glomerulonephritis
      3. Granuloma and fibrosis of lung
      4. Liver: cirrhosis, hepatitis
      5. Lupus profundus (mammary gland and skin)
      6. Pemphigus: bullous
      7. Ulcer, gastric

fluorescence (Busch et al., 1979). Such studies, along with
evidence to be presented in the section on staining of gels,
indicated that the nucleolar antigens in the malignant tumor

might reflect activation of the fetal genes which could be important in the over-all neoplastic process.

Breast Cancer

Because of the need for a "preliminary" evaluation of the possible diagnostic use of the fluorescence assay for the human tumor antigens, it was important to find a series of a particular tumor type that would lend itself to a "blind" evaluation. It was fortunate that at the Michigan Cancer Foundation, a prospective study on human breast cancer was in progress. As part of this study, a large series of patients with breast cancer are being analyzed for relationships between the pathology of the neoplasm and the course of the disease (Busch et al., 1981). Sections of normal breast tissue as well as benign and malignant tumors were analyzed for bright nucleolar fluorescence by the indirect immunofluorescence technique. These investigations were all approved by the Human Research Committee of Baylor College of Medicine and the Committee for Protection of Human Subjects of the Michigan Cancer Foundation.

The cryostat sections of the human tumors were kept at -20°; they were cut at 2μ and fixed for 12 min. in acetone at 4°. The tumors were evaluated histopathologically by a panel of five pathologists who provided a consensus diagnosis, designation of tumor grade, and other characteristics on the basis of H & E staining. The specimens were treated with either Ig or IgG fractions prepared from antisera absorbed with human placental nuclear extracts, fetal bovine serum, and human serum.

Before the "blind" study was initiated, known samples of breast carcinomas were examined. In 19/20 of these, bright nucleolar fluorescence was found to be distributed either throughout the sections or, in a few instances, in cell masses in particular portions of the sections. The 95% positive result for nucleolar fluorescence was similar to the first result (Busch et al., 1979) in which 81/84 samples (96%) were positive in the variety of malignant tumors.

In some cases, the whole specimen consisted of cells with irregular, large brightly fluorescent nucleoli (Busch et al., 1981). In others, the neoplastic cells were either in focal lesions or randomly distributed, and in some, chords of tumor cells were distributed throughout the specimens. The background fluorescence ranged from negligible to moderately intense.

In some sections, the neoplastic cells were confined to small areas or were not visible. In some "false negatives," the antibodies did not penetrate the cells, as a result of sample thickness, proteolysis, or "waxy deposits." In other instances, the region containing the tumor cells was lost or only at the periphery of the specimen. To avoid such problems, examination of several slides from a single specimen was necessary to define sharply the area of the neoplastic cells.

What are the Nucleolar Antigens?

Because of the necessity for more complete information on the numbers and types of antigens, studies were undertaken to characterize the nucleolar antigens in these human tumors chemically. Although it would be highly desirable and ulti- mately possible to isolate and purify the antigens from a variety of tumors, it was first necessary to develop techniques for their purification from a satisfactory source. The initial attempts at characterization were made with nucleolar products from HeLa cells, but unfortunately there is no satis- factory commercial source and the cell masses required are extremely expensive.

It was most fortunate that during this period, the Fred- erick Cancer Research Center was in the process of large-scale production of interferon from Namalwa cells, a Burkitt tumor line. Through the cooperation of Drs. Vincent DeVita, John Douros, and Fred Klein, quantities of such cells from 100- 250 grams were made available. Although not completely satis- factory, in that the nuclear preparations from these frozen cells were less elegant than those from fresh cells, these cells were a satisfactory source of the nucleolar antigens for purification and for further characterization (Chan et al., 1980).

Isoelectric Focusing of the Nucleolar Antigens

The studies on the nucleolar antigens of the Novikoff hepatoma showed that multiple antigenic determinants and multiple antigens might exist in the human tumor nucleoli. To initiate studies on these human antigens (with the recog- nition that some methods might preclude identification of a number of other antigens) isoelectric focusing of the antigens was undertaken (Chan et al., 1980). For this purpose, the proteins were incorporated into the gels so that antigens would not be lost by loading on either the basic or acidic side, and, secondly, 8M urea was added to the ampholine solution to enhance the resolution of the bands. However, it seemed likely that the urea and the ampholines might react with or modify some of the antigens and make them unrecognizable.

For visualization of the antigens, the gels were washed 3 times with isotonic saline, immersed in acetone briefly to shrink the gel, and then soaked in the antitumor nucleolar antibodies (antiserum, Ig fraction or IgG fraction). Excess antiserum was then removed from the gel by washing 6 times with the buffered saline solution, and the fluorescein- or peroxidase- conjugated goat-antirabbit antibody was added to the preparation. With this procedure, it was possible to visualize the antigen in the gel either by fluorescence or by the peroxidase staining methods.

Identification of the pI 6.3 and 6.1 Antigens

In the isoelectric focusing gels, two antigens were identified both by fluorescence and peroxidase staining methods. The major antigen focused at pI 6.3 and the minor band focused at pI 6.1. Later studies showed these antigens had molecular weights of approximately 68,000 and 61,000 respectively, and accordingly they were referred to as HuAg 68/6.3 and 61/6.1 (M.W.$\times 10^{-3}$/pI). These antigens were not detected with preimmune serum and were not found in the normal liver cells, nuclei, or nucleolar proteins focused on corresponding gels.

In addition to these two bands which were regularly observed in such preparations, weakly immunostained bands were occasionally observed at pI 6.6, 5.5, 5.7, and 5.9. However, they were also observed following incubation with preimmune serum.

Another set of bands which were nonspecifically bound to either the first or second antibody was on the basic side of the gels. These bands were also observed with preimmune serum, and they were generally present and also were in both normal human liver samples and HeLa and Namalwa samples. These bands may be of importance in nonspecific nucleolar staining reactions which have been a problem in some diagnostic studies. They may also be tissue specific, but this has not been shown yet.

It was important to run the gels for short periods in view of the possibility that some antigens might migrate rapidly off the acidic or basic sides. However, no reproducible antigens were found, other than the HuAg 68/6.3 and HuAg 61/6.1, even when the gels were run for very short periods. No additional antigens were demonstrable when higher concentrations of antibodies or proteins were used or when loading was done on the acidic or basic ends of the gels. Of course, none of these results eliminates the possibility that antigens are present that are denatured or are altered by the ampholines or the urea (Chan et al., 1980).

From the point of view of localization of the HuAg 68/6.3 and HuAg 61/6.1, it is notable that they were not present in the "nuclear sap" (75 mM NaCl/25 mM EDTA/0.1 mM PMSF/pH 8 extracts) of HeLa cells nuclei or in the cytosol fraction of these cells. They were found in the whole nucleolar protein extracts and in the 10 mM Tris extracts of nuclei after the nuclear sap was extracted with 75 mM NaCl/25 mM EDTA.

Densitometric Scanning of the Fluorescent Antigens

In the isoelectric focusing gel of the nucleolar proteins of the HeLa cells, there was a fluorescent-peak at pI 6.3 when the gel was treated with immune serum but not with the preimmune serum. Corresponding analysis of the nucleolar proteins of the normal liver did not show the presence of a corresponding antigen. Staining of the same gels with Coomassie Blue staining indicated that there were 36 protein bands which on 2-D gels separated into more than 60 peptides.

Similar studies on Namalwa nuclear Tris extracts demonstrated the presence of the same major and minor antigens. Because of the interest in whether fetal cells contain these antigens, a similar analysis was made of IMR-90 fetal human fibroblasts. Nucleolar antigens with pI values of both 6.3 and 6.1 were demonstrable in these cells. These results provide further support for the presence of oncofetal or "oncoembryonic" antigens in human malignant tumors. The question of what period in fetal life contains the "time window" at which these antigens are normally produced remains to be defined.

Purification of the Human Tumor Nucleolar Antigens

For characterization of these proteins, it was first necessary to develop a satisfactory purification procedure

with preservation of antigenicity and production of a homogeneous product. Initially, ammonium sulfate fractionation
was used. At a concentration of 40% ammonium sulfate, none
of the antigen was precipitated, and accordingly the 40%
sediment was discarded.

The 40-100% fraction contained the antigen, and after
sedimentation it was chromatographed on a DEAE-cellulose column. A stepwise NaCl gradient was used to elute the antigens
selectively at a concentration 0.15 M NaCl. This resulted in
approximately a 10-fold purification inasmuch as 10% of the
protein and most of the antigen were eluted in this fraction.
Analysis of the proteins in this fraction by isoelectric focusing gels indicated that only this fraction reproducibly
contained the HuAg 6.3 and HuAg 6.1 antigens. A Coomassie
Blue-stained band which corresponds to this fraction was
identified; this band was shown to be concentrated in the
0.15 M NaCl fraction but not in the other fractions.

To test whether the antigens in these fractions could
absorb the Ig fraction or the antiserum, the antibodies were
initially treated with the NaCl-eluted fractions and then
used for the double-antibody immunostaining of the gels. Only
the antibody fraction absorbed with the 0.15 M NaCl eluate
did not stain the antigen bands, an indication that the antigens in this fraction had bound the anti-HuAg antibodies.

Two-Dimensional Electrophoresis of the Antigens

Initially, the two antigens were detected on isoelectric
focusing gels; they were subjected to a second-dimensional
analysis on 12% SDS (sodium dodecyl sulfate) gels. Inasmuch
as only two faint spots were visible on the 2-D gel in the
6.3 and 6.1 region, these faint spots were suggested to be the
Coomassie Blue-stained antigens. Their molecular weights compared to known standards were approximately 68,000 and 61,000.
In further studies, these spots corresponded to the ^{125}I-
labeled antigens which were purified from the labeled proteins
in the 0.15 M NaCl eluates.

Affinity Gel Purification of the Antigens

In the previous studies on the nucleolar antigen of
Novikoff hepatoma (Marashi et al., 1979) affinity columns
containing the antibodies were successfully employed with the
Ig fraction of the antibodies to tumor nucleoli. Only small

amounts of the antigens were in the flow-through fraction; the fraction eluted with 3 M NaSCN contained highly purified antigens. To improve further the separation of the ^{125}I-labeled antigens from the nonspecifically binding proteins, the 0.15 M NaCl eluate was bound first to an affinity gel containing preimmune serum. The unbound fraction was then bound to the affinity gel containing the immune serum. Only two major spots were detected on the 2-D gel of the 3 M NaSCN eluate, namely, the 68/6.3 and 61/6.1 antigens.

Separation of the Antigens into Individual Components

To purify these antigens further, preparative isoelectric focusing gels were used. With these, "single spot" antigens were purified. The fact that the two spots of HuAg 68/6.3 remained together suggests they are minor modifications of the same protein. Isolation of the pI 6.3 antigen and the minor pI 6.1 antigen was achieved by preparative isoelectric focusing. Fractions designated A, B, and C were eluted from the gel and analyzed by the 2-D gel electrophoresis. The major pI 6.3 antigen was isolated to electrophoretic homogeneity in fractions A and B. Fraction C contained the minor antigen pI 6.1. The radioactive peak which focused at the acidic end (fractions 1-4) contained free ^{125}I-and nonspecific degraded materials. The recovery of the protein from the isoelectric focusing step was 85%. Without Tween 20 (0.05%) in the isoelectric focusing solutions, the recovery was reduced to 30%.

Amino Acid Composition of the Antigen

Table 3 presents the amino acid composition of the affinity-purified human tumor nucleolar antigen. The amino acids in highest amounts were glycine, 15%; glutamic acid, 11.6%; and serine, 9%. The ratio of the sum of the acidic to the sum of the basic amino acids was 2.

Maps of the Tryptic Digest of the pI 6.3 and 6.1 Antigens

The major and the minor antigen (three proteins) were separately digested with trypsin. The digests were fractionated by electrophoresis and chromatography on cellulose sheets as described. Fourteen ^{125}I-labeled peptides were obtained

Table 3. Amino Acid Composition of Human Tumor Nucleolar
pI 6.3 Antigen

	Mole Percentage
Lysine	5.4
Histidine	2.1
Arginine	3.3
Aspartic Acid	9.3
Threonine	5.7
Serine	9.1
Glutamic Acid	11.6
Proline	5.3
Glycine	15.0
Alanine	8.6
Valine	6.6
Methionine	1.4
Isoleucine	3.6
Leucine	7.3
Tyrosine	2.5
Phenylalanine	3.1
A/B*	1.95

*A/B=Molar ratio of the sum of aspartic acid and
glutamic acid to the sum of lysine, histidine,
and arginine.

from the trypsin digest of the major antigen. A very similar
peptide map was obtained from the pI 6.1 antigen in which
12 peptides (except the peptides 3 and 7 of the pI 6.3 antigen were missing) were identical to those obtained from the
pI 6.3 antigen. These results indicate that the major pI 6.3
antigen and the minor pI 6.1 antigen are related, and that the
pI 6.1 antigen is probably a related product from the pI 6.3
antigen.

Quantitative Analysis of the Nucleolar Antigens

    In further investigations on the nature of these tumor-
associated antigens, a quantitative assay was needed in addition to fluorescence microscopy and immunostaining of polyacrylamide gels. Enzyme immunoassays have recently become a useful tool for both research and clinical serodiagnosis (see
review by O'Beirne and Cooper, 1979).

Nuclei from HeLa or Namalwa cells were prepared by hypotonic shock/detergent lysis as described earlier (Busch et al., 1979; Chan et al., 1980; Davis et al., 1979; Smetana et al., 1979). The cells were swollen on ice in 10 mM Tris-HCl/10 mM NaCl/1.5 mM MgCl$_2$/pH 7.4 (RBS) for 10 min., centrifuged, and resuspended in RSB containing 0.5% Nonidet P-40 (Shell Chemical Co.). The cells were homogenized in a Teflon-glass homogenizer and the crude nuclei collected by centrifugation. The crude nuclei were further purified by homogenization in 0.25 M sucrose/10 mM MgCl$_2$ followed by centrifugation through a cushion of 0.88 M sucrose/0.5 mM MgCl$_2$.

The nuclei from liver or placenta were prepared by passing the tissues through a ginder and washing the ground tissue in 130 mM NaCl/5 mM KCl/0.8 mM MgCl$_2$. The washed tissue was homogenized in 10 volumes (w/v) of 2.2 M sucrose/10 mM MgCl2 with the use of a Teflon-glass homogenizer, filtered through cheesecloth, and centribuged at 17,000 g for 90 min. The pelleted nuclei were then washed once in 0.88 M sucrose/10 mM MgCl$_2$.

Preparation of Nuclear Extracts and Solid-Phase Absorbents

Purified nuclei were homogenized in 75 mM NaCl/25 mM EDTA/1 mM PMSF/pH 8.0 with the use of a Dounce homogenizer. After a 15 min. incubation on ice, the nuclei were centrifuged at 12,000 g for 10 min.; the extraction was repeated, and the two supernatants were combined (NaCl/EDTA extract). The nuclei and resulting chromatin were then extracted three times with 10 mM Tris-HCl/1 mM PMSF/pH 8.0 (Tris extract) for 15, 30, and 15 min. (Kelsey et al., 1981).

Enzyme Immunoassay (EIA)

Nuclear extracts were diluted in PBS, and 50 μl were added to the wells of polystyrene microtiter plates (Dynatech, Alexandria, Va.) and incubated at 4° overnight. The solutions were removed by aspiration, and the remaining protein-binding sites were blocked by the addition of PBS/Tween/BSA for 2 hrs. at room temperature. The plates were washed with PBS/0.5% Tween 20 (PBS/Tween), and 50 μl of IgG solution (40 μg/ml in PBS/Tween/BSA) was added to each well; incubation was done for 2 hrs. at room temperature. This solution was removed by aspiration and the plates were washed with PBS/Tween. Alkaline phosphatase-conjugated goat antirabbit IgG (diluted 1:1000 in

PBS/Tween) was added (50 μl/well), and the plates were incubated for 1 hr. at room temperature. After removal of this
solution, the plates were washed again with PBS/Tween, and
200 μl of 1 mg/ml p-nitrophenylphosphate (Boehringer Mannheim)
in 0.05 M NaCO$_3$/1 mM MgCl$_2$/pH 9.8 were added to each well.
After a 30 min. incubation at room temperature, color development was stopped by the addition of 50 μl of 4 N NaOH. The
color intensity in each well was measured at 405 nm by using
an ELIA reader (Fischer Scientific).

Quantitation of the Antigen

When various amounts of Namalwa Tris extracts were
assayed by EIA, a linear response was obtained over a portion
range of 100 to 500 ng. In each assay the data were fit by
linear regression analysis to a straight line with a correlation coefficient of >0.98. In addition to detecting antigens
in the extract of tumor nuclei, the unabsorbed antibodies also
reacted significantly with extracts from placental nuclei and,
to a lesser extent, with extracts from normal liver nuclei.
Because of the variability of the EIA with <100 ng of protein,
the lines are shown only in the linear range of 100-500 ng.
Increasing the amount of protein beyond 500 ng resulted in a
marked reduction in the slope of the response (Kelsey et al,
1981).

Possible Functions of the Nucleolar Antigen

Although there is no specific information yet on the
precise role of the nucleolar 68/6.3 antigen, its localization
has been analyzed both by light and electron microscopy. The
present evidence shows that it is present in the various soluble and formed elements of the nucleolus and is concentrated
in the "fibrillar" elements (approximately 70% of the antigen
is in RNP particles) of the fundamental nucleolonemal structure of the nucleolus. Its localization is quite similar to
the "silver-staining protein C23" of rat tumor nucleoli,
although evidence has not been obtained that the antigen is
a silver-staining or an NOR protein. However, this is one
possibility that needs further examination.
Another nucleolar element that is distributed in a
similar fashion is the U3 RNP particle. Although the function
of the U3 RNA of the nucleolus is not defined, it may serve
a role similar to the "splicing" function of the U1 RNA and

possible other small nuclear RNAs. The U3 RNA is in a small RNP particle which is intimately associated with the large 60S and 80S subunit elements of the nucleolar preribosomal RNP particles. Inasmuch as the antigen is concentrated in the particulate elements of the nucleolus, one possibility being explored is that it constitutes a structural element of these small particles.

An intriguing recent problem is the finding, by ELISA analysis for the antigen, of a particle which is approximately 100 A in diameter and has a donut- or ring-shaped appearance. This particle was found in large amounts in saline extracts of Namalwa cells and in corresponding extracts of HeLa cells. It represents a possible contaminant of these cells, although it seems unlikely that such a contaminant would exist in two cell lines of such diverse origin (a Burkitt lymphoma and a uterine carcinoma). Whether the antigen is on its surface is not yet clear.

This type of "miniparticle" was found earlier by Narayan and Rounds (1973) who observed them in tissue culture fluids of KB, HeLa, and CMP (a human adenocarcinoma). The particles were reported to contain approximately 5% DNA and 10% RNA. Whether they are U3 RNP particles, unique molecular elements, or some rhino or other virus is not known.

Recently evidence has been adduced that nuclei of human cancer cells contain a novel DNA polymerase, Cm (Lowenstein, et al., 1980), which differs from the normal DNA polymerases of human cells. Inasmuch as the antigen might serve a special role in the replication of rDNA, it is conceivable that it is either the same DNA polymerase or possibly an rDNA polymerase. Studies on this point will be done.

Another possibility that requires study is that the antigen may reflect the presence of an unusual or "fetal" subunit of RNA polymerase I. It is well known that RNA polymerase I is a multisubunit enzyme, and little is known about it in human tissues. The antigen is present in such small amounts that it is likely to serve as an enzymatic function. A major function of the nucleolus is synthesis of rRNA, but one cannot rule out a role in any of the many synthetic, modification, or other functions that characterize the nucleolus. The "particles" may be a multiheaded enzyme.

Is the Antigen an Accelerator or a Gene-Control Element?

The almost ubiquitous presence of the antigen in human cancers certainly requires an explanation both in terms of function and reason for its presence. If it were transmitted epigenetically, as the data on the HeLa cells indicate (Busch et al., 1979), it might serve to "bypass" the usual gene controls on Gl entry. It might also serve to activate genes, either directly or through feedback mechanisms, that were normally not functional or were normally blocked and yet were essential for growth and cell division. It is clear that there is a "circus movement" of sorts in cancer cells which is insensitive to extrinsic or intrinsic controls. Accordingly, some system is activated to produce this antigen which is a common product of the activated genes of cancer cells. This system may be intimately related to the cancer process, or it may be involved in some essential function for the growth of these cells.

ACKNOWLEDGEMENTS

These studies were supported by the Cancer Research Grant CA-10893, awarded by the National Cancer Institute, DHEW, the Human Tumor Nucleolar Antigen Grant, CA-27534, the Farish Fund, the Pauline Sterne Wolff Memorial Foundation, the Michael E. DeBakey Medical Foundation, the Bristol-Myers Fund, the Sally Laird Hitchcock Memorial Fund, the Davidson Fund, and the Taub Fund.

REFERENCES

Busch, H. (1976). A general concept for molecular biology of cancer. Cancer Res. 36:4291

Busch, R.K., and Busch, H. (1977). Antigenic proteins of nucleolar chromatin of Novikoff hepatoma ascites cells. Tumori 63:347

Busch, R.K., Chan, P.K., Isenberg, W., Weigand, R., Russo, J., and Furmanski, P. (1981). Results of a "blind" study on the presence of the human tumor nucleolar antigen in breast carcinomas, benign breast tumors and normal breast tissues. Clinical Immunol. and Immunopath. 18:155

Busch, R.K., Daskal, I., Spohn, W.H., Kellermayer, M. and Busch, H. (1974). Rabbit antibodies to nucleoli of Novikoff hepatoma and normal liver of the rat. Cancer Res. 34:2362

Busch, H., Gyorkey, F., Busch, R.K., Davis, F.M., and Smetana, K. (1979). A nucleolar antigen found in a broad range of human malignant tumor specimens. Cancer Res. 39: 3024

Chan, P.K., Feyerabend, A., Busch, R.K., and Busch, H. (1980). Identification and partial purification of human tumor nucleolar antigen 54/6.3. Cancer Res. 40:3194

Davis, F.M., Busch, R.K., Yeoman, L.C., and Busch, H. (1978). Differences in nucleolar antigens of rat liver and Novikoff hepatoma ascites cells. Cancer Res. 38:1906

Davis, F.M., Gyorkey, F., Busch, R.K., and Busch, H. (1979). Nucleolar antigen found in several human tumors but not in nontumor tissue studies. Proc. Natl. Acad. Sci. USA 76:892

Kelsey, D.E., Busch, R.K., and Busch, H. (1981). An enzyme immunoassay for the detection of human tumor nucleolar antigens. Cancer Letters 12:295

Lowenstein, P.M., Lange, G.W., and Gerard, G.F. (1980). Distribution of DNA polymerase Cm in normal and malignant human tissues. Cancer Res. 40:4398

Marashi, F., Davis, F.M., Busch, R.K., Savage, H.E., and Busch, H. (1979). Purification and partial characterization of nucleolar antigen-1 of the Novikoff hepatoma. Cancer Res. 39:59

Narayan, K.S., and Rounds, D.E. (1973). Minute ring-shaped particles in cultured cells of malignant origin. Nature New Biology 243:146

O'Beirne, A.J., and Cooper, H.R. (1979). Heterogenous enzyme immuno-assay. J. Histochem. Cytochem. 27:1148

Smetana, K., Busch, R.K., Hermansky, F., and Busch, H. (1979). Nucleolar immunofluorescence in human hematological malignancies. Life Sci. 25:227

Yeoman, L.C., Jordan, J.J., Busch, R.K., Taylor, C.W., Savage, H.E., and Busch, H. (1976). A fetal protein in chromatin of Novikoff hepatoma and Walker 256 carcinosarcoma tumors that is absent from normal and regenerating rat liver. Proc. Natl. Acad. Sci. USA 73:3258

13th International Cancer Congress, Part E
Cancer Management, pages 247-258
© 1983 Alan R. Liss, Inc., 150 Fifth Avenue, New York, NY 10011

PROTEIN HORMONE-LIKE MATERIALS FROM NORMAL AND CANCER
CELLS -- "ECTOPIC" HORMONE PRODUCTION

William D. Odell, M.D., Ph.D., Eizo Saito, M.D.

Department of Medicine
University of Utah School of Medicine
Salt Lake City, Utah 84132

ECTOPIC HORMONE PRODUCTION

Cancers produce symptoms in two ways, either directly
by the presence of tumor mass <u>per se</u> or the production of a
humoral substance. The spectrum of humoral substances
produced or humoral syndromes caused by cancers is large
(Table 1).

TABLE 1

HUMORAL SYNDROMES ASSOCIATED WITH CANCER

1. ELABORATION OF HORMONES AND HORMONE PRECURSORS
2. ELABORATION OF ENZYMES (SOMETIMES FETAL ISOENZYMES E.G., ALKALINE,
   PHOSPHATASE, THYMIDINE KINASE)
3. PRODUCTION OF FETAL PROTEINS (E.G., CARCINOEMBRYONIC ANTIGEN, ALPHA
   FETAL PROTEIN)
4. NERVOUS SYSTEM EFFECTS:
   A) NEURONAL DEGENERATION OF DEMYELINATION (E.G., CORTICAL CEREBELLAR
      DEGENERATION, MULTIFOCAL LEUKOENCEPHALOPATHY, BULBAR ENCEPHALITIC
      PERIPHERAL NEUROPATHIES)
   B) MYOPATHIES OR MYOSITIS
   C) MYESTHENIC OR MYASTHENIC GRAVIS SYNDROMES
5. DERMATOLOGIC SYNDROMES (E.G., ACANTHOSIS NIGRICANS, DERMATOMYOSITIS,
   PACHYDERMIA)
6. DIGITAL CLUBBING AND ARTHROPATHIES
7. HEMATOLOGIC SYNDROMES (E.G., APLASTIC ANEMIA, THROMBOPHLEBITIS)
8. FEVER

Perhaps the best understood of these humoral syndromes
are the endocrine syndromes--syndromes of <u>Ectopic Hormone
Production</u>. Table 2 lists the hormones and related compounds reported to be produced by cancers.

TABLE 2

HORMONES REPORTED TO BE SECRETED BY CANCERS

PROACTH AND ACTH	CHORIONIC GONADOTROPIN (CG)
LIPOTROPIN	ALPHA PEPTIDE CHAIN OF CG
VASOPRESSIN	BETA PEPTIDE CHAIN OF CG
SOMATOMEDINS	HYPOGLYCEMIC PRODUCING FACTORS
PARATHYROID HORMONE	OSTEOCLAST ACTIVATING FACTOR
PROSTAGLANDINS	ERYTHROPOIETIN
GASTRIN	HYPOPHOSPHATEMIA PRODUCING FACTOR
GROWTH HORMONE	CHORIONIC SOMATOTROPIN
PROLACTIN	GROWTH HORMONE RELEASING HORMONE
CALCITONIN	SECRETIN
GLUCAGON	CORTICOTROPIN RELEASING HORMONE
NEUROPHYSINS	SOMATOSTATIN

Excepting the prostaglandins, the ectopic hormonal syndromes are caused by the tumor elaboration of bioactive proteins or peptides. Studies from our laboratories over the past five years include both prospective clinical studies (Odell et al. 1977, 1979; Wolfsen, Odell 1979; Schwartz et al. 1979) and more basic biochemical or endocrine characterization of such substances (Yoshimoto et al. 1977, 1979; Saito, Odell 1982; Odell, Evans 1980; Kyle et al. 1981).

We limit the data presented herein to discussion of the ectopic production of ACTH, lipotropin, and hCG. For such studies, it is essential to eliminate the possibility of assay artifacts and ensure that none exist. Methods used to extract tissues are of critical importance. We have found that glacial acetic acid extraction followed by lyophilization, then redissolving in assay buffer with careful final control of pH, osmolality, and protein content, results in artifact-free materials. To exemplify the necessity of such controls, Figure 1 shows the damage produced on ACTH by extracts prepared in several different ways. Only glacial acetic acid was satisfactory. Under these extract conditions, protein content was very low and the addition of several enzyme inhibitors did not change the results. Furthermore, incubation of labeled ACTH, βMSH, or hCG with glacial acetic acid extracts under assay conditions did not alter immunoactivity as assessed by excess antibody.

STUDIES OF ACTH

About 80% of patients with ectopic ACTH syndrome have small cell or oat cell carcinomas of the lung, thymomas, or pancreatic neoplasms (Odell 1981). However, taking oat cell

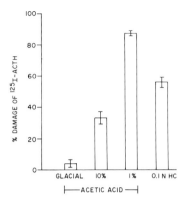

Fig. 1. Percent immunological damage to ^{125}I-ACTH produced by tissue extracts during 48 hr. incubation. Only glacial acetic acid extraction produced an extract that did not degrade label. From Saito and Odell, 1982.

carcinoma as a model, only 2.8% of patients with oat cell carcinoma have elevated plasma cortisol that fails to suppress with dexamethasone (Kato et al. 1969). Thus, some factor other than just the presence of oat cell carcinoma determines whether ectopic ACTH syndrome is present. Studies from our laboratory (Odell et al. 1977; Wolfsen, Odell 1979) and of Gewirtz and Yalow (1974) have shown that extracts of all carcinomas, regardless of histologic type, contain an ACTH-like material by radioimmunoassay (Table 3).

TABLE 3

IMMUNOACTIVE ACTH CONTENT - PG/GM WET WEIGHT

CARCINOMAS	22,359 ± 163	(N = 68)
NORMAL TISSUES	<1000	(N = 100)

The amounts extractable from carcinomas greatly exceed the amounts in normal tissues. Our studies also demonstrate that this material has a larger MW than standard ACTH and is not reactive in a radioreceptor assay, thus possessing little or no bioactivity.

We performed prospective clinical studies (Odell et al. 1977; Wolfsen, Odell 1979) of 100 consecutive patients admitted to the hospital with coin lesion or another abnormality on a chest X-ray. Twenty-four of the patients were found to have a benign disease; all had normal immunoactive ACTH. Seventy-four of the patients were found to have lung cancer; histological types included oat, squamous, alveolar, and undifferentiated cell types. Fifty-three (74%) of these patients with lung cancer had elevated plasma immunoactive ACTH. Figure 2 shows the concentration of immunoactive ACTH plotted against receptor assay ACTH in such plasma samples. This immunoactive ACTH-like material in the plasma of such cancer patients without clinically detectable ectopic ACTH syndrome also had a MW of over 20,000, greater than the 4500 standard bioactive ACTH, and showed little or no activity in the radioreceptor assay. In contrast, plasma from patients with clinically evident ectopic ACTH syndrome contained high levels of ACTH in the radioreceptor assay (indicating bio-activity) as well as in vivo bioassay activity.

CANCER PLASMA

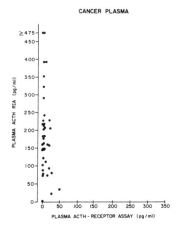

Fig. 2. Plasma ACTH meas-ured by RIA and radiorecep-tor assay in patients with cancer but no clinical dis-cernible ectopic ACTH syn-drome. 100 pg/ml is upper limits of normal in both assays. From Odell et al., 1977.

In earlier studies, the sensitivity of our ACTH radio-immunoassay was limited, permitting us to state only that ACTH was not detectable (<1000 pg/gm) in tissues of patients dying without cancer. However, in 1982, Saito and Odell have been able to greatly improve assay sensitivity, permit-ting the detection of as little as 5-10 pg of ACTH. Using this assay, extraction of normal (nonpituitary) tissues obtained from rats revealed that virtually all normal rat tissues contain an immunoactive ACTH. The MW of this mate-rial was 26,000 as measured by gel chromatography. This large MW ACTH by treatment is converted to 4500 MW ACTH by treatment with trypsin. Figures 3-6 illustrate these data.

Most recently, we have performed studies on human tis-sues obtained soon after traumatic death. The findings are similar to those shown for the rat (Saito, Odell 1982). Studies by Eipper and Mains (1980) of the biosynthesis of

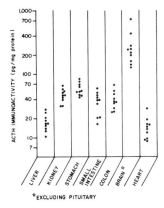

Fig. 3. ACTH content in extracts of normal rat tissues. From Saito and Odell, 1982.

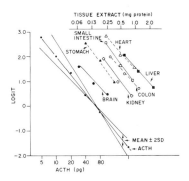

Fig. 4. Dose response lines of rat tissue ACTH-like material. From Saito and Odell, 1982.

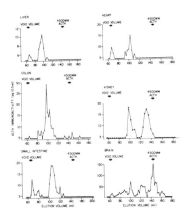

Fig. 5. Sephadex chromatography of rat tissue extracts Except for brain, no 4500 MW ACTH was found. The major peak has a MW of 26,000, except for brain. From Saito and Odell, 1982.

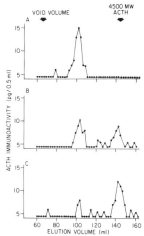

Fig. 6. Trypsin treatment tissue ACTH: A=control, B=3 min incubation, C=15 min incubation. The 26,000 MW is converted to 4500 MW ACTH. From Saito and Odell, 1982.

ACTH using AT-20 mouse pituitary tumor cells and primary pituitary cell cultures show that an ACTH-lipotropin common precursor exists as a molecular weight of 30,000. This MW is similar to the 26,000 of the big MW ACTH precursor we

find in normal rat tissues and further suggests that this
material is a precursor of ACTH.

LIPOTROPIN STUDIES

Lipotropin is a 91 amino acid protein that contains the
entire amino acid sequence of beta melanocyte stimulating
hormone (βMSH). We (Bachelot et al. 1977) and Bloomfield et
al. (1974) have shown that βMSH per se is not present in the
human pituitary nor is it normally secreted; it is an arti-
fact of the purification process originally used to prepare
it. Thus, lipotropin or the larger precursors to lipotropin
are probably the substances measured in radioimmunoassays
using antisera directed against synthetic βMSH. Using such
assays, we (Saito, Odell 1982) have shown that extracts of
all rat tissues, in addition to ACTH, contain an immunoactive βMSH-like material that coelutes with the 26,000 MW
precursor ACTH during gel chromatography (Figure 7).

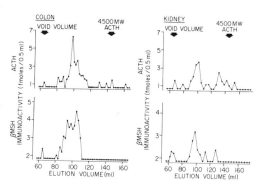

Fig. 7. G-75 Sephadex
chromatography of rat
colon and kidney ex-
tracts. MSH and ACTH
immunoactivities were
quantified; MW of both
activities = 26,000.
From Saito and Odell,
1982.

Antibodies against 4500 MW ACTH (anti-ACTH) were conjugated to Sepharose and used to prepare immunoabsorption columns. Such columns did not bind synthetic βMSH, [96.5 ±
6.0% (±SEM) recovered], but did bind 4500 MW ACTH (14.8 ±
3.5% recovered in eluate or 85.2 ± 3.5% bound to column).
However, such columns removed 85% of both ACTH and βMSH
activity in rat tissue extracts. The immunoabsorption and
gel chromatography studies suggest that both ACTH and MSH
immunoactivities reside on the same 26,000 MW molecule.

Based on these studies and the previously cited ACTH
biosynthetic data of Eipper and Mains (1980), this tissue
ACTH appears to be a ProACTH. In further support of this

hypothesis, we have shown that rat tissue ACTH-like material binds to concanavalin A and hence contains carbohydrate moieties similar to ProACTH (Saito, Odell 1982) (Figure 8).

Fig. 8. Concanavalin column studies of rat small intestine (A), kidney (B), and colon (C) ACTH-like material. Over 90% activity binds to Con A and is eluted with alpha methyl glucopyranoside. (D) (controls) Standard ACTH does not bind to Con A; ^{125}I-TSH added with extract binds to Con A. From Saito and Odell, 1982.

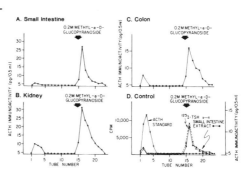

Identical studies have been completed on extracts of human tissues with similar results, except the ProACTH MW is slightly larger. We conclude: (1) A 26,00 to 30,000 MW precursor form of ACTH-lipotropin is extractable from all normal rat and human tissues. This material is converted to 4500 MW ACTH by incubation with trypsin and is probably an ACTH precursor. (2) Such a ProACTH is extractable in larger quantities from carcinomas, regardless of histological type. (3) The blood of patients with carcinomas not producing a clinical ectopic ACTH syndrome contains increased quantities of such a ProACTH material. It is immunoactive but has little biological activity. (4) The blood of patients with clinically evident ectopic ACTH syndromes contains increased quantities of smaller MW bioactive ACTH.

STUDIES OF HUMAN CHORIONIC GONADOTROPIN (hCG)

When the beta hCG radioimmunoassay was developed, increasing the ability to distinguish hCG from the biochemically related luteinizing hormone (LH), Braunstein et al. (1973) found that serum from 6-15% of patients with a variety of carcinomas had elevated blood hCG concentrations. We (Odell et al. 1977; Yoshimoto et al. 1977, 1979) reported that extracts of all carcinomas contained detectable hCG as determined in both beta hCG immunoassay and radioreceptor assay. We were also able to show that extracts of all normal human tissues contained hCG. The quantities of hCG in extracts of about 2/3 of the carcinomas were similar to those in normal tissues; the concentrations in about 1/3 were elevated above normal tissues. In contrast to placental hCG, normal tissue hCG showed little or no binding to concanavalin A, a plant lectin that binds certain carbohydrates. When we performed Con A studies on carcinoma extracts, in contrast to either normal tissue or placenta, BINDING WAS VARIABLE, ranging from as low as normal tissues to as high as normal placental tissues (Table 4).

TABLE 4

HCG BINDING TO CONCANAVALIN A

		% BOUND ± SEM	RANGE
NORMAL TISSUE	(10)	6.1 ± 1.6	(0.0 - 14.6)
CANCER TISSUE	(9)	31.2 ± 9.1	(4.0 - 86.0)
PLACENTA	(4)	92.5 ± 0.9	(90.1 - 94.0)
PREGNANT SERUM	(3)	100.0	
CANCER SERUM	(8)	54.7 ± 11.9	(3.1 - 92.5)

In recent studies, we partially purified human liver hCG and estimated MW using gel chromatography (Odell, Evans 1980). Liver hCG reacts in the entirely specific "tail" hCG assay, which uses antibodies directed against the beta chain tail region of hCG, a sequence of amino acids not present on LH (Figure 9). In the "tail" assay, liver hCG-like material did not "dose out" parallel to standard or placental hCG, indicating structural differences (Figure 10). It is uncertain whether differences only in carbohydrate composition cause this. Birkin et al. (1980) have shown that asialo or carbohydrate-free synthetic tail peptides react differently with tail antisera than when carbohydrate is present. The MW of normal liver hCG-like material was 27,000, smaller than estimates of carbohydrate-free hCG. Previously, Tsuruhara (1972) had shown that carbohydrate-free hCG possessed little in vivo biological activity. In vivo, the metabolic clearance rate increased, reducing the half time of disappearance to less than one minute.

In summary of the data on hCG, we conclude: (1) Extracts of all normal human tissues and carcinomas contain an hCG-like material. (2) This normal tissue hCG-like material is active in the entirely specific tail hCG assay, radioreceptor assays, and in vitro bioassays. (3) In contrast to placental hCG (93% Con A binding), normal tissue hCG-like material has little Con A binding (6%); the Con A binding of

carcinoma hCG varies (3-93%). (4) Those carcinomas associated with detectable blood hCG either glycosylate this hCG-
like material, prolonging its survival in blood, produce
much greater quantities, or both.

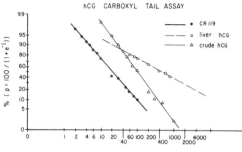

Fig. 9. Dose response
of hepatic CG in the
carboxyl tail assay of
hCG. From Odell and
Evans, 1982.

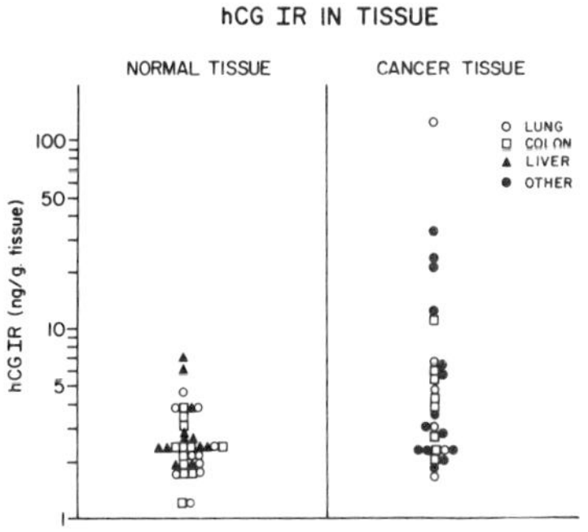

hCG IR IN TISSUE

Fig. 10. Content of CG in
human tissue extracts. From
Odell et al. 1977.

OTHER STUDIES

In addition to studies cited from our laboratories,
several protein hormone-like materials have been described
as being produced by nonendocrine tissue of mammals and some
by nonmammalian species. Rosenzweig et al. (1980) showed
that insulin was extractable from essentially all tissues of
humans and rats, as well as cultured lymphocytes and fibroblasts. LeRoith et al. (1981) showed that an insulin-like
material was present in nonvertebrates such as insects,
annelids, and bacteria. In 1974 Livingston showed that an
hCG material was produced by some bacteria; Acevedo et al.
(1978) confirmed these findings. We showed in 1980 that an
hCG material was extractable from tissues of codfish, chick-

ens, rats, rabbits, dogs, and cows (Yoshimoto et al. 1980).

These data have led us, as well as Roth et al. (Kolata 1982; Yoshimoto et al. 1980; Odell, Wolfsen 1980), to speculate that protein hormone-like materials are ubiquitous in nature and appear to precede vertebrate development in evolution. Pertinent to cancer, we hypothesize that: (1) All normal human tissues synthesize and secrete small amounts of protein hormone-like materials. Most are not biologically active or are weakly bioactive. (2) Cancers synthesize and secrete these same protein hormone-like materials, often in increased quantities. (3) Selected cancers metabolize these protein hormone-like materials to potent biologically active forms, causing a so-called ectopic hormone syndrome. This metabolic property correlates with the histological type of neoplasm. (4) "Ectopic" hormone syndromes are not ectopic.

REFERENCES

Acevedo HF, Slifkin M, Pouchet GR, Pardo M (1978). Immunohistological localization of a choriogonadotropin-like protein in bacteria from cancer patients. Cancer 41:1217.

Bachelot I, Wolfsen AR, Odell WD (1977). Pituitary and plasma lipotropins: Demonstration of the artifactual nature of βMSH. J Clin Endocrinol Metab 44:939.

Birken S, Canfield R, Laver R, Agosto G, Gobel M (1980). Immunochemical determinants unique to human chorionic gonadotropin: Importance of sialic acid for antisera generated to the human chronic gonodotropin β-subunit COOH-terminal peptide. Endocrinology 106:1659.

Bloomfield, GA, Holdaway IM, Corrin B, et al. (1977). Lung tumors and ACTH production. Clin Endocrinol 6:95.

Braunstein GD, Vaitukaitis JL, Carbone PP, Ross GT (1973). Ectopic production of human chorionic gonadotropin by neoplasms. Ann Int Med 78:39.

Eipper BA, Mains RE (1980). Structure and biosynthesis of pro-adrenocorticotropin/endorphin and related peptides. Endocrinol Review 1:1.

Gewirtz G, Yalow RS (1974). Ectopic ACTH production in carcinoma of the lung. J Clin Invest 53:1022.

Kato Y, Ferguson TB, Bennett DE, Burford TH (1969). Oat cell carcinoma of the lung. A review of 138 cases. Cancer 23:517.

Kolata G (1982). New theory of hormones proposed. Science 215:1383.

Kyle CV, Evans MC, Odell WD (1981). Growth hormone-like material in normal human tissues. J Clin Endocrinol Metab 53:1138.

LeRoith D, Lesniak MA, Roth J (1981). Insulin in insects and annelids. Diabetes 1:70.

LeRoith D, Shiloack J, Roth J, Lesniak MA (1981). Insulin on a closely related molecule is native to escherichia coli. J Biol Chem 10:256.

Livingston VW (1974). Some cultural, immunological, and biochemical properties of Progenitor cryptocides. Trans NY Acad Sci 36:569.

Odell WD (1981). Humoral manifestations of cancer. In Williams RH (ed): "Textbook of Endocrinology," Philadelphia: W. B. Saunders, p. 1228.

Odell WD, Evans MC (1980). Characterization of hepatic chorionic gonadotropin-like material. Fertil Steril 34:300 (abst).

Odell WD, Wolfsen AR (1980). Hormones from tumors: Are they ubiquitous? Am J Med 68:317.

Odell WD, Wolfsen AR, Bachelot I, Hirose FM (1979). Ectopic production of lipotropin by cancer. Am J Med 66:631.

Odell WD, Wolfsen A, Yoshimoto Y, Weitzman R, Fisher D, Hirose F (1977). Ectopic peptide synthesis. A universal concomitant of neoplasia. Trans Assoc Amer Phys 90:204.

Rosenzweig JL, Havrankova J, Lesniak MA, Brownstein M, Roth J (1980). Insulin is ubiquitous in extrapancreatic tissues of rats and humans. Proc Natl Acad Sci USA 77:572.

Saito E, Odell WD (1982). Universal presence of large molecular weight adrenocorticotropic hormone-like substances in normal rat extrapituitary tissues. Submitted.

Saito E, Odell WD (1982). Universal presence of large molecular weight adrenocorticotropic hormone-like substances in normal human extrapituitary tissues. Submitted.

Saito E, Odell WD (1982). ACTH-LPH common precursor-like material in normal rat extrapituitary tissues. Submitted.

Schwartz KE, Wolfsen AR, Forster B, Odell WD (1979). Calcitonin in nonthyroidal cancer. J Clin Endocrinol Metab 49:438.

Tsuruhara T, Dufau ML, Hickman J, et al. (1972). Biological properties of hCG after removal of terminal sialic acid and galactose residues. Endocrinol 91:296.

Yoshimoto Y, Odell WD, Fugita T (1980). Human chorionic gonadotropin-like substance in non-mammalian vertebrates and mammalians other than humans. Program of 6th International Congress of Endocrinology (Abstract).

Yoshimoto Y, Wolfsen A, Hirose F, Odell WD (1979). Human chorionic gonadotropin-like material: Presence in normal human tissue. Am J Obstet Gynecol 134:729.

Yoshimoto Y, Wolfsen A, Odell WD (1977). Human chorionic gonadotropin-like substance in nonendocrine tissues of normal subjects. Science 197:575.

Yoshimoto Y, Wolfsen AR, Odell WD (1979). Glycosylation: A variable in hCG production by cancers. Am J Med 67:414.

Wolfsen AR, Odell WD (1979). ProACTH: Use for early detection of lung cancer. Am J Med 66:765.

CONGRESS SYMPOSIA

BIOLOGICAL RESPONSE MODIFIERS Yamamura, Y.,
Japan, Chairman; Hersh, E., USA, Co-Chairman;
Opera House

Potential Use of Muramyl Peptides in Cancer
Therapy. *Chedid, L. A., Paris, France.

Chemically Defined Immunotherapeutic Agents.
*Hadden, J. W., Tampa, FL USA.

Interferons: In Pursuit of the Promise.
*Borden, E. C., Madison, WI USA.

Prospective Uses of Thymic Hormones in Cancer.
*Trainin, N., Handzel, Z. T. and Zaizov, R.,
Rehovot, Israel.

Modification of Tumor Cell Antigen.
*Kobayashi, H., Sapporo, Japan.

Current Clinical Status of Interferon and
Management of Cancer In Man. *Horoszewicz, J. S.
and Mirand, E. A., Buffalo, NY USA.

The Stability of Human Fibroblast Interferon
(HuIFN-β). *Leong, S. S., Horoszewicz, J. S. and
Mirand, E. A., Buffalo, NY USA.

Please note: Papers that are listed as "By Title
Only" were presented at the 13th International
Cancer Congress, but are not included in these
volumes.

13th International Cancer Congress, Part E
Cancer Management, pages 261–271
© 1983 Alan R. Liss, Inc., 150 Fifth Avenue, New York, NY 10011

POTENTIAL USE OF MURAMYL PEPTIDES IN CANCER THERAPY

Louis A. Chedid

Experimental Immunotherapy, Institut Pasteur,

Paris, France.

Microbial products represent some of the most potent exogenous activators of the immune systems. They have been repeatedly used as immunoregulating agents in view of enhancing non specific immunity. They have also been used in association with tumor antigens to enhance specific immuni ty. However the following less ambitious strategies should be considered for the use of such biological response modifiers (BRM) in tumor immunology:

1. Enhancement of non specific immunity against pathogens liable to produce intercurrent infections by administering them alone or associated to antibiotics.

2. Specific immunization against opportunistic organisms or against pathogens which seem to be involved with the etiology of certain tumors.

3. Specific immunization against endogenous products such as hormones which may prove to be an additional useful therapeutic approach for certain hormone-dependent cancers.

The use of whole microorganisms endowed with immuno-modulating properties, such as BCG or *C.parvum*, can elicit a variety of side effects such as granuloma formation, lymphoid hyperplasia, adjuvant arthritis, sensitization to bacterial antigens and potentiation of toxic effects of endotoxins (Chedid *et al.* 1978). Isolation and characterization of the minimal bacterial cell wall structure necessary for biological activity but which is devoid of most of these undesirable effects has therefore represented a major advance in the field of biological adjuvants deriving from

bacteria (Johnson *et al.* 1978). The smallest biological active cell wall moiety has been shown to be a simple glycopeptide containing a bacterial specific carbohydrate and
two amino-acids (Ellouz *et al.* 1974). This glycopeptide
(Muramyl Dipeptide or MDP) has been synthesized and to date
several hundred analogs have been prepared from which a
large number have been tested in various *in vivo* and *in
vitro* immunological systems (Dukor *et al.* 1979; Lederer
1980; Lefrancier, Lederer 1981).

   In several experimental models MDP derivatives, alone
or associated with trehalose diesters, have been shown to
enhance non specific immunity to tumors. Since many of
these aspects have been reviewed recently (Lederer, Chedid
1981; Chedid, Morin 1982) we will summarize briefly the
results concerning most of the above mentioned topics and
will deal in more detail with their potential use as adjuvants in relation to immunization against pathogens or
against hormones.

ENHANCEMENT OF NON SPECIFIC TUMOR IMMUNITY

   In most cases, muramyl peptides have been used in
water and mineral oil emulsions such as Freund's complete
adjuvant (FCA), or with more metabolisable oils such as
squalane. Under such conditions and in combination with
trehalose dimycolate (TDM), a glycolipid also derived from
mycobacterial cell wall, MDP and several analogs have been
shown to inhibit the growth of hepatocarcinoma intradermally transplanted in guinea pigs (McLaughlin *et al.* 1980;
Yarkoni *et al.* 1981). Mineral oil vehicles can be avoided
however, by the use of various procedures. Inclusion of
MDP within liposomes resulted in non specific tumor activity as has been reported by Fidler *et al.* (1981) using a
metastatic murine melanoma model. In addition Sone and
Fidler (1981) have observed that a combination of some
threshhold amounts of MDP and macrophage activating factor
(MAF) can act synergistically inducing alveolar macrophages
to become tumoricidal for syngeneic, allogeneic and xenogeneic target cells. Specific immunization against tumor
cells using lipophilic MDP analogs such as 6-0-acyl esters
and quinonyl has also been studied (Yamamura *et al.* 1977;
Azuma *et al.* 1979). These compounds have been shown to be
highly effective even when administered in an aqueous
medium and should be considered as very promising agents.

Inhibitory activity of muramyl dipeptides on the growth of murine lymphoid tumors has recently been observed *in vivo* and also studied *in vitro* (Phillips *et al.* 1982; Phillips *et al.*, submitted). The ability of MDP and its adjuvant-inactive stereoisomer MDP(D-D) to inhibit the growth of a number of murine ascitic cell lines of both T- and B-lymphocyte lineage was evaluated *in vivo*. The ascitic growth of the cell line expressing the LYT-1^+2^- "helper" phenotype was not inhibited by MDP or MDP(D-D) in the dose range studied (0.06 to 5 mg/kg/day via the ip route). The growth of two out of three cell lines expressing the LYT-1^-2^+ "cytotoxic/suppressor" phenotype and both cell lines expressing the LYT-1^+2^+ "precursor" phenotype was inhibited by MDP whereas MDP(D-D) had no effect. Control groups treated with cyclophosphamide in the dose range 1.25 to 20 mg/kg/day showed a significant inhibition of growth of all the thymoma cell lines. In contrast to the results obtained with the thymoma cell lines, MDP had no significant effect on the growth of the B-cell or plasmacytoma cell lines. However, significant inhibition of the growth of these cell lines was observed with MDP(D-D).

In vitro, the following results were found: MDP inhibited the growth of all three thymoma cell lines studied expressing different LYT phenotypes. MDP(D-D) inhibited the two cell lines expressing LYT-1^+2^- or LYT-1^+2^+ phenotypes, but not the third cell line which expressed the LYT-1^-2^+ phenotype. The ability of MDP or MDP(D-D) to inhibit thymoma growth was lost when the ascitic cell populations were depleted of macrophages. MDP could be replaced by a supernatant derived from an ascitic LYT-1^+2^- cell population exposed to MDP. To be active this supernatant also required the presence of macrophages. The inhibition by MDP of the growth of the LYT-1^-2^+ cell line was prostaglandin synthetase dependent: the presence of indomethacin antagonized the inhibitory activity of MDP. The inhibition by MDP of the LYT-1^+2^- cell line was partially antagonized by indomethacin and no antagonism was observed with the LYT-1^+2^+ cell line.

A number of interesting observation s have arisen from this study. Firstly, where a tumor cell line is responsive to treatment with MDP or MDP(D-D), the muramyl dipeptide is some 7 to 10-fold more effective than cyclophosphamide in inhibiting its growth. Secondly, the ability of MDP to inhibit the growth of the thymoma cell lines does not appear to correlate with the LYT-phenotype expressed by these cells but rather with their low degree of maturity. Thirdly, the results would suggest that specific inhibition of lymphoma growth relative to the lineage of the tumor cell (T- or B-lymphocyte) may be possible using different muramyl dipeptides, offering the potential of selective chemotherapy. Whilst it is difficult to extrapolate to other tumor systems, such selectivity and efficacy may have advantages over the use of established chemotherapeutic agents in the treatment of lymphoid tumors. Whilst the mechanisms by which the muramyl dipeptides exert their anti-tumor effect is not known, preliminary studies have indicated that the resident macrophage population within the ascites plays a central role in the expression of activity.

ENHANCEMENT OF SPECIFIC TUMOR IMMUNITY

For the time being, enhancement has been obtained by administering with BCG or FCA irradiated tumor cells or immunostimulants intralesionally. This approach may become extremely important when neo-antigens will be identified and both immunogenic preparations and acceptable adjuvants may become available. The following possibilities seem to be more easily attainable.

ENHANCEMENT OF NON SPECIFIC IMMUNITY TO INTERCURRENT INFECTIONS

The protective capacity of MDP was first demonstrated in normal adult mice infected with *Klebsiella pneumoniae* (Chedid *et al*. 1977). Interestingly, a non specific enhancement of resistance could be observed even when MDP was administered orally. Moreover, MDP and some of its derivatives have been shown to exert a protective effect in neonate mice challenged with antibiotic-resistant strains (Parant *et al*. 1978). MDP was found capable of augmenting non specific resistance to a variety of organisms commonly found in immunocompromised hosts. Such effects have also been observed in animal models of immunosuppression which are relevant to certain clinical situations. In addition both in normal and in immunocompromised infected mice a synergetic effect between muramyl peptide and antibiotics has been demonstrated (Dietrich *et al*. 1980; Fraser-Smith *et al*. 1981).

SPECIFIC IMMUNIZATION AGAINST PATHOGENS

Adjuvant properties of MDP has been demonstrated with
several vaccines. The incidence of pseudomonas infections
in patients accounts for about 50% of all bacterial septi-
cemia. A large number of such patients still die in spite
of improved anti-infectious management and with *P.aeruginosa*
pneumonia, fatality may be as high as 80% (Reynolds *et al.*
1975). MDP has been shown to be a suitable adjuvant when
associated with *P.aeruginosa* toxoid which is weakly immunogenic when injected alone (Cryz *et al.* 1981). Since an
adjuvant active analog has been shown to be well tolerated
in clinical trials, such an agent may be of use for a
future pseudomonas vaccine.

Specific immunization against organisms which seem to
be etiologically involved with the appearance of tumors such
as hepatitis B virus may lead to the first anti-cancer
vaccine, a number of epidemiological studies have demonstrated a striking correlation between the occurrence of primary hepatocellular carcinoma (PHC) and the presence of hyper-
endemic hepatitis B virus (HBV). Uncommon in Europe and the
USA (1.3/100,000), this cancer has a high incidence in
Tropical Africa and the Far East (up to 150/100,000). In
all population samples, the incidence of HBV infection is
considerably higher in PHC patients (Maupas, Melnick 1981).
It is therefore reasonable to suppose that active immunization in early life against HBV infection would allow some
control of PHC in such high risk populations. Because of the
cost and scarcity of the HBV surface antigen (HBS), a reduction in the amount of material required for immunization by
association with a potent adjuvant would be attractive.
Better still would be to obtain synthetic antigens administered with a synthetic adjuvant. The first example of a
successful immunization against a bacterial infection
(diphtheria) using an entirely synthetic vaccine has recently been reported (Audibert *et al.* 1981). Several other
synthetic bacterial or viral antigens have been described
including HBsAg peptides (Lerner *et al.* 1981; Dreesman *et
al.* 1982; Prince *et al.* 1982). These antigens are weakly
immunogenic, as could be expected, and have been administered usually with FCA, which is not clinically acceptable.
However, Dreesman *et al.* (1982) were able to immunize mice
with synthetic HBsAg peptides in the presence of MDP.

SPECIFIC IMMUNIZATION AGAINST ENDOGENOUS PRODUCTS SUCH AS
HORMONES

Peptidic and even synthetic hormones such as the terminal fragment of human β-chorio-gonadotropin (β-HCG) or the
hypothalamic factor LH-RH have been used as immunogens in
view of either controlling fertility (Stevens 1975; Ramakrishnan *et al*. 1979) or of increasing body weight of cattle
by immunological castration (Robertson *et al*. 1979). Similar
vaccines may, however, have a potential in cancer therapy.

Effect of Antibodies to Choriogonadotropin (CG) in Neoplasias

Such antibodies could be of use not only as a diagnostic tool, but also as a therapeutic agent in cancers associated with an excess of β-HCG production such as chorio-
epitheliomas. Moreover there is increasing evidence that
CG-like polypeptides are synthesized by a variety of non-
trophoblastic malignant neoplasms, when more sensitive and
more specific methods of detection are used. Kellen *et al*.
(1982) have recently shown that preimmunization of rats with
a conjugate of the β-HCG subunit and tetanus toxoid retarded
significantly the growth of a mammary adenocarcinoma or of
an implanted hepatoma. Antibodies to human β-HCG have also
been obtained with MDP associated to a synthetic β-HCG
fragment (Stevens *et al*. 1981). Whether a natural or a
synthetic antigen is used it can be reasonable assumed that
the addition of an adjuvant to these weak immunogens will
be desirable.

Immunization against LH-RH

Chronic administration of two potent LH-RH antagonists
was shown to inhibit significantly the growth of two chemically induced rat prostate tumors (Redding *et al*. 1982).
These results suggest the possibility of new types of therapy for prostate carcinoma and other endocrine dependent
neoplasias. Since the elevated levels of anti-LH-RH antibodies correlated reciprocally with a decrease in the level
of circulating LH, the effect observed is likely to be due,
at least in part, to an inhibition of pituitary LH-release,
Recently, studies in mice have shown that the coupling of
MDP-lysine derivative with LH-RH produced high antibody

titers and immunological castration of male mice, as
judged by histological changes occurring in testicular inter-
stitial cells and seminiferous tubules, and by the disappearance of germ cells (Carelli *et al*. 1982). These results
were observed even though the conjugate was administered in
an aqueous medium. Moreover, coupling of the muramyl dipeptide derivative resulted in a loss of its pyrogenic activity
and did not elicit MDP antibodies. In those malignancies
where an excess of hormonal production, dependent on an
hypersecretion of hypothalamic LH-RH, is thought to be involved, synthetic hormone vaccines could thus be of use in
performing a selective immunological hypophysectomy rather
than a total one through surgery or irradiation.

CONCLUSION

The possible mechanisms of action of MDP have been
studied in a large variety of *in vitro* systems. Certain
derivatives of muramyl peptides have been shown to be potent and very selective macrophage activators (For an extensive review see Leclerc and Chedid 1982). For instance,
certain analogs were found devoid of pyrogenicity although
they had retained the adjuvant and stimulating activities of
the original molecule. One of these non pyrogenic derivatives, N-acetyl-muramyl-L-alanyl-D-glutamine-α-butyl ester
also called Murabutide (Chedid *et al*. 1982), has been shown
to produce lymphocyte activating factor (LAF) without leukocytic pyrogens (LP) (Damais *et al*. 1982). Murabutide was
also found to differ from MDP since it did not induce leukopenia, or enhance the production of serum amyloid. Also,
contrarily to MDP, it was devoid of toxic synergism with
gram negative lipopolysaccharides. The retention of the biological properties without associated pyrogenic activity in
some muramyl peptides, notably Murabutide, has opened up the
possibility of their therapeutic use in man (Oberling *et al*.
1981). Besides macrophage activation, it seems that muramyl
peptide can stimulate cytotoxic effects observed in systems
which are thought to be involved in host anti-tumor defenses
such as antibody-dependent cell mediated cytotoxicity,
T cell-dependent cytotoxicity or natural killer activity in
spleen cells (See Leclerc and Chedid 1982).

In conclusion, the multi-faceted activity of structurally well-defined agents such as muramyl peptides, coupled
with the absence of toxic side-effects observed with the use

of whole microorganisms, offers the potential for their employment in a controlled, safe and specific manner. Their
anti-tumor activity, both specific and non specific anti-
infectious and immunomodulatory properties, present a number
of possibilities for the treatment and in certain cases for
the prevention of cancer.

REFERENCES

Audibert F, Jolivet M, Chedid L, Alouf JE, Boquet P,
    Rivaille P, Siffert O (1981). Active antitoxic immuniza-
    tion by a diphtheria toxin synthetic oligopeptide. Nature
    289:593.
Azuma I, Yamawaki M, Uemiya M, Saiki I, Tanio Y, Kobayashi S,
    Fukida T, Imada I, Yamamura Y (1979). Adjuvant and anti-
    tumor activities of quinonyl-N-acetylmuramyl dipeptides.
    Gann 70:847.
Carelli C, Audibert F, Chedid L, Gaillard J (1982). Immuno-
    logical castration of male mice by a totally synthetic
    vaccine (LH-RH conjugated to MDP) administered in saline.
    Proc Natl Acad Sci USA, in press.
Chedid L, Parant M, Parant F, Lefrancier P, Choay J,
    Lederer E (1977). Enhancement of nonspecific immunity to
    Klebsiella pneumoniae infection by a synthetic immunoadju-
    vant (N-acetyl-muramyl-L-alanyl-D-isoglutamine) and seve-
    ral analogs. Proc Natl Acad Sci USA 74:2089.
Chedid L,Audibert F, Johnson AG (1978). Biological activi-
    ties of muramyl dipeptide, a synthetic glycopeptide ana-
    logous to bacterial immunoregulating agents. Progr
    Allergy 25:63.
Chedid L, Morin A (1982). Current status of muramyl pepti-
    des. In Serrou B, Rosenfeld C, Daniels J (eds): "Inter-
    national Symposium on Current Concepts in Human Immunology
    and Cancer Immunomodulation", Amsterdam: Elsevier/North
    Holland Biomedical Press, in press.
Chedid LA, Parant MA, Audibert FM, Riveau GJ, Parant FJ,
    Lederer E, Choay JP, Lefrancier PL (1982). Biological
    activity of a new synthetic muramyl peptide adjuvant
    devoid of pyrogenicity. Infect Immun 35:417.
Cryz SJ, Friedman RL, Pavlovskis OR, Iglewiski BH (1981).
    Effect of formalin toxoiding on *Pseudomonas aeruginosa*
    Toxin A: Biological, chemical and immunochemical studies.
    Infect Immun 32:759.
Damais C, Riveau G, Parant M, Gerota J, Chedid L (1982).

Production of lymphocyte activating factor in the absence of endogenous pyrogen by rabbit or human leukocytes stimulated by a muramyl dipeptide derivative. Int J Immunopharm, in press.

Dietrich FM, Sackmann W, Zak O, Dukor P (1980). Synthetic muramyl dipeptide immunostimulants: protective effects and increased efficacy of antibiotics in experimental bacterial and fungal infections in mice. In Nelson JD, Grassi C (eds): "Current Chemotherapy and Infectious Diseases, Proc. 11th ICC and 19th ICAAC," Washington: American Society for Microbiology 2:1730.

Dreesman GR, Sanchez Y, Ionescu-Matiu I, Sparrow JT, Six HR, Peterson DL, Hollinger FB, Melnick JL (1982). Antibody to hepatitis B surface antigen after a single inoculation of uncoupled synthetic HBsAg peptides. Nature 295:158.

Dukor P, Tarcsay L, Baschang G (1979). Immunostimulants. Annu Rep Med Chem 14:146.

Ellouz F, Adam A, Ciorbaru R, Lederer E (1974). Minimal structural requirements for adjuvant activity of bacterial peptidoglycan derivatives. Biochem Biophys Res Commun 59:1317.

Fraser-Smith EB, Matthews TF (1981). Protective effects of muramyl dipeptides analogs against infections of *Pseudomonas aeruginosa* or *Candida albicans* in mice. Infect Immun 34:676.

Johnson AG, Audibert F, Chedid L (1978). Synthetic immunoregulating molecules: a potential bridge between cytostatic chemotherapy and immunotherapy of cancer. Cancer Immunol Immunother 3:219.

Kellen JA, Kolin A, Mirakian A, Acevedo HF (1982). Effects of antibodies to choriogonadotropin in malignant growth. II. Solid transplantable rat tumors. Cancer Immunol Immunother 13:2.

McLaughlin C, Schwartzman SM, Horner BL, Jones GH, Moffatt JG, Nestor Jr JJ, Tegg D (1980). Regression of tumors in guinea pigs after treatment with synthetic muramyl dipeptides and trehalose dimycolate. Science 208;415.

Leclerc C, Chedid L (1982). Macrophage activation by synthetic muramyl peptides. Lymphokine Reports 3, in press.

Lederer E (1980). Synthetic immunostimulants derived from the bacterial cell wall. J Med Chem 23:819.

Lederer E, Chedid L (1982). Immunomodulation by synthetic muramyl peptides and trehalose diesters. In Mihich E (ed): "Immunological Approaches to Cancer Therapeutics," New York: Wiley Interscience 4:107.

Lefrancier P, Lederer E (1981). Chemistry of synthetic

immunomodulant muramyl peptides. Prog Chem Org Natur Prod 40:1.

Lerner RA, Green N, Alexander H, Liu FT, Sutcliffe JG, Schinnick TM (1981). Chemically synthesized peptides predicted from the nucleotide sequence of the hepatitis B virus genome elicit antibodies reactive with the native envelope protein of Dane particles. Proc Natl Acad Sci USA 78:3403.

Maupas P, Melnick JL (1981). Hepatitis B infection and primary liver cancer. Prog Med Virol 27:1.

Oberling F, Bernard C, Chedid L, Choay J, Giron C, Lang JM (1981). Phase I study of MDP in man. In "International Symposium on Immunomodulation by Microbial Products and Related Synthetic Compounds", Osaka, Japan, Abst. IX.6:41.

Parant M, Parant F, Chedid L (1978). Enhancement of the neonate's non specific immunity to Klebsiella infection by muramyl dipeptide, a synthetic immunoadjuvant. Proc Natl Acad Sci USA 75:3395.

Phillips N, Paraf A, Bahr G, Modabber F, Chedid L (1982). Modulation of murine lymphoma growth by MDP, MDP(D-D) and cyclophosphamide. I. Inhibition of growth in vivo. Submitted.

Phillips N, Bahr GM, Modabber FZ, Chedid L. Modulation of murine lymphoma growth by MDP, MDP(D-D) and cyclophosphamide. II. Inhibition of growth in vitro. Submitted.

Prince AM, Ikram H, Hopp TP (1982). Hepatitis B virus vaccine: identification of HBsAg/a and HBsAg/d but not HBsAg/y subtype antigenic determinants on a synthetic immunogenic peptide. Proc Natl Acad Sci USA 79:579.

Ramakrishnan S, Das C, Dubey SK, Salahuddin M, Talwar GP (1979). Immunogenicity of three C-terminal synthetic peptides of the beta subunit of human chorionic gonadotropin and properties of the antibodies raised against 45-aminoacid C-terminal peptide. J Reprod Immunol 1:249.

Redding TW, Coy DH, Schally AV (1982). Prostate carcinoma tumor size in rats decreases after administration of antagonists of luteinizing hormone-releasing hormone. Proc Natl Acad Sci USA 79:1273.

Reynolds HY, Levine AS, Wood RE, Zierdt CH, Dale DC, Pennington JE (1975). Pseudomonas aeruginosa infections: persisting problems and current research to find new therapies. Ann Intern Med 82:819.

Robertson IS, Wilson JC, Fraser HM (1979). Immunological castration in male cattle. Veterinary Record 105:556.

Sone S, Fidler IJ (1981). In vitro activation of tumoricidal properties in rat alveolar macrophages by synthetic muramyl dipeptide encapsulated in liposomes. Cell Immunol 57:42.

Stevens VC (1975). Female contraception by immunization with HCG. Prospects and status. In Nieschlag (ed): "Female Contraception by Immunization with HCG. Prospects and Status. Immunization with Hormones in Reproduction Research," Amsterdam: North-Holland Publishing Co., p 217.

Stevens VC, Cinader B, Powell JE, Lee AC, Koh SW (1981). Preparation and formulation of a human chorionic gonadotropin antifertility vaccine: selection of adjuvant and vehicle. Amer J Reprod. Immunol. 1:315.

Yamamura Y, Azuma I, Sugimura K, Yamawaki M, Uemiya M, Kusumoto S, Okada S, Shiba T (1977). Immunological and anti-tumor activities of synthetic 6-O-mycoloyl-N-acetyl-muramyl dipeptides. Proc Japan Acad 53:63.

Yarkoni E, Lederer E, Rapp HJ (1981). Immunotherapy of experimental cancer with a mixture of synthetic muramyl dipeptide and trehalose dimycolate. Infect Immun 32:273.

13th International Cancer Congress, Part E
Cancer Management, pages 273–286
© 1983 Alan R. Liss, Inc., 150 Fifth Avenue, New York, NY 10011

CHEMICALLY DEFINED IMMUNOTHERAPEUTIC AGENTS

John W. Hadden, M.D.

Immunopharmacology Program
University of South Florida Medical College
Tampa, Florida 33612

The list of drugs in development for immunotherapy
has grown in the last few years. A partial list includes
levamisole, DTC, NPT 16416, isoprinosine, NPT 15392,
muramyl dipeptides, azimexon, bestatin, pyran copolymers,
polynucleotides, dipyrimidinoles, allylysophospholipids,
lipoidal amines, thiobenzimidazoles, polyglucoses,
glycans, tuftsin, lynestrenol and cyclomunine. A more
general discussion of these compounds can be found in
Advances in Immunopharmacology (Hadden et al., 1981) and
in *Augmenting Agents in Cancer Therapy: Current State
and Future Prospects (Hersh et al., 1981)*. For the
present discussion, I will restrict my general comments
to those compounds with sufficient immunopharmacology
background to warrant consideration for cancer immunotherapy
(see figure).

Levamisole (Renoux, 1978; Symoens, Rosenthal, 1977;
Amery, 1979)

Levamisole (2, 3, 4, 6-tetra-hydro-6-phenylimidazo
(2 1-b) thiazole) was first observed by Renoux in 1972
to be an immunostimulant. The last 10 years of its
development has provided us with interesting perspectives
on this compound. Short of aspirin, no compound has
seen experimental application in as many disease states
as levamisole. To recapitulate the profile of its
immunopharmacology, levamisole acts directly on lymphocytes,
macrophages and granulocytes to modify their mobility,
secretion and proliferation. It can be augmenting or
depressing in its effect depending on the dose and the

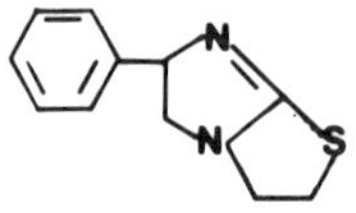

LEVAMISOLE 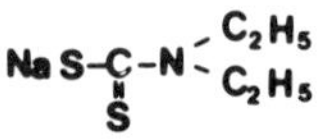   DTC 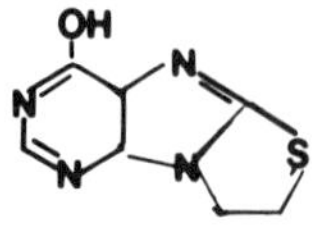   NPT 16416

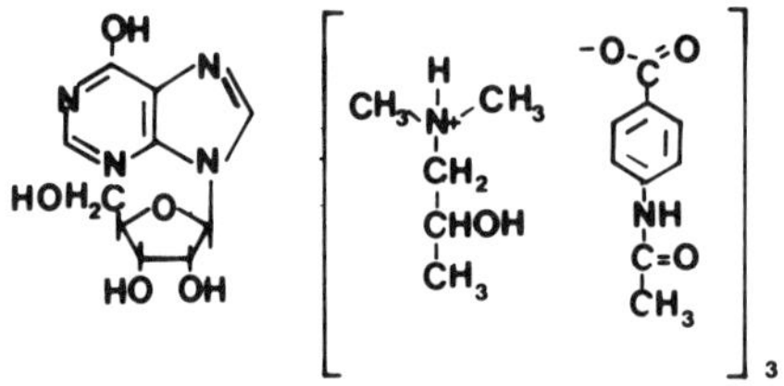

ISOPRINOSINE 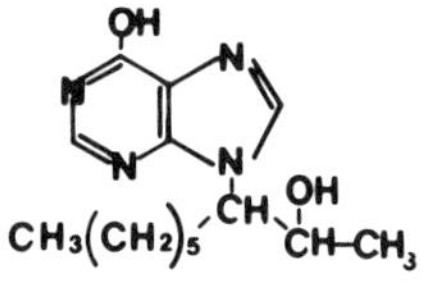   NPT 15392

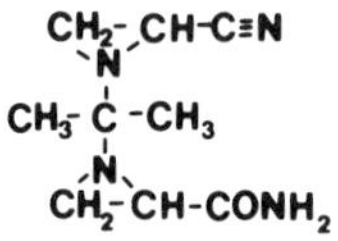

AZIMEXON 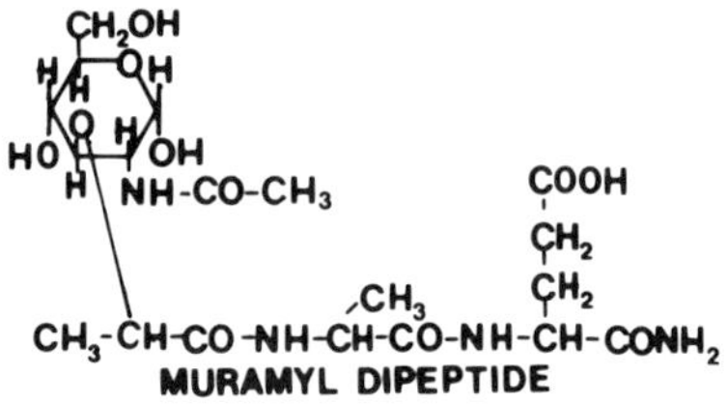   MURAMYL DIPEPTIDE

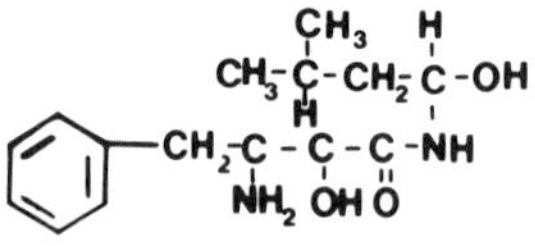

BESTATIN 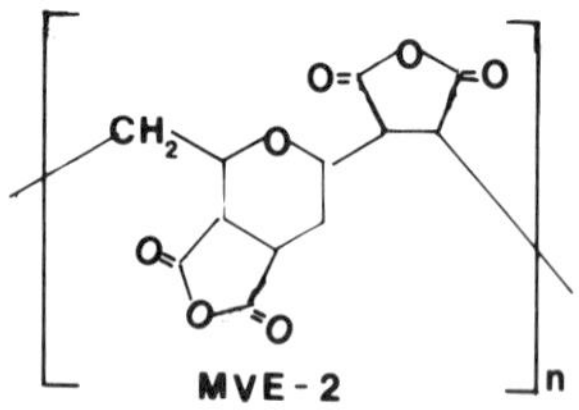   MVE-2

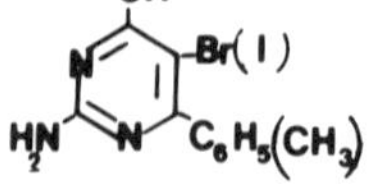

PYRIMIDINOLES

Thr- Lys - Pro -Arg

TUFTSIN

timing of administration. In vivo levamisole (1-25
mg/kilo) augments the expression of cellular more than
humoral immunity, and the latter effect is probably
dependent on its action on T cells and macrophages. Its
action is generally that of an immunopotentiator in that
demonstrable positive effects usually require the concomitant administration of a primary stimulus such as antigen.
The magnitude of effects appears to depend on the degree
to which the stimulus is optimal and the normality of the
responding immune system. For this latter characteristic,
levamisole has been termed an 'immunonormalizing' agent.
In general, its action is weak and non-responder strains
of mice and individual humans exist for reasons which are
not yet clear. Its use has been safe with mild side
effects of metallic taste, nervousness, nausea and vomiting;
however, occasional more severe side effects are dermatitis
and agranulocytosis (particularly in individuals with HLA
B 27 and rheumatoid arthritis).

Levamisole has not shown activity in some thirty four
different murine tumor systems when used alone; however,
in thirteen of twenty one adjunctive protocols in which
the primary tumor was decreased by chemotherapy, radiation
or surgery, levamisole showed some increase in mean survival time or the number of animals surviving. The tumors
included leukemias, fibrosarcomas, mammary carcinoma, and
melanoma. Some degree of clinical efficacy of levamisole
(150 mg three times a week, every other week) has been
reported in 'remission stabilization' of a variety of
double-blinded human cancer studies including breast,
lung, head and neck, leukemia, and multiple myeloma. The
effect in humans with cancer, when observed, has been to
increase the number of patients remaining in remission
following primary tumor reduction by other therapies. On
the average approximately a 15% increase in survival has
resulted in the majority of studies. Clinical efficacy in
rheumatoid arthritis comparable to penicillamine has been
reported by a number of investigators. Numerous reports
have appeared of efficacy in such diverse disorders as
chronic and recurrent viral infections, particularly
Herpes, chronic and recurrent bacterial infections including leprosy, aphthous stomatitis, erythema multiforme and
lupus erythematosus. These many applications may startle
those schooled in the traditional development of pharmaceutical agents. The comprehension of their appropriate-
ness relies upon an understanding that all disorders are

immune based and, almost without exception in each, immunological disturbance has been demonstrated which can be
interpreted as contributing to its pathogenesis. The idea
of treating a dysfunctional or failing immune system,
while a relatively new notion, has direct parallel to each
of the other organ systems for which we have therapy for
dysfunction (e.g. the heart, pulmonary, renal, gastrointestinal and CNS, etc.). While the clinical applications can be justified and supported, the issues of less
than moderate efficacy, prolonged periods to achieve a
response, approximately a 30% non-responder frequency in
any particular disease category, and our inability to
monitor effects of drugs on the immune system simply and
consistently, has accounted and will continue to account
for slow acceptance of the agent by physicians and regulatory agencies.

Other Sulphur Containing Agents

NPT 16416 (7,8-dihydrothiazole 3,2-e hypoxanthine)
was synthesized by us to produce a nontoxic drug similar
in structure and action to levamisole (Hadden et al.,
1982). NPT 16416 is nontoxic with an LD50 by the oral
route in mice in excess of 500 mg/kilo. Immunopharmacologic
effects to increase active rosetting of T lymphocytes and
to induce T cell differentiation in the Komuro and Boyse
assay are evident in vitro at .01 μg/ml. Like levamisole,
only small effects are observable on T cell lymphoproliferative responses; however, at 5-200 μg/ml B cell
responses to LPS and pokeweed mitogen are augmented. In
mice, antibody responses to sheep erythrocytes are augmented
by NPT 16416 (.05-5 mg/kilo). Preliminary studies indicate
that the in vitro effects of NPT 16416, like those of
levamisole, are accompanied by elevations in cellular
levels of cyclic GMP. The immunotherapeutic effects of
this compound remain to be determined.

DTC (sodium diethyldithiocarbamate) has been developed
by Renoux as a less toxic sulphur-containing compound
based on the premise that part of levamisole's in vivo
activity results from its sulphur moiety (see Renoux in
Hersh et al., 1981). Like levamisole, DTC induces in vivo
a thymic hormone-like factor (hepatosin) which is thought
to derive from the liver rather than the thymus. DTC
(30 - 50 mg/kilo) has been used safely as a treatment of
human patients with metal poisoning. In addition to

pharmacologic effects to protect animals against certain
carcinogens and ionizing radiation, DTC (.5 - 25 mg/kilo)
augments both humoral and cellular immune responses. The
cellular targets of action are presumed to be T cells
based upon effects of DTC to induce hepatosin and, in
turn, of this substance to induce T cell differentiation
in vitro. Other actions remain to be investigated. In
vivo administration to humans has been demonstrated to
modify T cell proliferative responses to mitogens and to
restore depressed T cell rosetting to sheep erythrocytes.
The therapeutic effects of this compound remain to be
determined.

Thiazolobenzimidazole (WY 18251-(3-(p-chlorophenyl)
thiazolo(3,2-a)benzimidazole-2-acetic acid) shares some of
the activities of levamisole in modifying T cell responses
and delayed hypersensitivity in vivo at 25 - 150 mg/kilo
(see Gregory et al in Hersh et al., 1981). In addition,
this compound shows some anti-inflammatory activity
distinct from the levamisole type of action. Antimetas-
tatic activity of this compound in the Lewis lung model
has been reported but no reports of human data are available.

Cimetidine (N"-cyano-N-methyl-N'-{2 (5-methylimidazol-
4-yl) methylthio ethyl} guanidine) is a histamine H_2
blocker in clinical use as an antipeptic ulcer drug. A
number of studies indicate this agent has activity on the
immune system (see Friedman in Hersh et al., 1981). The
mechanism of this action is thought to be the blockade of
H_2 receptors and consequently of histamine-induced T
suppressor cell function; however, the presence of a
sulphur moiety as well as a free imidazole group predicts
this compound may have levamisole-like actions. Our
preliminary studies (Castellazi & Hadden, unpublished
observation) indicate that cimetidine (10^{-6}M) augments
active T cell rosettes and increases cyclic GMP levels of
T cells, an action paralleled by imidazole. It would be
of interest to know whether cimetidine induces a thymic
hormone-like serum factor in vivo, as does levamisole and
DTC. Two studies indicate that cimetidine is active in
the EL4 and the Lewis lung murine tumor systems. As a
licenced drug with demonstrated safety, cimetidine is of
interest for possible immunotherapy applications, particularly in those forms of cancer where overactive suppressor cells have been demonstrated.

Isoprinosine (see Hadden, Giner-Sorolla in Hersh et al., 1981; Ginsberg, Hadden, 1982)

Isoprinosine (a complex of p-acetoamidobenzoic acid, N,N-dimethyl-amino-2-propanol and inosine (3:1 molar ratio)) is under development as an antiviral agent. The components of isoprinosine form a complex by a variety of physicochemical criteria and as a complex display biological activities either not apparent or weakly so when the components are employed alone. The complex shows a degree of inhibition of replication of several viruses in vitro by a variety of tests of antiviral activity; however, rather high concentrations are required and the maximal antiviral activity does not, in general, approach antimetabolite antiviral compounds in degree. Modifications of RNA metabolism, perhaps akin to how interferon works, have been invoked as the mechanism. Isoprinosine is virtually non-toxic with only hyperuricemia reported consistently as a side effect. It has been applied in several thousand humans for the treatment of viral or virus-related disorders. In carefully controlled or double blinded studies, significant, mild to moderate efficacy to reduce symptoms and/or shorten disease period or recurrences have been reported in subacute sclerosing panencephalitis (SSPE), and in Herpes simplex types II, influenza and rhinovirus infections.

While antiviral activity might be involved to explain these clinical results, it seems much more likely that known effects of this compound on the immune system make a more plausible explanation. The immunopharmacology of isoprinosine (1-100 µg/ml) includes actions to induce lymphocyte differentiation in a way comparable to thymic hormones and actions to augment lymphocyte, macrophage, and natural killer cell functions in a potentiator mode of action. In general, the activity, both in vitro and in vivo, of isoprinosine has been more consistently reproducible and of greater magnitude than that of levamisole. While virtually all the clinical studies have been for viral infections, a substantial amount of data supports effects of isoprinosine to augment, in patients, virus-specific immune parameters of both cellular and humoral response and non-specific immune parameters including mitogen and lymphokine responses, active rosettes and skin test responses.

Isoprinosine (50-600 mg/kilo) has been shown to be

active in murine tumor systems to potentiate vaccine protection in L1210 Leukemia, to potentiate interferon
therapy in sarcoma 180, and to reduce tumor development in
rabbits infected with Shope virus and NZB mice with auto-
immune disease. Isoprinosine therapy has promoted restoration of depressed immunologic responses in humans with
gynecological cancer treated with radiation and decreased
infections in chemotherapy-treated leukemia patients.
These data, in addition to animal studies, should justify
the clinical application of isoprinosine in an adjuvant
mode in immunosuppressed cancer patients and perhaps some
of the other clinical entities in which levamisole has been
applied.

NPT 15392 (see Hadden and Giner-Sorolla in Hersh et al.,
1981; McKensie, Hadden, 1982)

A structurally similar (non complex) coumpound, NPT
15392, (9-erythro-2-hydroxy-3-nonylhypoxanthine) has been
developed by us. This compound shares each of the immunopharmacological activities of isoprinosine; however, it is
effective at 1/10th - 1/100th of the concentration of
isoprinosine. A number of differences in the degree of
activities suggests that NPT 15392 may have clinical
activities which will be complementary to those of isoprinosine. Specifically, NPT 15392 at .01-1 µg/ml induces
differentiation and augments active rosettes of T cells and
modulates their proliferative, helper, and suppressor
functions. It also potentiates lymphokine effects on
macrophages. At therapeutic doses of .1-1 mg/kilo side
effects in animals and man have been negligible and animal
toxicity studies indicate an oral LD50 of more than 500
mg/kilo. In vivo immunopharmacologic effects have included
significant augmentation of antibody and cellular immune
responses in mice. NPT 15392 augments natural killer cell
activity in mice in vivo but not in vitro. This affect is
apparently not mediated by interferon and the effect of the
combination of interferon and NPT 15392 is additive.

In murine models NPT 15392 (.1 mg/kilo) has shown
effects to reverse, partially, tumor, virus, and chemother-
apy-induced immunosuppression in 8/9 studies.

Correlation of immunorestoration with increased survival or decreased metastasis formation has been observed
in T241 fibrosarcoma, sarcoma 180, Lewis lung carcinoma,

AH4lc, 44, 66 and 130 tumors, and P388 leukemia. No effect
alone was observed in Ll210 leukemia or NF sarcoma. In
immunopharmacologic trials in humans with cancer under the
aegis of the EORTC, NPT 15392 showed effects to augment
lymphocyte counts, active rosettes, and natural killer
cells in some but not all patients. Clinical studies with
this agent in cancer immunotherapy are under consideration.

Muramyl Dipeptide (Lederer, Chedid, 1982; Chedid in Hadden
et al., 1981)

     Muramyl dipeptide (N-acetylmuramyl-L-alanyl-D-isoglut-
amine, MDP) was found by Lederer to be the smallest active
component of the mycobacterial cell wall, having adjuvant
activity characteristic of complete Freunds Adjuvant (CFA)
Since it is water soluble, MDP can be administered by
mouth. A large series of analogs have been prepared,
particularly by French and Japanese investigators, and it
appears that the immunopharmacology of the MDP analogs
depends on their particular structure. Full adjuvancy
equivalent to CFA is not, however, achieved unless MDP is
incorporated into oil or a liposome or is linked as it is
naturally to a lipid-like mycolic acid. 6-0 acyl derivatives of MDP, polymerization with glutaraldehyde, coupling
with carrier-borne antigens have all shown increased
adjuvant activity. MDP itself has both adjuvant potential
when administered with antigen and protective potential in
bacterial challenge when given before and, to an extent,
after antigen. Based upon structure-function studies with
the analogs these two activities appear to be unrelated.
MDP also induces fever and prostaglandin production by
macrophages both of which are prevented by indomethacin, a
prostaglandin (PG) synthetase inhibitor. In the face of an
indomethacin block of PG synthesis, MDP loses no adjuvant
or protective activity indicating that the responses of
fever and PG production are irrelevant side effects. These
effects have been obviated by analog formation and by
polymerization. The n-butyl ester derivative under development by Chedid and co-workers shows both adjuvant and
protective activity but does not induce fever. Many of the
published immunopharmacological studies have been performed
with MDP itself and the critical features of action include
promotion of macrophage activation for tumoricidal and
bactericidal activity and for secretion of enzymes and
monokines. The effect of MDP is a direct one not requiring
lymphokine or other influence. With oil and antigen, MDP

can augment both humoral and cellular immunity. In vitro
studies indicate action of MDP on T helper and suppressor
function and on B cell proliferation as well. The participation of monokines and other macrophage-derived mediators
in these functions has not been completely ruled out.

As a 3-substituted sugar, MDP is interesting in offering
insight into the immunostimulating mechansim of polyglucoses and glycans. The various immunologically active
glycans (lentinan, krestin, levan, shizophyllan, etc.)
require a β-1-3 link to be active, suggesting that the
chemical modification at the 3 position is critical. The
various glycans appear to act via their effects on the
macrophage. The MDP's may, therefore, offer a more specific
approach to macrophage-oriented immunotherapy without the
problems of persistent retention of high molecular weight
antigens and without prolonged reticuloendothelial system
expansion. While the major focus on the MDP's has been on
uses related to adjuvancy with vaccines, their immunopharmacology strongly suggest useful application in cancer
immunotherapy to prevent both tumor re-occurrance and
infections to which the macrophage plays a role in the
resistance. A complementary therapeutic role might well be
observed with levamisole or isoprinosine. MDP's have been
only recently introduced into humans for toxicological
evaluation so clinical trials may be expected relatively
soon.

Azimexon (Chirigos, Mastrangelo, 1982)

Azimexon (BM12,531),2-(2-cyanaziridinyl)-(1)-1-(2-
carbamoylaziridinyl)-(1)-propane, is an orally active
immunostimulating compound under development for use in
cancer. Its immunopharmacology from in vitro studies shows
direct action on both lymphocytes and macrophages. In vivo
studies show augmented cell-mediated immunity, T cell-
dependent humoral immunity and natural killer cell activity.
It also induces an expansion of the reticuloendothelial
system with splenomegaly. It induces leukocytosis and
hastens recovery from leukopenia. Its only significant
side effect known to date is a dose-related toxic hemolytic
anemia which may limit clinical indications to malignant
diseases. In animal studies with cancer, the drug is more
active in increasing survival and longevity in adjuvant
protocols with irradiation and chemotherapy than is levamisole. In human patients, a variety of depressed immune

parameters were improved following clinical administration
of azimexon. It remains to be determined whether clinical
response in cancer can be achieved in the absence of the
complication of anemia.

Bestatin (Umezawa, 1981)

Bestatin ((2S, 3R)-3-amino-2 hydroxy-4 phenyl butyryl-
l-Leucine) is a substance extracted from Streptomyces
olivoreticuli by Umezawa and co-workers. It is a non
toxic, orally active immunostimulating compound thought to
act by binding to lymphocytes and macrophages and inhibiting
aminopeptidase B and leucine aminopeptidase. Cellular
targets of its action appears to be the macrophage, the
bone marrow precursors for granulocytes (CFUc), natural
killer cells, and possibly T lymphocytes. In vivo injection in mice of 5-50 mg/kilo increases DNA synthesis in
spleen, thymus, and bone marrow but not in other organs
tested. Associated were increases in terminal deoxynucleo-
side transferase and DNA polymerase α in T lymphocytes.
Metabolic conversion of bestatin to p-hydroxy bestatin was
observed in vivo and the half lives of each were less than
4 hr. P-hydroxy bestatin was also shown to be immunologically active. In vivo treatment of mice (doses ranging
from .05-5 mg/kilo) is associated with up to 3 fold increases in antibody production to sheep erythocytes (SRBC)
and delayed hypersensitivity to SRBC or oxazalone. Immunorestoration in tumor bearing or chemotherapy-treated mice
was also observed. Some tumor growth inhibition was observed
by bestatin treatment in animals bearing the slow growing
tumors IMC and Gardner's lymphosarcoma but no effect was
observed in Ll210 leukemia or Erhlich ascites tumor. In
the latter two tumors bestatin therapy following chemotherapy with adriamycin or bleomycin, respectively, increased survivals as well as mean survival times. Prophylactic therapy reduced spontaneous tumor development in
aged mice in association with immunorestoration. Uncon-
trolled trials in limited numbers of human patients have
been reported to be encouraging. Human toxicity has been
negligible and efforts to increase NK cell activity and E
rosette forming T cells have been observed in some patients.
Clarification of cell targets, particularly T cells, and of
immunopharmacologic mechanisms is needed but additional
controlled clinical studies appear warranted.

Tuftsin (Najjar, Schmidt, 1981; Nishioka etal., 1981)

Tuftsin (Thr-Lys-Pro-Arg) represents residues 289-292 of the heavy chain of α-globulin and is thought to be liberated by selective cleavage with tuftsin-endocarboxy-peptidase. Following cleavage it binds to leukokinin and requires a cell surface leukokininase to liberate free tuftsin. Tuftsin (.2-25 µM) acts to stimulate motility, phagocytosis, processing of antigen, and tumoricidal activity of macrophages. Tuftsin increases neutrophil chemotaxis, phagocytosis, and killing. Reportedly natural killer cell activity is increased. Its effects appear to be mediated in part by elevations of cyclic GMP levels and depression of cyclic AMP levels in macrophages. As a biologic peptide, it is nontoxic and without significant side effects. In vivo administration of tuftsin in mice (20 mg/kg) produces macrophages activated for tumoricidal activity and increases in T cell dependent or independent antibody production and antibody-dependent cytotoxicity. In murine tumor models, tuftsin (10-50 mg/kilo) prolonged survival in Ll210 leukemia and in the Cloudman S-91 melanoma. In addition, immunoprophylactic therapy in aged mice reduced the incidence of spontaneous neoplasms. Therapeutic application of tuftsin in humans with cancer remains to be performed.

Pyran Copolymer (Chirigos, Mastrangelo, 1982)

Maleic anhydride-divinyl ether copolymer (MVE) exists as a series of copolymers with varying molecular weights. MVE-2 (15,500 daltons) has been selected for clinical evaluation based upon its minimal toxicity. This prepration has been well tolerated in animals by both oral and parenteral routes. Dose dependent toxicity at sublethal levels was associated with hepatosplenomegaly resulting from expansion of reticuloendothelial elements in the absence of cell damage. Doses of less than 20 mg/kg appears to be acceptable in mice. With doses less than 20 mg/kg, reticuloendothelial expansion is observed and is reflected in increased clearance rates for ^{51}CR labeled erythrocytes persisting up to one week. 28 days following injection of labeled MVE-2, over 20% of the copolymer or its metabolites were retained; the long term significance of this retention has not been assessed. The implication of this retention for human use is disturbing. The primary cell target of MVE-2 action appears to be the macrophage. Following in vivo and in vitro administration, macrophages cytotoxic for tumor cells have been observed. The mechanism of macro-

phage activation has not been clearly elucidated. Interferon has been implicated, as MVE-2 does induce macrophage
interferon production in vitro and in vivo. Alternatively
nuclear effects of phagocytized MVE-2 have been implicated.
Consistent with interferon induction, increased natural
killer cell activity has been noted in vivo. In vivo
effects to increase lymphocyte numbers and functions have
been observed; however, in the absence of the appropriate
in vitro studies, the determination of whether these are
direct or indirect effects cannot be made. In vivo administration enhanced delayed hypersensitivity to sheep erythrocytes and augmented cellular immunity as assessed by augmentation of the protective effect of a tumor vaccine. Effects
of MVE-2 have been described in virus challenge systems.
Pretreatment was required as is the case with the interferon
inducers such that no direct antiviral action is thought to
be involved. An interferon inducer has been reported.
MVE-2 alone has been active in several animal tumor models
(BL-2, Mammary CA IC/E, P815 Mastocytoma, B 15 melanoma)
with a moderate effect to prolong survival by 25% on the
average. It has been inactive in the LSTRA leukemia system.
MVE-2 in chemoimmunotherapy with cytoxan increased both
survival time and the number of survivors in the MBL-2
system. A small increase in mean survival time in the
Lewis lung model was observed following surgical ablation
of the primary tumor. Significant effect of MVE-2 alone
was observed in mouse fibrosarcomas (NFSA + Fsa) and in one
mammary carcinoma (MDAH - MCa-4) but not another (MCa-k)
(Milas, Hersh, Hunter, 1981). The effects involved decrease
metastases and increased life span, but not cures. Clinical
studies in humans with cancer using the mixed copolymers
(4-16 mg/kilo) showed interferon induction, fever, chills,
malaise, coagulation defects, in one case thrombocytopenia,
leukopenia and acute tubular necrosis of the kidney. Other
toxicities included hypertension and CNS effects. Phase I
trials with MVE-2 are in progress to determine if its
toxicities are acceptable.

Pyrimidinoles (see Stringfellow in Hersh et al., 1981)

In general, interferon inducers have been limited in
their development by their toxicity and the refractory
state to interferon induction which develops following
their administration. The 6-phenyl pyrimidinoles represent
an interesting group of compounds in this regard. Two
compounds of this group 2-amino-5-bromo-6-phenyl 4-pyrimi-

dinol (ABPP) and 2-amino-5-iodo-6 phenyl-4-pyrimidinol
(AIPP) both show antiviral and antitumor activity. While
both agents activate macrophages and natural killer cells,
only ABPP is an inducer of interferon; the mechanisms of
their protective effects remains, therefore, to be fully
clarified. On the basis of its ability to induce interferon
ABPP has been emphasized and Stringfellow has recently
reported that the refractory response to interferon induction following its administration can be circumvented by
less frequent administration, (i.e. once a week) while
still not losing protection. ABPP is currently in Phase I
trials at the MD Anderson Hospital, U.S.A. The comparative
effects of AIPP remain of great interest since it apparently
has potent immunomodulating effects without interferon
induction as a side effect.

Conclusion

The foregoing represents only a partial list of chemically defined agents potentially useful in the immunotherapy
of cancer. No single agent in this group, nor for that
matter among the biologicals or the bacterial or fungal
products, offers an immunotherapeutic potential capable of
curing cancer as a monotherapy. These agents can presently
be envisioned to be employed in combination with chemotherapy, surgery or radiation to reduce the frequency of
recurrence and frequency of infection resulting from immunosuppression. Their successful use in active, progressive
cancer will depend upon the development of new strategies.
Already it is apparent that combinations of immunotherapeutic agents offer potentiative interactions (e.g. isoprinosine and interferon, MDP or endotoxin and lymphokines,
endotoxin and cell wall skeleton, etc.). These potentiative
interactions need to be more fully explored. With more
potent immunorestoration and activation and strategies to
overcome tumor-related immunosuppression and to enhance
tumor immunogenicity, more broadly based and successful
immunotherapies will develop.

References

Amery, W. (1979) Time in chemo-immunotherapy models. Int.
  J. Immunopharmacol. 1:65.
Chirigos, M., Mastrangelo, M. (1982) Immunorestoration by
  chemicals In Milich (ed) "Immunological Approaches to
  Cancer Therapeutics", New York, John Wiley & Sons,
  p. 191.
Ginsberg, T., Hadden, J. (1982) Immunopharmacology of
  methisoprinol In Fudenberg, Ambrogi (eds.) "Frontiers
  in Immunomodulation", New York, Plenum Press (in press).
Hersh, E., Chirigos, M., Mastrangelo, M. (1981) "Augmenting
  agents in Cancer Therapy" New York, Raven Press.
Hadden, J., Chedid, L., Mullen, P., Spreafico, F. (1981)
  "Advances in Immunopharmacology" New York, Pergamon Press.
Hadden, J., Giner-Sorolla, A., Hadden, E., Ikehara, S.,
  Pahwa, R., Coffey, R., Castellazzi, A., Jones, C.,
  Maxwell, K., Simon, L. (1982) NPT 16416: A levamisole-
  like purine with immunomodulatory effects. Int. J.
  Immunopharmacol. 4: 287.
Lederer, E., Chedid, L. (1982) Immunomodulation by synthetic
  muramyl dipeptides and trehalose esters In Mihich (ed.)
  "Immunological Approaches to Cancer Therapeutics", New
  York, J. Wiley & Sons, P. 107.
McKensie, D., Hadden, J. (1981) Immunopharmacologic actions
  of isoprinosine & NPT 15392 In Friedman (ed.) "Biological
  Response Modifiers In Human Oncology and Immunology", New
  York, Plenum Press (in press).
Milas, K., Hersh, E., Hunter, N. (1981) Therapy of artificial
  and spontaneous metastases of murine tumors with maleic
  anhydride-divinyl ether-2, Cancer Res. 41: 2378.
Najjar, V., Schmidt, J. (1980). The chemistry and biology of
  tuftsin, Lymphokine Reports 1: 157.
Nishioka, K., Amoscoto, A., Babcock, G. (1981) Tuftsin: A
  hormone-like tetrapeptide with antimicrobial and antitumor
  activities, Life Sci. 28: 1081.
Renoux, G. (1978) Modulation of immunity by levamisole,
  Pharmac. Ther. 2: 397.
Symoens, J., Rosenthal, M. (1977) Levamisole in the modula-
  tion of the immune response, J. Retic Endothel Soc 21: 175.
Umezawa, H. (1981) "Small Molecular Immunomodifiers of
  Microbial Origin" New York, Pergamon Press.

13th International Cancer Congress, Part E
Cancer Management, pages 287–296
© 1983 Alan R. Liss, Inc., 150 Fifth Avenue, New York, NY 10011

INTERFERONS: IN PURSUIT OF THE PROMISE

Ernest C. Borden, MD

Departments of Human Oncology and Medicine
Wisconsin Clinical Cancer Center
University of Wisconsin
Madison, Wisconsin 53792

Interferons of all three major classes, α, β, and γ, increasingly seem to be biological molecules which regulate cellular function. These effects undoubtedly underlie their therapeutic activity in neoplastic diseases. Since their original discovery as antivirals, the pleiotropic biological effects of interferons have been a subject of ever-increasing research and clinical interest. Over the past three years, marked by the beginning of the American Cancer Society interferon program, an extraordinary expansion in our understanding of interferons, particularly those of human origin, has occurred. This review will briefly summarize some of that progress.

STRUCTURE AND PURIFICATION

By use of recombinant DNA techniques, a complete nucleotide sequence for interferons α and β has been defined (Mantei et al., 1980; Taniguchi et al., 1980a; Derynck et al., 1980). The amino acid sequence has been derived from the DNA codon. Human interferons α and β are 166 amino acids in length. A comparison of the sequences of inter-ferons α and β revealed 45% homology of nucleotides and 29% homology of amino acids (Taniguchi et al., 1980b). Nucleo-tide sequencing of interferon cDNA inserts in E. coli clones confirmed directly the existence of multiple interferons α (Goeddel et al., 1980, Nagata et al., 1980a). Each of these non-allelic human genes differed by approximately 10% in nucleotide sequence and 15 to 25% in amino acid sequence. Thus a family of more than a dozen physicochemically-related interferon α proteins has been defined (Streuli et al., 1980; Goeddel et al., 1981). Differences in amino acid composition probably explain, the chromatographic heterogeneity of naturally-produced leukocyte and lymphoblastoid interferons. The relative proportion of subclasses of interferons in naturally-produced preparations is not yet defined.

A gene for interferon γ has recently been expressed in E. coli (Goeddel, et al., 1982). Like interferon β, only one interferon γ has been identified. This protein is 146 amino acids in length, with an additional 20 amino acid secretory peptide present on the amino terminal end. It has approximately a 12% amino acid sequence homology with α interferons (Epstein, 1982).

Recombinant-produced interferons α and β have been purified to homogeneity. Their amino acid composition, predicted by nucleotide sequence, has been confirmed. Methods for scale-up of the purification have been identified. This has also made possible production of bulk quantities of pure interferon molecules for clinical trials.

BIOLOGICAL RESPONSE MODIFICATION

The diverse cellular actions of interferons (Borden and Ball, 1981) have been confirmed to reside in the same proteins which induce the antiviral effects. Human interferons α and β have been purified to homogeneity with retention of all effects on immunologic function and cellular proliferation (Knight, 1976; Evinger et al., 1980). Expression of diverse biological activities by an interferon produced from a single human gene cloned in E. coli also strongly substantiates that the activities reside in a single molecule (Masucci et al., 1980). Interpretation of non-antiviral effects of naturally-produced interferon γ preparations, which contain lymphokines and are, at present, less purified, must be viewed more cautiously.

A number of biochemical alterations have been identified in interferon-treated cells (Table 1). Three enzymes, which probably play a major role in effecting action of interferons, are an oligoadenylate synthetase, a protein kinase, and a 2'phosphodiesterase. Except for the

Table 1

Biologic Response Modification
by Interferons

Enzymatic changes
    Induction of 2-5A synthetase*
    Activation of latent endonuclease by 2-5A
    Induction of protein phosphokinase
    Induction of 2' phosphodiesterase
    Increased arylhydrocarbon hydroxylase
    Depressed ornithine decarboxylase induction
    Depressed hepatic cytochrome p450-linked mono-oxygenases
    Depressed induction of glucocorticoid-inducible enzymes

Immunomodulatory effects
    T cells
        depressed proliferation*
        depressed leukocyte migration inhibition
        enhanced cytotoxicity
        enhanced suppressor cell function
    B cells
        depressed proliferation
    NK cells
        enhanced effector cell function*
        depressed target cell sensitivity
    K cells
        enhanced cytotoxicity*
    Macrophages
        depressed monocyte differentiation
        enhanced phagocytosis

Cell surface changes
    Protein hormone binding decreased
    Ligand binding increased
    Membrane compositional changes
    Enhanced β_2 microglobulin release*
    Decreased membrane transport
    Increased histocompatibility antigen synthesis and
      expression*
    Cytoskeletal alterations

---

*Changes also identified in patients treated with
interferons.

Further reviewed and referenced in Borden and Ball,
1981.

latter, these enzymes require double-stranded RNA for activity. Oligoadenylate synthetase levels increased 3-8 fold in patients receiving interferon α (Schattner et al., 1981b; Merritt, Ball, Borden, in preparation).

Alterations in immunologic function may not only explain the antitumor effects of interferons but also may be useful for measurement of biological changes in treated patients (Table 1). Interferons influence generation of immune effector cells with cytotoxic reactivity to tumor cells such as T cells, NK cells, K cells and macrophages. Moreover, membrane changes resulting from interferons may alter immunogenicity of tumor cells. Preclinical effects of interferons sometimes depend upon which arm of an immune response, afferent or efferent, is in progress at the time of interferon addition. Thus, clinical effects of interferons upon some host immune responses may depend upon the pre-existing immunological relationship between host and tumor.

Whether membrane changes result in the antiproliferative effects of interferons remains to be determined. Interferons inhibit the mitotic cycle by prolongation of all cell cycle phases. In general, tumor cells have been more inhibited in growth than normal cells.

CLINICAL TRIALS

Solid Tumors

A study of metastatic breast cancer, evaluated the effects of buffy coat leukocyte (α) interferon in 17 female patients treated with interferon (Gutterman et al., 1980). Six of the treated patients achieved a partial response. Median duration of remission was 27 weeks (range 8 to 60+ weeks) (Gutterman et al., 1980). To confirm these findings, the American Cancer Society initiated a multi-center trial with interferon α (Borden et al., 1982a). Five of 23 patients treated had objective regression of measurable tumor. The duration of partial responses ranged from 14 to 121 days. In this trial, patients had evidence of significant elevations of NK and K cell cytotoxicity and β_2 microglobulin (Borden et al., 1982). Although no correlation with disease response could be made, these findings suggest interferons truly act in vivo as biologic response modifiers.

Loco-regional administration sometimes supplemented by limited periods of systemic administration of leukocyte interferons has resulted in significant tumor regressions in other recurrent tumors sometimes refractory to conventional therapies. Interferon has been administered intravesically to patients with low grade bladder carcinomas (Ikic et al., 1981; Osther et al., 1981). Eight of 14 had complete disappearance of tumor and three additional patients had partial regressions. In 10 patients with recurrent glioma, fibroblast interferon (β) was administered by Rickham catheter placed directly into tumor (Nagai, 1982). Six of 10 patients had evidence of significant tumor regression documented on CAT scan.

The only adjuvant clinical trial with interferons is in osteosarcoma. This trial, which utilized interferon (α) was initiated in 1972 at the Karolinska Institute in Stockholm (Strander et al., 1978). Life table analyses project that 60% of the interferon-treated group will remain free of metastatic disease three years following their diagnosis. The effects of interferon in this trial are thus comparable to those reported for adriamycin and high-dose methotrexate adjuvant therapy for osteosarcoma.

Hematologic Malignancies

Decreases in objectively measurable parameters of multiple myeloma have been reported (Mellstedt et al., 1979; Gutterman et al., 1980). Decreases in serum monoclonal protein concentration, Bence Jones protein excretion in the urine, size of objectively measurable plasmacytomas, and improvement in performance status have all been documented. To evaluate further the activity of interferon α in multiple myeloma, the American Cancer Society initiated a clinical trial which involved twenty-one patients (Osserman et al., 1981). Four of these patients had disease regression.

In initial trials in malignant lymphoma, two patients with previously untreated nodular poorly differentiated lymphoma achieved a complete response. A third patient relapsed six months after treatment was stopped. Three patients with previously treated diffuse histiocytic lymphoma treated in the same manner did not respond (Merigan et al., 1978). Activity of interferon α in malignant lymphoma was confirmed in a subsequent trial (Gutterman

et al., 1980). Marked decreases in peripheral blasts with
occasional marrow improvement have been observed in Phase I
trials in acute leukemia (Hill et al., 1981; Rohatiner
et al., 1982).

Toxicity

Both subjective and objective side effects occur with
pure leukocyte interferons. Lymphoblastoid interferons,
purified by monoclonal antibody affinity chromatography,
resulted in the same side effects as impure lymphoblastoid
interferons (Scott et al., 1981). A human leukocyte
interferon subspecies (α_2), prepared by recombinant DNA
techniques and then purified to homogeneity, resulted in
qualitatively similar side effects as impure buffy coat
leukocyte interferons (Gutterman et al., 1982).
Recombinant α_2 leukocyte interferon also resulted in a
similar frequency of side effects as the crude buffy coat
interferons (Table 2).

Table 2

Comparative Side Effects of Impure
and Pure Leukocyte Interferons*

Side Effect	Leukocyte Interferon			
	Buffy Coat		Recombinant α_2	
	n	%	n	%
Anorexia/nausea	16/21	76	11/14	76
Malaise/fatigue	12/21	57	6/14	43
Fever (>100.5°F) d 1	17/21	81	11/14	79
WBC (<4000)	10/17	59	11/14	79
Weight loss (>1 kg)	8/17	47	6/14	43

*Studies at Wisconsin Clinical Cancer Center.
Number (n) patients with side effects of number treated.

CONCLUSION

The cloning and expression of human interferon genes
into E. coli with subsequent protein purification has
resulted in confirmation of previous data that pleiotropic

biological effects of interferons result from the interferon molecule _per se_. Recombinant DNA technology has also made possible clinical trials with interferons purified to homogeneity. The fermentation methods will make feasible the commercial production of interferons at reasonable cost.

The emphasis in current trials with recombinant interferons is upon identification of the maximally-tolerated clinical dose. This approach is based upon the postulate, derived from application of cancer chemotherapeutic agents, that the maximal dose will have the greatest antitumor effect. This assumes that the antiproliferative effects of interferons are primary in their antitumor action and is a critical hypothesis to test.

As biologic response modifiers (Borden _et al_., 1982b), one must approach interferon use in cancer with a different perspective from conventional cytotoxic therapy. For rational design of Phase II and III trials, initial studies will need to define both a biologically-effective dose and a maximally-tolerated dose. Biological changes, such as alteration in T cell proliferative and cytotoxic responses, augmentation of NK cell cytotoxicity, and changes in 2-5A synthetase levels, may be effective probes for determining an optimal dose. Correlation of basic pharmacokinetic data such as peak serum levels, estimation of serum half life, and duration of detectable serum levels at intermediate and maximal doses with desired biologic responses may provide a scientific rationale for schedule and dose modification. Previous approaches to development of cancer drugs may require modification in clinically evaluating interferons. The generally-accepted standard of 50% reduction in cross-sectional area may not be apparent if growth of tumor is only inhibited. In planning for adjuvant trials, it may become important to look for consistent modulation of biologic effects.

The therapeutic promise of interferons for cancer remains to be fulfilled. Phase II clinical trials in many malignancies are only now underway. In nodular lymphomas and multiple myeloma, the most responsive tumors in initial trials, randomized Phase III studies are in only the planning stages. Adjuvant randomized trials in melanoma and colorectal carcinoma, to test effectiveness of interferons resulting in eradication of micrometastases in patients at high risk for recurrence, are also just beginning. These studies will allow more definitive predictions as to the potential usefulness of interferons with other treatment modalities for neoplastic diseases.

It seems probable, based upon results to date, that interferons will prove an important new approach to cancer management. If so, a number of problems remain to be resolved. However, if findings over the next three years only partially match the understandings that have emerged in the past three, substantial progress will have occurred.

ACKNOWLEDGEMENTS

Studies with interferons at the University of Wisconsin Clinical Cancer Center have been supported by NIH P01 CA20432, NIH R26 CA 27436, NIH N01-CM 07434, the American Cancer Society, Hoffman LaRoche Inc., and Burroughs-Wellcome Inc. The continued support and collaboration of colleagues in my laboratory and in the Division of Clinical Oncology were instrumental to completion of studies.

REFERENCES

Borden EC, Ball LA (1981). Interferons: biochemical, cell growth inhibitory and immunological effects. In Brown EB (ed): "Progress in Hematology," Vol XII, New York: Grune and Stratton, Inc, p 299.
Borden EC, Holland JF, Dao TL, Gutterman JU, Wiener L, Chang Y-C, Patel J (1982a). Leukocyte-derived interferon (α) in human breast carcinoma. The American Cancer Society Phase II Trial. Ann Int Med 97(1):1.
Borden EC, Edwards BS, Hawkins MJ, Merritt JA (1982b). Interferons: biological response modification and pharmacology. In Mihich E (ed): "Biological Responses in Cancer: Progress Toward Potential Applications," New York: Plenum Publishing, in press.
Derynck R, Content J, DeClercq E, Volckaert G, Tavernier J, Devos R, Fiers W (1980). Isolation and structure of a human fibroblast interferon gene. Nature 285:542.
Epstein LB (1982). Interferon-gamma: success, structure and speculation. Nature 295:454.
Evinger M, Rubinstein M, Pestka S (1980). Growth-inhibitory and antiviral activity of purified leukocyte interferon. Ann NY Acad Sci 350:399.

Goeddel DV, Yelverton E, Ullrich A, Heyneker HL, Miozzari G, Holmes W, Seeburg PH, Dull T, May L, Stebbing N, Crea R, Maeda S, McCandliss R, Sloma A, Tabor JM, Gross M, Familletti PC, Pestka S (1980). Human leukocyte interferon produced by E. coli is biologically active. Nature 287:411.

Goeddel DV, Leung DW, Dull TJ, Gross M, Lawn RM, McCandliss R, Seeburg PH, Ullrich A, Yelverton E, Gray PW (1981). The structure of eight distinct cloned human leukocyte interferon cDNA's. Nature 290:20.

Gray PW, Leung DW, Pennica D, Yelverton E, Najarian R, Simonsen CC, Derynck R, Sherwood PJ, Wallace DM, Berger SL, Levinson AD, Goeddel DV (1982). Expression of human immune interferon cDNA in E. coli and monkey cells. Nature 295:503.

Gutterman JU, Fein S, Quesada J, Horning SJ, Levine JL, Alexanian R, Bernhardt L, Kramer M, Spiegel H, Colburn W, Trown P, Merigan T, Dziewanowska Z (1982). Recombinant human leukocyte interferon (IFLrA): a clinical study of pharmacokinetics, single dose tolerance, and biologic effects in cancer patients. Ann Int Med 96:549.

Gutterman JU, Blumenschein GR, Alexanian R, Yap H-Y, Buzdar AV (1980). Leukocyte interferon induced tumor regression in human metastatic breast cancer, multiple myeloma and malignant lymphoma. Ann Intern Med 93:399.

Hill NO, Pardue AS, Khan A (1981). Phase I human leukocyte interferon trials in cancer and leukemia. J Clin Hematol Oncol 11:23.

Ikic D, Nola P, Maricic Z, Smudj K, Oresic V, Knezevic M, Rode B, Jusic D, Soos E (1981). Application of human leukocyte interferon in patients with urinary bladder papillomatosis, breast cancer and melanoma. Lancet 1:1022.

Knight E (1976). Interferon: purification and initial characterization from human diploid cells. Proc Natl Acad Sci (USA) 73:520.

Mantei N, Schwarzstein M, Streuli M, Panem S, Nagata S, Weissmann C (1980). The nucleotide sequence of a cloned human leukocyte interferon cDNA. Gene 10:1.

Masucci MG, Sziegeti R, Klein E, Klein G, Grueset J, Montagnier L, Taira H, Hall A, Nagata S, Weissmann C (1980). Effect of interferon-α_1 from E. coli on some cell functions. Science 209:1431.

Mellstedt H, Abre A, Bjorkholm M, Holm G, Johansson B, Strander H (1979). Interferon therapy in myelomatosis. Lancet 1:245.

Merigan TC, Sikora K, Breeden JH, Levy R, Rosenberg SA
(1978). Preliminary observations on the effect of human
leukocyte interferon in non-Hodgkin's lymphoma. N Engl J
Med 299:1449.

Nagai M, Arai T, Kohno S and Kohase M (1982). Interferon
therapy for malignant brain tumors in Kono R and Vilcek J
(eds). The Clinical Potential of Interferons. Treatment
of Viral Diseases and Malignant Tumors. Tokyo: University
of Tokyo Press, p. 257.

Osserman EF, Sherman WH, Alexanian R, Gutterman JU,
Humphrey RL (1981). Human leukocyte interferon in
multiple myeloma: The American Cancer Society-sponsored
trial. DeMaeyer E, Galasso G, Schellekens H (eds). The
Biology of the Interferon System. Amsterdam:
Elsevier/North Holland, p. 409.

Osther K, Salford LG, Hornmark-Stenstam B, Flodgren P,
Christophersen IS, Magnusson K (1981). Local versus
systemic human leukocyte interferon treatment. In
DeMaeyer, et al., ibid, p 415.

Rohatiner AZS, Balkwill F, Griffin DB, Malpas JS, Lister TA
(1982). A Phase I study of human lymphoblastoid
interferon administered by continuous intravenous
infusion. Cancer Chemotherapy Pharmacology, in press.

Schattner A, Merlin G, Levin S, Wallach D, Hahn T, Revel M
(1981). Assay of an interferon-induced enzyme in white
blood cells as a diagnostic aid in viral diseases. Lancet
2:497.

Strander H, Adamson U, Aparisi T, Brostrom LA, Cantell K,
Einhorn S, Hall K, Ingimarsson S, Nilsonne V, Soderberg G
(1978). Adjuvant interferon treatment of human
osteosarcoma. Recent Results Cancer Res 68:40.

Streuli M, Nagata S, Weissmann C (1980). At least three
human type α interferons: structure of α2. Science
209:1343.

Taniguchi T, Mantei N, Schwarzstein M, Nagata S, Muramatsu
M, Weissmann C (1980a). Human leukocyte and fibroblast
interferons are structurally related. Nature 285:547.

Taniguchi T, Ohno S, Fujii-Kuriyama Y, Muramatsu M
(1980b). The nucleotide sequence of human fibroblast
interferon cDNA. Gene 10:11.

13th International Cancer Congress, Part E
Cancer Management, pages 297–304
© 1983 Alan R. Liss, Inc., 150 Fifth Avenue, New York, NY 10011

PROSPECTIVE USES OF THYMIC HORMONES IN CANCER

Nathan Trainin, M.D.*, Zeev T. Handzel, M.D.**,
and Rina Zaizov, M.D.***

*Department of Cell Biology, Weizmann Institute
of Science, Rehovot, **Clinical Immunology Unit,
Kaplan Hospital, Rehovot, ***Department of Pediatric Hematology and Oncology Beilinson Medical
Center, Petah-Tikva, Israel

The thymus plays a critical role in establishing the
integrity of the lymphoid system and is essential in the
maintenance of immune competence throughout life. Some of
the thymic functions are mediated by hormone-like products
which have been traced back to the epithelial component of
this organ. Earlier, we observed that neonatally thymectomized mice bearing thymus-containing diffusion chambers
were protected from the effects of thymus deprivation only
in those cases in which the chambers contained viable epithelial thymic cells continuously (Levey, Trainin & Law
1963). More recently, immunoelectromicroscopic studies
(Schmitt et al. 1980), indirect fluorescence antibody procedures (Hirokawa, McClure & Goldstein 1982) and monoclonal
antibody technology (Dardenne et al. 1982) have detected,
separately, the presence of some of these hormones in the
cytoplasm of thymic reticuloepithelial cells.

A series of substances with well defined chemical properties have been isolated and purified by now starting from
calf thymus extraction. They include thymosins (Hooper et
al. 1975) thymopoietins (Goldstein 1974) and THF, thymic
humoral factor (Kook, Yakir & Trainin 1975). A serum thymic
factor, FTS, was originally isolated from pig serum (Bach
and Carnaud 1976). Since this principle is absent from the
serum of thymectomized or nude animals and reappears after
thymus grafting, its strict thymic dependence has apparently
been established (Bach & Dardenne 1973). Thymostimulin or

TP-1 (Bergesi & Falchetti 1977), also extracted from calf
thymus, is a more recent member of the family of thymic hormones.

From the chemical point of view, all share a peptidic
composition though none of the products studied show structural homology among themselves. Their molecular weights
vary from 900 for FTS (Pleau et al. 1977) and 3220 for THF
(Kook, Yakir & Trainin 1975), to 5560 for thymopoietins I
and II, two closely related polypeptides (Goldstein 1974).
It has been found that a pentapeptide (TP-5) retains all the
biological activities of thymopoietin II (Goldstein et al.
1979). Thymosin fraction 5 is actually a mixture of polypeptides with molecular weights varying from 1,000 to 15,000
daltons. Some of these polypeptides are specifically produced by thymic epithelial cells and are properly termed
thymic hormones. Thymosin fraction 5 contains also lymphokines and other ubiquitous cellular components. The polypeptides obtained from thymosin fraction 5 were classified
upon their isoelectric focusing pattern in the pH range of
3.5 to 9.5 into 3 regions: the α region consists of polypeptides with PI below 5.0, the β region between 5.0 and
7.0, and the γ region above 7.0. By combination of ion exchange chromatography and gel filtration 16 polypeptides
were isolated from the α region and 4 from the β region.
Thymosin α_1, which has a molecular weight of 3108 seems to
be the most representative of thymosin fraction 5 activities. Thymosin α_5 and α_7 have molecular weights of 3,000
and 3,200 respectively (Marshall et al. 1980). Thymostimulin (TP-1) consists of a group of polypeptides of less
than 12,000 MW and on polyacrylamide gel electrophoresis it
contains two characteristic bands (Klein and Shoham 1981).
Some of the thymic hormones like thymosin fraction 5, THF
and thymostimulin are at present obtained from native calf
thymus, while others, such as FTS, thymopoietin II, TP-5
and thymosin α_1 are prepared by synthetic procedures.

Many years of research have permitted to establish that
thymic hormones act upon cells which belong to the lymphoid
system. The chain of events which leads to activation, di-
ferentiation and maturation of target cells by thymic hormones includes a) the binding of these peptide molecules to
specific receptors on the surface of cells; b) the activation of membranal enzymes, such as adenylcyclase; and
c) the intracellular synthesis of cyclic nucleotides. Some
steps of this sequential process have been demonstrated with

certain hormones (Kook & Trainin 1975), while not yet sub-
stantiated with others. It seems that the basal levels of
cAMP are definitely increased by some thymic hormones (Kook
& Trainin 1975; Yakir et al. 1978; Trainin et al. 1979),
while others rather activate cGMP (Goldstein et al. 1980;
Sunshine et al. 1978)

At any rate, though the precise biochemical *modus
operandi* is not totally understood for each thymic preparation, their biological functions are well established.
Thymic hormones are involved in T-cell ontogenesis at the 3
levels known for these cells, thus including the bone
marrow, the thymus gland and the peripheral lymphoid system.
The evaluation of biological activity of thymic hormones is
based on assessment of induction of T-cell specific membranal markers and functions expressing cellular immune competence. The parameters studied at the membranal level
entailed those antigenic markers related to T-cell differentiation including Thy-1, Lyt and TL in mice and E-rosettes
(E), active E-rosettes (AE), T-lymphocyte antigen (HTLA) and
OKT subsets in humans. Enzymes associated with stages of
cell differentiation, such as terminal deoxynucleotidyl-
transferase (TdT) and functional assays including the proliferative responses to T-mitogens (PHA and Con-A), allogeneic stimulation in the mixed lymphocyte culture (MLC),
cell-mediated lymphocytotoxicity (CML) and the graft-versus-
host (GvH) reactivity have further extended our knowledge.
Secretory functions of lymphocytes, such as the production
of leucocyte or macrophage migration inhibition-factor (LIF,
MIF), T-cell growth factor (TCGF, IL-2), immune interferon
(IF) and lymphocytotoxin (LTx) have also been used for the
measurement of thymic hormone activity in in vitro and,
moreover, in in vivo models, thus understressing their physiological role.

Patients suffering from malignancies in general and
from lympho or myeloproliferative disorders in particular,
live now longer, as the result of improved combined chemotherapy or radiochemotherapy. One of the major side-effects
of these therapeutic modalities consists, however, of severs
immune suppression, affecting mainly cell-mediated immunity,
which becomes more protracted, as the treatment proceeds.
This serious side-effect restricts frequently the extension
and the efficacy of the current antineoplastic protocols.
The awareness towards these iatrogenic immunodeficiency
states is justified since this clinical condition is

accompanied by a marked enhancement of the susceptibility of the treated patients to potentially fatal ubiquitous infections, such as Herpes group viruses, Pneumocystis carinii, etc.

Thymic hormones, having the potential for enhancement of cell-mediated immune functions and possibly for restoration of impaired immunological balance seem to be ideal candidates for cancer adunct immunotherapy. This attitude is strengthened by some preliminary data of therapeutic trials with thymic hormones, pointing at these substances as devoid of undesirable side-effects along or following their use. Treatment with relatively high doses of thymosin fraction 5 has shown a beneficial effect as an adjuvant in a group of patients with small cell carcinoma of the lung. This was manifested in a reversal of depressed levels of circulating T-cells and a prolongation of survival, compared to a similar group of patients receiving chemotherapy alone (Cohen et al. 1979). An other recent study suggests a similar trend in a trial on head and neck cancer patients treated with thymosin fraction 5 and local irradiation (Wara et al. 1981). The immunostimulating effect of thymostimulin on peripheral blood lymphocytes and its favorable effect on Varicella-Zoster infections occurring in immune compromised cancer patients has been reported (Tovo & Nicola 1980). In more than 50 patients affected with lymphoproliferative or myeloproliferative disorders, THF has been shown to consistently restore a battery of severely suppressed cell-mediated immune functions and to combat effeciently herpetic and Varicella-Zoster viral infections (Zaizov et al. 1979; Handzel et al. 1981). THF triggers the proliferation of lymphocytes towards the T-cell lineage. This is expressed in a chain of events starting with lymphocytosis followed by an increase in E-rosettes and later by an augmentation of T-cell functions manifested by higher reactivity against T-mitogens, delayed hypersensitivity tests and antiviral activity. In addition, THF has expressed an immune regulating effect in some leukemic patients and in one patient with Histiocytosis-X, restoring the balance between T-cell suppressor/cytotoxic and helper/inducer subpopulations as judged by monitoring with anti T-cell monoclonal antibodies (Trainin et al. 1982). A restoration of NK activity to normal values seems to occur as the later stage in this sequential process. In children with AML, THF as immuno-adjuvant to chemotherapy in remission maintenance, have enabled to maintain immunocompetency and to reduce the

incidence of opportunistic infections. Although the contribution of THF in the improved survival observed, is not yet
conclusive, THF therapy provided the adequate conditions to
adminster the optimal scheduled intensive chemotherapy.
(Zaizov et al. unpublished results).

Since tumor cells are characterized, among many other
features, by antigenic changes, the possibility of a direct
effect of thymic hormones on local tumor growth and metastatic spread should be considered. Trainin and Small (1978)
have demonstrated inhibition of growth of transplanted
tumors in mice by THF. They have suggested that this effect
could be mediated by a shift in T-cell subpopulations from
immature-enhancing to mature-inhibiting tumor growth cells.
Preincubation of lymphocytes with a crude thymic preparation
also reduced the rate of growth of Lewis tumor cells in a
Winn test in mice (Cupissol et al. 1981). Human prealbumin,
which is considered by some authors as responsible for more
than 95% of the total thymic hormone-like activity present
in human blood, was shown recently to augment secondary
cell-mediated immune responses in vitro and to increase the
capacity of mice to reject a transplantable mammary tumor
(Leung et al. 1982). Similarly, treatment with thymostimulin retarded the rate of growth of primary tumors and
increased survival of tumor-bearing mice by delaying the
appearance of distant metastases. Moreover, a marked
synergistic effect of thymostimulin with chemotherapy was
noted (Klein & Shoham 1981). Also, thymosin fraction 5 has
been shown to improve the effect of cyclophosphamide on the
growth of a MOPC-315 plasmacytoma in mice (Serrou et al.
1981). It has been suggested that thymosin fraction 5
blocks the expression of suppressor activity of lymphocytes
more abundant in cancer bearing patients, thus possibly
acting as an immunomodulator which increases antitumor
helper function (Zatz et al. 1981). Finally, in a beautiful
experimental model, Small (1982) has demonstrated that
immature T-lymphocytes with tumor enhancing potential have,
by the same token, suppressor properties on other lymphoid
cells and bear Fc receptors, thus enabling the binding of
immune complexes to their surface.

This experimental and clinical body of information
points to the possibility of the use of thymic hormones as
biological modifiers in immune suppressed cancer patients.
By driving immature T-cells towards differentiation and
maturation, thymic hormones may affect the balance between

cytotoxic/suppressor and helper/inducer T-cell supopula-
tions. Alternatively, it is also plausible that different
thymic hormones act selectively and more specifically on
certain T-cell subsets. The disclosure of the exact mode
of action of each of the members of the thymic hormone
family on the numerous components of the lymphoid system
is certainly a required aim for their appropriate use in
cancer patients.

Bach JF, Carnaud C (1976). Thymic Factors. Prog Allergy
    21:342.
Bach JF, Dardenne M (1973). Studies on thymic products. II
    Demonstration and characterization of circulating thymic
    hormone. Immunology 25:353.
Bergesi G, Falchetti R (1977). Caratterizione chimica ed
    attivita biologica d'un nuovo estratto timico. Folia
    Allergol Immunol Clin 24:204.
Cohen MH, Chretien PB, Ihde DC, Fossieck BE, Jr, Makuch R,
    Bunn PA, Jr, Johnston AV, Shackney SE, Matthews MJ,
    Lipson SD, Kenady DE, Minna JD (1979). Thymosin fraction
    V and intensive combination chemotherapy. JAMA 241:1813.
Cupissol D, Touraine JL, Serrou B (1981). Ability of lympho-
    cytes treated with thymic factor to decrease lung metas-
    tasis in tumor-bearing mice. Thymus 3:9.
Dardenne M, Pleau JM, Savino W, Bach JF (1982). Monoclonal
    antibody against the serum thymic factor (FTS). Immunol
    Letters 4:79.
Goldstein AL, Low TLK, Thurman GB (1980). Thymosin: Basic
    properties and clinical application in the treatment of
    immunodeficiency diseases and cancer. In Beers RF, Jr.,
    & Bassett EG (eds):"Polypeptide Hormones" N.Y.: Raven
    Press, p. 449.
Goldstein G (1974). Isolation of a bovine thymic, a poly-
    peptide hormone of the thymus. Nature 247:11.
Goldstein G, Sheid MP, Boyse EA, Schlesinger DH, Van Wauwe
    J (1979). A synthetic pentapeptide with biological acti-
    vity characteristic of the thymic hormone thymopoietin.
    Science 204:1309.
Handzel ZT, Zaizov R, Varsano I, Levin S, Pecht M, Trainin
    N (1981). The influence of thymic humoral factor on immu-
    noproliferative disorders and viral infections in humans.
    Advances in Immunopharmacology P. 83.
Hirokawa K, McClure JE, Goldstein AL (1982). Age-related
    changes in localization of thymosin in the human thymus.
    Thymus 4:19.
Hooper JA, McDaniel MC, Thurman GB, Cohen CH, Schulof RS,

Goldstein AL (1975). Purification and properties of bovine thymosin. Ann N.Y. Acad Sci 249:125.

Klein AS, Shoham J (1981). Effect of the thymic factor, thymostimulin (TP-1), on the survival rate of tumor-bearing mice. Cancer Res 41:3217.

Kook AI, Trainin N (1975). Intracellular events involved in the induction of immune competence in lymphoid cells by a thymus humoral factor. J Immunol 114:151.

Kook AI, Yakir Y, Trainin N (1975). Isolation and partial chemical characterization of THF, a thymus hormone involved in immune maturation of lymphoid cells. Cell Immunol 19:151.

Leung KH, Ehrke MJ, Bercsenyi K, Mihich E (1982). Human prealbumin fraction: Effects on cell-mediated immunity and tumor rejection. Immunopharmacology 4:55.

Levey RH, Trainin N, Law LW (1963). Evidence for function of thymic tissue diffusion chambers implanted in neonatally thymectomized mice. Preliminary report. J Natl Cancer Inst 31:199.

Marshall GD, Jr, Thurman GB, Low TLK, Goldstein AL (1980). Thymosin: Basic properties and clinical application in the treatment of immunodeficiency diseases and cancer. Recent Results Cancer Res 75:100.

Pleau JM, Dardenne M, Blouquit Y, Bach JF (1977). Structural study of circulating thymic factor: A peptide isolated from pig serum. II. Amino acid sequence. J Biol Chem 252:8045.

Schmitt D, Monier C, Dardenne M, Pleau JM, Deschaux P, Bach JF (1980). Cytoplasmic localization of FTS (facteur thymique serique) in thymic epithelial cells. An immunoelectromicroscopic study. Thymus 2:177.

Serrou B, Cupissol D, Caraux J, Thierry C, Rosenfeld C, Goldstein AL (1980). Ability of thymosin to decrease in vivo and in vitro suppressor cell activity in tumor bearing mice and cancer patients. Recent Results Cancer Res 75:110.

Small M (1982). Tumor enhancing T-lymphocytes in mice: Further studies on characteristics and mechanism of activity. Int J Cancer 29:465.

Sunshine GH, Bash RS, Coffey RG, Cohen KW, Goldstein G, Hadden JW (1978). Thymopoietin enhances the allogeneic response and cyclic GMP levels of mouse peripheral, thymus-derived lymphocytes. J Immunol 120:1594.

Tovo PA, Nicola P (1980). TP-1 therapy in patients with secondary immunodeficiencies. In Aiuti F & Wigzell H (eds): "Thymus, Thymic Hormones and T lymphocytes" London:

Academic Press, p. 307.

Trainin N, Handzel ZT, Pecht M, Netzer L, Elmalek M, Zaizov R (1982). The role of THF, a thymic hormone, as a regulator of T-cell differentiation in humans. In Serrou B et al. (eds): "Current Cocepts in Human Immunology and Cancer Immunomodulation" Elsevier Biomedical Press B.V. p. 85.

Trainin N, Rotter V, Yakir Y, Leve R, Handzel ZT, Shohat B, Zaizov R (1979). Biochemical and biological properties of THF in animal and human models. Ann N.Y. Acad Sci 333:9.

Trainin N, Small M (1978). T-lymphocytes and modulation of tumor growth. Comprehensive Therapy 4:31.

Wara WM, Neely MH, Ammann AJ, Wara DW (1981). Biologic modification of immunologic parameters in head and neck cancer patients with thymosin fraction V. Limphokines and thymic hormones: Their potential utilization in cancer therapeutics. p. 257.

Yakir Y, Kook AI, Trainin N (1978). Enrichment of in vitro and in vivo immunologic activity of purified fractions of calf thymic hormone (THF). J Exp Med 148:71.

Zaizov R, Vogel R, Wolach B, Cohen IJ, Varsano V, Shohat B, Handzel ZT, Rotter V, Yakir Y, Trainin N (1979). The effect of THF in lymphoproliferative and myeloproliferative diseases in children. N.Y. Acad Sci p. 172.

Zatz MM, Glaser M, Seals CM, Goldstein AL (1981). Effects of combined cyclophosphamide and thymosin treatment on tumor growth and host survival in mice bearing a syngeneic tumor. Lymphokines and thymic hormones: Their potential utilization in cancer therapeutics. p. 249.

13th International Cancer Congress, Part E
Cancer Management, pages 305–314

MODIFICATION OF TUMOR CELL ANTIGEN

Hiroshi Kobayashi, M.D.
Professor Laboratory of Pathology
Cancer Institute
Hokkaido University School of Medicine
Sapporo 060, Japan

The term Biological Response Modifiers, or "BRM", is a general term for agents which modify tumor-host relationships, resulting in longer survival of the host not by the direct killing of tumor cells but by the modification of biological responses. The term "BRM" includes not only immunological approaches as the use of microbial adjuvant, polysaccharides, synthetic agents but also approaches for modifying biological responses such as the use of Interferon, Interferon inducers, thymic hormones and other agents, all of which may lead to a better situation for the host and to a worse situation for the tumor cell. However, the concept of "bRM" also involves tumor factors such as the idea of differentiating tumor cells from undifferentiated to highly differentiated, by which differentiation tumors in the host may become more benign in a broad biological sense.

It ought to be emphasized further that the increase in the immunogenicity of tumor cells may also improve the tumor-host relationship for the host while worsening it for the tumor cell. The complete definition of BRM, therefore, involves not only all agents active against the host, but also various means active against tumor cells, in which an increase in the immunogenicity of tumor cells or modification of tumor antigen is a major factor involved here.

There are number of ways to modify tumor antigens by means of viruses, chemicals, mutagen, enzymes, interferon and other agents. In this article, a couple of experiments for modifying tumor cell antigen by viruses is shown.

Table 1. Biological Response Modifiers

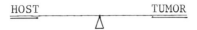

HOST	TUMOR

1) Immunopotentiators

    Microbiol
    adjuvant
      BCG
      Nocardia
      CWS
      OK432
      etc
    Polysaccharides
      PSK
      Lentinan
      etc

    Synthetic agents
      Levamisole
      Bestatin
      etc

2) Interferon

3) Thymic hormones

1) Differentiation

2) Increase in
   immunogenicity
   (Modification
   of tumor
   antigen)

    Virus
    Chemicals
    Mutagen
    Enzyme
    Interferon
    etc

When a murine leukemia virus such as Friend, Rauscher or Gross is injected into newborn rats, virus-induced leukemias or lymphomas develop 100-200 days after birth. It is interesting that these tumors are all unable to grow in syngeneic normal rats, while they grow and kill all virus-tolerant rats neonatally injected with the corresponding virus (table 2).

The same is true in MCA-induced tumors developed in virus tolerant rats. When MCA is sc injected into Friend virus tolerant rats which have been neonatally injected with Friend virus, the developed MCA-induced tumors are also unable to grow in syngeneic normal rats, while they grow and kill Friend virus tolerant rats or immunologically suppressed rats.

Table 2. Regression of various tumors developed in murine leukemia virus-tolerant WKA rats.

Tumors	Lethal growth in	
	Normal syngeneic rat	Each virus tolerant rat
Friend virus induced tumors (13 lines)	3/168 (1.8%)	455/465 (97.8%)
Rauscher virus-induced tumors (7 lines)	0/48 (0%)	99/99 (100%)
Gross virus-induced tumors (10 lines)	0/50 (0%)	98/101 (97.0%)
MCA-induced tumors in Friend virus-tolerant rats (2 lines)	0/18 (0%)	18/18 (100%)

The reason for this curious transplantation result is that the tumor cells developed in each virus tolerant rat possess a new foreign antigen derived from the virus which was obtained from the spleen of "mice". Rats and mice are of different species, so that if rat tumor cells possess an antigen derived from the virus which was obtained from mice, the tumor cells are unable to grow in syngeneic normal rats, because the tumor cells which possess such a foreign antigen are recognized by the rat as foreign and will thus be rejected. But in the virus-tolerant rats the tumor cells possessing such an antigen are able to grow and kill these rats, because these rats are immunologically tolerant to such a new foreign antigen.

Next, attempts have been made to produce spontaneous regression of the tumor by infection of tumors with a virus artificially. The ordinary types of virus-unrelated transplantable tumors such as spontaneously developed sarcomas, MCA-induced sarcomas, 4NQO-induced lung cancer, NBU-induced breast cancers and leukemia, and DAB-induced hepatomas were all artificially infected with foreign antigenic virus (in this experiment, for example, with Friend virus) to make rat tumor cells of these lines foreign by attaching foreign antigenic viruses to them (table 3).

Table 3. Regression of various tumors artificially infected with Friend virus into syngeneic and autochthonous rats

Tumor infected with virus		Lethal growth (%)	
Spont-sarcoma:	WST-5	0/26	(0)
	Takeda	6/25	(26.1)
	KST-1	0/25	(0)
MCA-sarcoma:	KMT-17	0/443	(0)
	KMT-19	0/80	(0)
	KMT-50	0/17	(0)
	AMC-60	0/10	(0)
		0/2	(0)*
4NQO-lung cancer:	DLT	0/28	(0)
NBU-breast cancer:	KBT-1	0/12	(0)
	KBT-2	0/8	(0)
DAB-hepatoma:	AH109	2/8	(25.0)
	KDH-8	0/58	(0)
NBU-leukemia:	KNL-1	0/15	(0)**
In total:		8/755	(1.1)

* Autochthonous host.   ** Tumors recurred 2-3 months after the regression in all cases.

Various types of rat tumors which are capable of killing all normal syngeneic hosts are unable to grow in syngeneic and autochthonous hosts, when these tumors have previously been infected with a foreign antigenic virus. Even if they grow initially, they eventually regress. A thousand rats have been used for this type of experiment using other types of foreign antigenic viruses as well with the indication that all types of rat tumors including carcinomas and sarcomas are unable to grow in syngeneic or autochthonous hosts, if they have been artificially infected with foreign antigenic viruses. This should be the first model of so-called "spontaneous regression" of these tumors.

In this experiment, there is no need for the total population of tumor cells to be infected with viruses. Depending on the original immunogenicity in each tumor line, 30 to 80% of viral antigen-positive tumor cells will be sufficient to cause all tumor tissues to regress.

In the above model system, virus infection generates a foreign antigen on the surface of the tumor cell. It is also possible that a new foreign antigen could be generated on the surface of a tumor cell by treating the tumor cell with a mutagen. This would mean that the previously mentioned immunologicall regression of tumors could also be obtained following the production of new foreign antigens with chemicals as well. Dr. Tierry Boon of Belgium, treated various types of tumor cells with the chemical mutagen MNNG, and obtained cell variants that are unable to grow in syngeneic mice. This work suggests that the procedure of using a mutagen to generate nontumorigenic variants carrying new foreign transplantation antigens may be applicable to modifying tumor cell-immunogenicity.

Here, we see two possibly different ways of alienating or modifying tumor cells in the host. One is to increase the immunogenicity of formerly existing tumor specific or associated TAA antigen. Cancer immunology has till now focused on how to increase the immunogenicity of TAA. The main aim of increasing TAA-immunogenicity is to obtain potential TAA-vaccine from tumor cells. However, there may be a certain limit to the increasing of the immunogenicity of TAA antigen, since its immunogenicity is originally very weak.

Instead, a new approach has arisen, to produce new foreign antigen on the tumor cell surface artificially. In other words, the tumor cells having such a new foreign antigen —— a virus specific or associated VAA antigen in this case —— are comparatively highly immunogenic, so that the tumors regress spontaneously.

Therefore, these two ways of increasing the immunogenicity of TAA, and of producing new foreign VAA antigen on the cell surface are involved in increasing the entire foreignness of tumor cells.

We have coined the word "Xenogenization" of tumor cells for all such trials. Xenos means foreign in Latin, and the

concept of Xenogenization is to make a tumor cell foreign as
a new model of Biological Response Modifiers.

It is of interest that TAA-immunogenicity also increases
after the production of new foreign antigen. It is also of
interest that tumor cells having a new foreign VAA antigen
are unable to grow lethally in the host. Therefore, such
tumor cells may be used as a potentioal viable tumor cell-
vaccine.

Table 4 indicates the result of immunotherapy with
viable xenogenized tumor cells in order to inhibit metastasis after surgery of the original tumor. 28 out of 65
rats (43%) died of metastasis in the host immunized with
viable xenogeniged tumor cells, while in a control group,
38 out of 56 rats (68%) died of metastasis if subsequent
immunotherapy was not performed. The effect of immunotherapy
using such viable tumor cell-vaccine is not so dramatic in
inhibiting the development of metastasis, but the difference
between the immunotherapy and control groups is statistically
significant. It has been concluded, therefore, that viable
xenogenized tumor cells may be used as a potential specific
tumor cell-vaccine in the experimental therapeutics of
cancer.

Table 4. Immunotherapy with viable xenogenized tumor cells
(KMT-17) against the metastasis of original tumor cells

Treatment	Metastasis*
Immunotherapy with viable xenogenized tumor cells after surgery	28/65 (43%) P< 0.01
Surgery alone	38/56 (68%)

* Two-month observation.

For the past several decades, many investigators have
attempted to increase the TAA-immunogenicity. However, it
seems now that tumor cells persistently infected with nonlytic foreign virus are the most appropriate candidates for
the elucidation of TAA-immunogenicity. As shown in table 5,

the LTD50 of transplanted KMT-17 tumor in a host immunized
with viable xenogenized tumor cells was remarkablly increased.

Table 5. TAA-immunogenicity of high and low immunogenic
tumor cells with various treatment

Treatment of tumor cells for immunization	LTD50 of tumors	
	High immunogenic (KMT-17)	low immunogenic (KDH-8)
Virus-infection* (1X)	1,000X (sc) 10,000X (id)	40X (id)
Formalin, Mitomycin C (0.2%, 3X)	5-10X	1-3X
Crude membrane	1-5X	
Oncolysate	5-10X	
Irradiation (6,000 rad, 3X)	200X	20X
None	1X	1X

* Persistently infected nonlytic foreign antigenic virus.

    The LTD50 in normal host was 1X, or approx 1,000 cells
while the LTD50 in a host immunized with xenogenized tumor
cells was 1,000X or 1,000,000 cells with sc-immunization and
more than 10,000X or 10,000,000 cells with intradermal
immunization. This is a remarkable difference in rechallenge
resistance. The increase in LTD50 in those immunized with
tumor cell-vaccine inactivated by formalin, MMC was 5-10X,
and that in those immunized with crude membrane and oncoly-
sate was 1-10X. The LTD50 in a host immunized 3 times with
irradiated tumor cells was 200X. Therefore, viable xenogenized tumor cells infected with foreign virus do seem to
produce the strongest anti-tumor specific immunity. One
reason that such xenogenized tumor cells can produce the
strongest immunogenicity may be caused by the fact that the
vaccine used for immunization consists of viable intact
tumor cells which may produce massive effector T-cells.

However, there is an appropriate condition for production of higher immunogencity in virus-infected xenogenized tumor cells. In a word, an excessive amount of VAA may often decrease TAA-immunogenicity, and the passage of tumor cells through a virus-tolerant host for 2-4 generations (having 80% VAA-positive cells) may be the most appropriate condition for the production of the highest TAA-immunogenicity with only one intradermal immunization.

Comparison has been made between the TAA-immunogenicity of viable xenogenized tumor cells and tumor cells mixed with living BCG under the optimal conditions. The immunogenicity of the viable xenogenized tumor cells is definitely higher than that of the viable tumor cells mixed with living BCG in general. For example, when 1,000 - 100,000 viable tumor cells were used for immunization and $10^7 - 10^8$ tumor cells were challenged, a marked differences between xenogenized tumor cell-immune group and BCG-tumor mixture-immune group is observed. Although it is difficult to generalize these results with regards to all other types of tumor, it seems that viable xenogenized tumor cells are more highly immunogenic than the BCG-tumor mixture.

It is said that tumor cells mixed with bacteria are sometimes strongly immunogenic. In fact, the immunogenicity of the BCG-tumor mixture is very strong in our experiment as well. However, if the immunogenicity of xenogenized tumor cells was actually stronger than that of a BCG tumor cell-mixture, it would be explained by the fact that the vicinal association of TAA and VAA on the cell surface results in stronger immunogenicity than that achieved by the mixture, which does not have such antigenic vicinity, since in the mixture there may be no changes in the tumor cell-membrane.

Unfortunately, we have to recognize that the KMT-17 tumor cells used in these experiments have a comparatively high antigenic property, while in a low and non-immunogenic tumors such as KDH-8 liver cell cancer, the inhibitory effect against the challenge of the tumor is limited, even if viable xenogenized tumor cells are used for immunization. The increase in LTD50 by id immunization with viable xenogenized KDH-8 tumor cells is only 40X, which is lower than that in the KMT-17 of the former experiment (Table 5)

Therefore, there might be a certain limit to the application of the cencept of xenogenizing or modifying tumor cells for the active specific immunotherapy of human cancers, since most human cancers seem to be low or non-immunogenic. However, attempts should be made to produce a new foreign antigen for the spontaneous regression of such non-immunogenic tumors, instead of attempting to increase the weak TAA-immunogenicity.

Table 6. Modification of tumor cell antigen

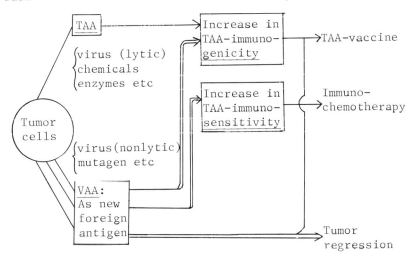

In summary, TAA-immunogenicity may be increased by viruses, chemicals, enzymes and other agents, but the grade of its increase in general is not so dramatic. However, when new foreign antigen, particularly foreign virus-related VAA-antigen is produced on the cell surface, tumors regress by themselves immunologically regardless of their original TAA-immunogenicity. TAA-immunogenicity also increases concomitantly if tumor cells are xenogenized by viruses, so that such viable tumor cells possessing foreign VAA antigen can be used experimentally as a potential TAA-vaccine as already stated.

Furthermore, it is interesting that the TAA-immuno-sensitivity of tumor cells also increases when a new foreign antigen is produced. It is possible to measure the immuno-sensitivity of tumor cells, since in this case tumor cells may survive under certain conditions without cytolysis. Nonlytic foreign virus-infected tumor cells are more sensitive to immunoreactions such as complement-dependent

cytotoxicity and lymphocyte-mediated cytotoxicity when
compared to noninfected tumor cells, and also possiblly more
sensitive to immunochemotherapy as well even if tumors do
not regress by themselves.

REFERENCES

Hosokawa M, Okayasu T, Ikeda K, Katoh H, Suzuki Y, Kobayashi
H (submitted). Variable expression of immunogenicity of
xenogenized tumor cells in syngeneic rats with special
reference to existing-time of immunizing cells in hosts.
Cancer Res.
Kobayashi H, Hosokawa M, Takeichi N, Sendo F, Kodama T
(1969). Transplantable Friend virus-induced tumors in
rats. Cancer Res 29:1385.
Kobayashi H, Sendo F, Kaji H, Shirai T, Saito H, Takeichi N,
Hosokawa M, Kodama T (1970). Inhibition of transplanted
rat tumors by immunization with identical tumor cells in-
fected with Friend virus. J Nat Cancer Inst 44:11.
Kobayashi H, Kodama T, Gotohda E (1977). "Xenogenization of
Tumor Cells." (Hokkaido University Medical Library Series,
Vol. 9) Sapporo: Hokkaido University School of Medicine.
Kobayashi H, Takeichi N, Kuzumaki N (1978). "Xenogenization
of Lymphocytes, Erythroblasts, and Tumor Cells." (Hokkaido
University Medical Library Series, Vol. 10) Sapporo:
Hokkaido University School of Medicine.
Kobayashi H, Sendo F (1979). Immunogenicity of viable xeno-
genized tumor cells. In Kobayashi H (ed): "GANN Monogr
Cancer Res Vol. 23" Tokyo: Japan Scientific Societies
Press, P 27.
Kobayashi H (1979). Viral xenogenization of intact tumor
cells. Adv Cancer Res 30:279.
Kobayashi H (1982). Modification of tumor antigenicity in
therapeutics: Increase in immunologic foreignness of tumor
cells in experimental model systems. In Mihich E (ed):
"Immunological Approaches to Cancer Therapeutics", New
York: Johan Wiley & Sons, Inc, P 405.
Yamaguchi H, Moriuchi T, Hosokawa M, Kobayashi H (1982).
Increased or decreased immunogenicity of tumor-associated
antigen according to the amount of virus-associated antigen
in rat tumor cells infected with Friend virus. Cancer
Immunol Immunother 12:119.

13th International Cancer Congress, Part E
Cancer Management, pages 315–325
© 1983 Alan R. Liss, Inc., 150 Fifth Avenue, New York, NY 10011

CURRENT CLINICAL STATUS OF INTERFERON AND MANAGEMENT OF CANCER IN MAN

Julius S. Horoszewicz, M.D., D.M.Sc. and
Edwin A. Mirand, Ph.D., D.Sc.
Department of Biological Resources
Roswell Park Memorial Institute
Buffalo, N.Y.

Better management of several cancers in man requires the introduction of new therapeutic approaches rigorously evaluated in controlled clinical trials. Natural products capable of physiological modulation of biological events are rapidly moving toward the top of the list of potentially useful anti-cancer drugs. Several years of basic laboratory studies accompanied by progress in technology of production and purification led to the current availability of some of these substances for testing in human neoplasia. This brief review will focus on human interferons.

Human interferons are a group of secretory glycoproteins produced by human cells following appropriate stimulation. Interferon molecules are carriers of potent biological activities. The antiviral, antiproliferative and immunomodulatory interferon functions could benefit the cancer patient and are of obvious interest to the clinician.

The discovery of interferon dates back to 1957, when Isaacs and Lindenmann (1957) found that viruses could trigger secretion by an infected cell of a substance which in turn can render other cells resistant to infection not only by the same virus, but a variety of other viruses as well. It was also recognized that interferon activity was considerably restricted by species barriers existing between cells of different origin. In addition to viruses, a wide array of natural and synthetic molecules could stimulate cells to produce interferon. So far, no obvious structural similarities common to all interferon inducers were found. The "interferon system" consists of inducer which derepresses the cellular interferon genes, leading to the transcription of an appropriate messenger RNA. This RNA is translated into the interferon polypeptide chain which subseqently is subjected to epigenetic glycosylation and secretion into the extracellular fluid. The secreted interferon molecules interact then with specific receptor present on cellular membrane of surrounding and distant cells. Subsequently, a whole cascade of events activates genes responsible for antiviral resistance and a multitude of changes in cell physiology and structure. The amount of interferon synthesized by a single cell is less than 10 femtograms. However, the biologic activity compares favorably with the most potent polypeptide hormones, and could be detected at concentrations below 10^{-13} molar. Measurments of interferon popotency are based on biological assay of its antiviral activity in cell culture systems calibrated with an appropriate standard preparation and expressed in International Units (IU).

The classification and nomenclature of interferons is based in part on antigenicity, chemical structure and cellular origin (Stewart et al., 1980). HuIFNα, known as leukocyte interferon is produced by B-lymphocytes, lymphoblasts, null lymphocytes and macrophages in response to viruses, foreign cells and B-mitogens. HuIFNβ, known as fibroblast interferon originates from fibroblasts or epithelial cells stimulated with natural or synthetic double stranded ribonucleic acid. HuIFNγ, known as immune interferon is elaborated by T-lymphocytes upon induction-sensitization by T-mitogens or foreign antigens.

Recent advances in recombinant DNA technology led to cloning and expression of individual human interferon genes in either bacteria or yeasts Derynck et al., 1980, Hitzeman et al., 1981, Rubinstein et al., 1979). This overcomes in principle limitations on basic and clinical studies imposed by the excessive cost and insufficient amounts of interferon protein available. Over 10 human genes which code for the production of different interferon species were recognized and their DNA sequences determined. Recombinant DNA products lack sugar moieties, which are bound to interferons secreted by human cells. Strong evidence, however, is mounting that such carbohydrates are dispensable for either antigenicity or the recognized spectrum of interferon biological activities (Rubenstein et al., 1979).

Regardless of source all interferons intended for clinical application must be purified several thousand-fold to remove, or at least reduce the accompanying bio-products. This is accomplished by sophisticated chromatographic procedures utilizing a variety of ligants (eg: lectins,

hydrophobic molecules, monoclonal antibodies, etc.
(Berg et al., 1981-82, Secher et al., 1980, Sulkowski 1981-82). The specific activity of pure human interferon α has been estimated at between 2 and 4 x 10^8 IU per mg protein, molecular weight at 16,500-21,000 and the sequence of all 165 amino acids determined (Rubenstein et al., 1979, Streuli et al., 1980). Human interferons β and γ have higher molecular weights (up to 25,000) due to more extensive glycosylation (Moschera et al., 1981-82).

The details of molecular mechanism of interferon actions are not completely understood. The modulation of protein synthesis in interferon treated cells could be linked to activation of protein kinase phosphorylating eIF-2, one of the initiation factors of protein translation. Interferon also enhances the level of (2'-5') oligoiso-adenylate synthetase. The products of this enzyme action on ATP trigger a latent endoribonuclease which in turn degrades messenger RNA, thus further impairing protein synthesis (Lengyel, 1981).

In addition to antiviral effects, other functions of interferon were extensively studied since 1962. Interferon inhibits directly cell multiplication in vitro and in vivo of both normal and malignant cells (Bradley et al., 1981, Paucker et al., 1962). The inhibition is reversible and in only few instances cytopathic effect or killing occurs. Susceptibility to interferon could vary among human cells derived from histologically similar tumors of different individuals. Rapidly proliferating cell populations appear to be less sensitive, than cells in a quiescent state (Horoszewicz et al., 1979). Reversible arrest of normal myeloid cells differentiation (Verma et al., 1979) is the presumed mechanism responsible for leukopenia in patients treated with interferon.

The effects of interferon on the immune system are apparent, but only partially understood. Low doses increase antibody production, while large doses have a suppressive effect (Braun et al., 1972). Hypersensitivity reactions are potentiated, but graft versus host response is diminished (DeMaeyer et al., 1980). Activation of macrophages and enhancement of phagocytosis are readily demonstrable (Imanishi et al., 1975). Natural killer (NK) cells are rapidly stimulated by minute concentrations of interferon (Zarling et al., 1979). However, the extrapolation of this phenomenon to anti-tumor effect is far from simple. Initial augmentation of NK activity during interferon therapy gives way on prolonged administration to suppression of NK cells

(Pape, et al., 1981). To complicate the matter further, it was reported that exposure of tumor cells to interferon renders them less susceptible to the action of NK cells (Trinchieri et al., 1978). Moreover, new observations indicate that interferon activation of lymphocytes enhances lytic potential against allogeneic, but not autologous biopsy derived tumor cells (Vanky et al., 1982). A controversy also exists whether interferon can augment antibody dependent cell mediated cytotoxicity (ADCC). At least some of the effects of interferon on the immune system, as well as modulation of the cellular proliferation and differentiation, could result from alterations of the plasma membrane-cytoskeletal complex. Following exposure to interferon, greater rigidity of plasma membrane, changes in microfilament organization and increased organization of cell surface fibronectin is evident (Pfeffer et al., 1980). It should be pointed out that the general trend of such changes appears to counteract some of the recognized phenotypic properties of neoplastic and transformed cells. This would imply that interferon might be capable of suppressing the malignant potential of tumors.

Basic studies on interferon provided evidence of multiple biological effects suggestive of clinical potential. Thus strong scientific rationale was established for controlled clinical trials to seek pertinent data and to reach conclusions about safety, pharmacokinetics and therapeutic efficacy in human disease (Borden EC, 1979, Merigan TC, 1981). Phase I clinical studies have demonstrated that treatment with high doses of interferon is safe: in excess of 100 million units of recombinant DNA interferon α, and 10 to 30 million IU of natural interferons α or β were tolerated when injected I.M. or I.V. 3X a week for a prolonged time (Hawkins et al., 1982, Horoszewicz et al., 1980, Oldham et al., 1982). Dose-dependent side effects such as fever, headache, chills, malaise, fatigue, anorexia, moderate alopecia, leukopenia, transient elevation of hepatic transaminases in serum and occasional mental confusion (Gutterman et al., 1980, Hawkins et al., 1982, Scott et al.,1981) occur with variable frequencies. None of these side effects, however are life threatening and they disappear rapidly upon cessation of interferon treatment. It is increasingly apparent that systemic toxic manifestations in man are inherently linked to the biological properties of interferon molecules and are not abolished by extensive purification.

Pharmacokinetics studies (Gutterman et al., 1980, Hawkins et al., 1982, Horoszewicz et al., 1980) show that

interferon is rapidly cleared from the circulation and high
serum levels are difficult to maintain. The catabolism
of interferon appears to take place in the liver and kidneys,
but interferon is not excreted in urine. Instead, it is
broken down in the lysosomes of tubular cells following
reabsorption from the glomerular filtrate (Bocci V, 1981-82).
The clinical significance of circulating interferon is unclear. For example: human interferon β after intramuscular injection is practically not detectable in the serum,
despite demonstrable systemic, anti-tumor and immunological
effects (Horoszewicz et al., 1980, Quesada et al., 1982).
In contrast, high concentrations of interferon in the cere-
bro-spinal fluid are preserved for several hours by the
blood-brain barrier after direct injections into Ommaya
reservoir or intrathecal space (Horoszewicz et al., 1980).

Pharmacologic potency of interferon therapy was
confirmed by positive responses in the treatment of respiratory virus infections (Merigan et al., 1973), chronic
viral hepatitis B (Greenberg et al., 1976), disseminated
varicella-zoster (Arvin et al., 1978, Merigan TC, 1978),
cytomegalovirus infections (Cheescman et al., 1979), herpes
simplex (Pazin et al., 1979), and keratitis caused by
herpes simplex, adenovirus and vaccinia viruses (Romano
et al., 1980, Sundmacher et al., 1978).

Clinical trials in cancer demonstrated an apparent
therapeutic activity against osteogenic sarcome (Strander
H, 1977), multiple myeloma(Mellstedt et al., 1979), Hodgkin's
disease (Blomgren et al., 1976), lymphoma (Merigan et al.,
1978), acute leukemia (Hill et al., 1979), melanoma
(Borgström et al., 1982, Horoszewicz et al., 1978), breast
cancer (Gutterman et al., 1980, Murphy GP, 1981, Quesada
et al., 1982), renal cell carcinoma (Murphy GP, 1981,
Quesada et al., 1983), laryngeal papilloma (Dunnick et al.,
1979) and certain brain tumors (for review see Merigan TC,
1981). This long list of responding tumors ought to be
viewed with the clear understanding that only a fraction
of patients benefited from interferon and that so far
neither optimal dosage, length and frequency of treatment,
mode of parenteral delivery, nor definition of therapeutic
indications have been established. It also is uncertain
which of the known human interferons could offer the
greatest therapeutic advantage. Laboratory data suggest
the existence of differences in biological effects not
only between interferons α , β and γ but also the possibility that each product of the several interferon genes
may have a distinct activity. In addition, the synergistic

potentiation of antitumor and antiviral action of interferons α and β by small amounts of interferon γ (Schwarz
et al., 1981-82), introduces a challenging problem to the
design of future clinical trials with interferon mixtures.
The results of simple in principle predictive assays of
interferon sensitivity of clonogenic cells from individual
tumors (Bradley et al., 1981) may not be sufficiently
enlightening, since such assays do not provide informations
on the responses of the host immune system. Stronger
effects on human tumors might be obtained by combining
interferon with drugs that impair cell cycling activity
and result in a population enriched in resting tumor cells.
Interferon and chemotherapeutic drugs might be expected
to have a synergistic effect when used in an appropriate
sequence. It would be required that the chemotherapeutic
drug selected have a mode of action compatible with interferon induction of its various intracellular mediators
(Horoszewicz et al., 1979). For example: vincristin,
adriamycin and 6-mercaptopurine significantly decrease
in vitro biological activity of interferon (Cesario et al.,
1981-82). Conversely, interferon affects drug metabolism
by suppressing the cytochrome P-450 system which is the
major enzyme system in the liver for metabolism of drugs
(Sonnenfeld et al., 1981-82). A recent report that
cimetidine combined with interferon treatment (Borgström
et al., 1982) leads to a regression of human metastatic
melanoma, indicates that other than anticancer compounds
may potentiate clinical response and are worthy to consider.
Radiation injury is also enhanced by small concentrations
of interferon (Dritschilo et al., 1982), therefore
careful monitoring of dosage and timing of both modalities
may lead to improved combined treatment strategies.
    In women, interferon suppresses concentrations of
circulating estradiol and progesterone (Kauppila et al.,
1982) suggesting a modulation of follicle stimulating
and luteinizing hormones functions in vivo. In vitro,
interferon enhances estrogen receptor activity in cytosols
from normal tissue, as well as from breast and uterine
cancer (Dimitrov et al., 1982). Such observations provide
an additional incentive to examine the potential of
interferon therapy in steroid sex hormones responsive
versus non-responsive tumors.
    The first systematic phase II study of interferon
in prostate carcinoma is now in progress under the joint
sponsorship of the National Prostatic Cancer Project and
the American Cancer Society (ACS). The participants are:

Roswell Park Memorial Institute (RPMI) in Buffalo, N.Y., University of Iowa Hospital in Iowa City and California University Hospitals of University of California in San Diego. The objective of this study is to determine the efficacy of human fibroblast interferon against advanced, hormone refractory prostate cancer. Twenty orchiectomized patients with progressive metastatic disease, not treated previously with radiation or cytostatic drugs, will receive intravenous infusions of 6 million IU of fibroblast interferon (HuIFNβ), 3 times per week for 12 weeks and responses to treatment will be evaluated. The interferon is produced at RPMI in human diploid fibroblasts by the superinduction procedure, purified by sequential affinity chromatography to a specific activity in excess of 10^7 IU/mg protein, freeze dried and safety tested (Leong et al., 1981, Murphy GP, 1981). It is used under an investigational new drug permit (BB-IND 1325) issued by the Bureau of Biologics of the U.S. Food and Drug Administration. Its potency, safety, pharmacokinetics and clinical efficacy were demonstrated by numerous studies at RPMI (for review see Murphy GP, 1981) and under ACS sponsored clinical trials elsewhere (Hawkins et al., 1982).

It is impossible today to predict the ultimate benefit of interferon therapy to the patient with prostatic cancer. Proper caution should be exercised and premature optimism avoided. During clinical trials in other neoplastic diseases of man, objective anti-tumor responses were observed at best in 15 to 30% of patients treated. So far, strong evidence is lacking that interferon alone is superior to conventional methods of tumor management. Indications for the judicious use of interferon against cancer in adjuvant or combination therapy should emerge from additional controlled clinical trials. Increased availability of interferon and a better awareness of its potential by the clinician augur well for future progress.

REFERENCES

Arvin A, Feldman S, Merigan TC: Human leukocyte interferon in the treatment of varicella in children with cancer: A preliminary controlled trial. Antimicrob Agents and Chemother 13: 605, 1978.

Berg K, Secher D, Heron I: Purification and characterization of the HuIFNα species. Texas Rep Biol Med 41: 225, 1981-1982.

Blomgren H, Cantell K, Johansson B, Lagergren C, Ringborg U, Strander H: Interferon therapy in Hodgkin's disease. Acta Med Scand 199: 527, 1976.

Bocci V: Pharmacokinetics of interferon. A reappraisal. Texas Rep Biol Med 41: 336, 1981-1982.

Borden EC: Interferons: Rationale for clinical trials in neoplastic disease. Ann Int Med 91: 472, 1979.

Borgström S, von Eyben F, Flodgren P, Sjögren O: Regression of metastatic malignant melanoma induced by combined treatment with α interferon and cimetidine. Proc 13th International Cancer Congress, Abstract #2930, 1982.

Bradley EC, Ruscetti FW: Effect of fibroblast, lymphoid and myeloid interferons on human tumor colong formation in vitro. Cancer Res 41: 244, 1981.

Braun W, Levy MB: Interferon preparations as modifiers of immune responses. Proc Soc Exp Biol Med 141: 769, 1972.

Cesario TC, Tilles JG: Interactions between body fluids, chemotherapeutic agents and interferon. Texas Rep Biol Med 41: 359, 1981-1982.

Cheeseman S, Rubin R, Steward J, Tolkoff-Rubin N, Cosimi AB, Cantell K, Gilbert J, Winkle S, Herrin J, Black P, Russell P, Hirsch M: Controlled clinical trial of pro- phylactic human leukocyte interferon in renal transplan- tation. N Eng J Med 300: 1345, 1979.

DeMaeyer E, DeMaeyer-Guignard J: Immunoregulatory action of type 1 interferon in the mouse. Ann NY Acad Sci 350: 1, 1980.

Derynck R, Remaut E, Saman E, Stranssens P, DeClercq E, Content J, Fiers W: Expression of human interferon gene in Escherichia coli. Nature 287: 193, 1980.

Dimitrov NV, Myer C, Strander H, Einhorn S, Cantell K: Interferon as modifier of estrogen receptors in breast and uterine cancers. Proc 13th International Cancer Congress, Abstract #2929, 1982.

Dritschilo A. Mossman K, Gray M, Sreevalsan T: Potentiation of radiation injury by interferon. Am J Clin Oncol 5: 79, 1982.

Dunnick JK, Galasso G: Clinical trials with exogenous interferon: Summary of a meeting. J Infect Dis 139: 109, 1979.

Greenberg HB, Pollard RB, Lutwick LI, Gregory PB, Robinson WS, Merigan TC: Human Leukocyte interferon and hepatitis B virus infection. N Eng J Med 295: 517, 1976.

Gutterman JU, Blumenschein GR, Alesanian R, Yap HY, Buzdar AV, Cabanillas F, Hortobagyi GN, Hersh EM, Rasmussen SL, Harmon M, Kramer M, Pestka S: Leukocyte interferon-induced tumor regression in human metastatic breast cancer, multiple myeloma and malignant lymphoma. Ann Int Med 93: 399, 1980.

Hawkins MJ, Krown SE, Borden EC, Real F, Krim M, Cunningham-Rundles S, Oettgen H, Fox RW, Stock CC, Rauscher Jr FJ: American Cancer Society Phase I trial of human interferon beta. AACR Proc 23: 246, 1982.

Hill NO, Loeb E, Pardue AS, Dorn GL, Khan A, Hill JM: Response of acute leukemia to leukocyte interferon. J Clin Hematol Oncol 9: 137, 1979.

Hitzeman AR, Hagie FE, Levine HL, Goeddel DV, Ammerer G, Hall D: Expression of a human gene for interferon in yeast. Nature 293: 717, 1981.

Horoszewicz JS, Leong SS, Carter WA: Noncycling tumor cells are sensitive targets for the antiproliferative activity of human interferon. Science 206: 1091, 1979.

Horoszewicz JS, Leong S, Dolen J, Brecher M, Tebbi C, Freeman A, Aungst W, Mirand E: Human Fibroblast interferon as a potential anti-cancer drug: Phase I studies on intravenous and intrathecal administration. In: International Symposium on New Trends in Human Immunology and Cancer Immunotherapy, B. Serrou and C. Rosenfeld (eds). Doin Editeurs, Paris 1980, p 908.

Horoszewicz JS, Leong SS, Ito M, Mikulski AJ, Buffett RF, Karakousis C, Holyoke E, Job L, Dolan JG, Carter WA: Human fibroblast interferon in human neoplasia: Clinical and laboratory study. Cancer Treat Rep 62: 1899, 1978.

Imanishi J, Yokota Y, Kishida T, Mukainaka T, Matsuo A: Phagocytosis enhancing effect of human leukocyte interferon preparation on human peripheral monocytes in vitro. Acta Virol 19: 52, 1975.

Isaacs A, Lindenman J: Virus interference. I. The interferon. Proc R Soc Lond B147: 258, 1957.

Kauppila A, Cantell K, Jänne O, Kokko E, Vihko R: Serum sex steroid hormone concentrations and endometrial estrogen and progestin receptor levels during administration of human leukocyte interferon. Int. J. Cancer 29: 291, 1982.

Lengyel P: Enzymology of interferon action. Meth in Enzymol 79: 135, 1981.

Leong SS, Horoszewicz JS: Production and preparation of human fibroblast interferon for clinical trials. Meth in Enzymol 78: 87, 1981.

Mellstedt H, Bjorkholm M, Johansson B, Ahre A, Holm G, Strander H: Interferon therapy in myelomatosis. Lancet i: 245, 1979.

Merigan TC: Present appraisal of and future hopes for the clinical utilization of human interferons. In "Interferon 1981" I. Gresser (ed): Academic Press (Publ) 3: 135, 1981.

Merigan TC, Rand KH, Pollard RB, Abdallah PS, Jordan GW, Fried RP: Human leukocyte interferon for the treatment of Herpes zoster in patients with cancer. N Eng J Med 298: 981, 1978.

Merigan TC, Reed SE, Hall TS, Tyrrel DAJ: Inhibition of respiratory virus infection by locally applied interferon. Lancet i: 563, 1973.

Merigan TC, Sikora K, Breeden JH, Levy R, Rosenberg SA: Preliminary observations on the effect of human leukocyte interferon in non-Hodgkin's lymphoma. N. Eng J Med 299: 1449, 1978.

Moschera JA, Hobbs DS, Levy WP, Stein S, Rubinstein M, Pestka S: Purification and structure of the interferons. Texas Rep Biol Med 41: 250, 1981-1982.

Murphy GP: Current report on the interferon program at Roswell Park Memorial Institute. J Surg Oncol 17: 99, 1981.

Oldham R, Sherwins, Fein S, Whisnat J: Phase I trials of recombinant and lymphoblastoid alpha interferons in patients with disseminated cancer. Proc 13th International Cancer Congress, abstract #2927, 1982.

Pape GR, Hadam MR, Eisenburg J, Reithmüller G: Kinetics of natural cytotoxicity in patients treated with human fibroblast interferon. Cancer Imm Immunoth 11: 1, 1981.

Paucker K, Cantell K, Henle W: Ouantitative studies on viral interference in suspended L-cells. III. Effect of interfering viruses and interfering viruses and interferon of the growth rate of cells. Virology 17: 324, 1962.

Pfeffer LM, Wang E, Tamm I: Interferon effects on microfilament organization, cellular fibronectin distribution and cell motility in human fibroblasts. J Cell Biol 85: 9, 1980.

Pazin G, Armstrong J, Lam MT, Tarr G, Jannetta P, Ho M: Prevention of reactivated Herpes simplex infection by human leukocyte interferon after operation on the trigeminal root. N Eng J Med 301: 225, 1979.

Quesada JR, Gutterman JU, Hersh E: Clinical and immunological study of beta interferon by intramuscular route in patients with metastatic breast cancer. J Interferon Res 2: 593, 1982.

Quesada JR, Swanson DA, Trindade A, Gutterman JU: Renal cell carcinoma: Antitumor effects of leukocyte interferon. Cancer Res 43: 940, 1983.

Romano A, Revel M, Guarari-Rotman D, Blumenthal M, Stein R: Use of human fibroblast-derived (beta) interferon in the treatment of epidermic adenovirus keratoconjunctivitis. J Interferon Res 1: 95, 1980.

Rubinstein M, Rubinstein S, Familetti, PC, Miller RS, Waldman AA, Pestka S: Human leukocyte interferon: Production, purification to homogeneity and initial characterization. Proc Natl Acad Sci USA 76: 640, 1979.

Schwarz LA, Fleischmann WR Jr: Potentiation of interferon action. Texas Rep Biol Med 41: 298, 1981-1982.

Scott GM, Secher DS, Flowers D, Bate J, Cantell K, Tyrrell DAJ: Toxicity of interferon. Brit Med J 282: 1345, 1981.

Secher DS, Burke DC: A monoclonal antibody for large scale purification of human leukocyte interferon. Nature 285: 446, 1980.

Sonnenfeld G, Harned CL, Nerland DE: Effects of interferon on durg metabolism. Texas Rep Biol Med 41: 363, 1981-1982.

Stewart WE, Blalock JE, Burke DC et al. Interferon Nomenclature. Cancer Res 40: 3860, 1980.

Strander H: Interferons: Antineoplastic drugs? BLUT 35: 277, 1977.

Streuli M, Nagata S, Weissmann C: At least three human type α interferons: Structure of $\alpha 2$. Science 209: 1343, 1980.

Sulkowski E: Purification and characterization of interferons. Texas Rep Biol Med 41: 234, 1981-1982.

Sundmacher R, Cantell K, Neumann-Haefelin D: Combination therapy of dendritic keratitis with trifluorothymidine and interferon. Lancet ii, 687, 1978.

Trinchieri G, Santoli D: Anti-viral activity induced by culturing lymphocytes with tumor derived or virus-transformed cells. Enhancement of human natural killer cell activity by interferon and antagonistic inhibition of susceptibility of target cells to lysis. J Exp Med 147: 1314, 1978.

Vanky F, Klein E: Alloreactive cytotoxicity of interferon-triggered human lymphocytes detected with tumor biopsy targets. Immunogenetics 15: 31, 1982.

Verma DS, Spitzer G, Gutterman JU, Zander AR, McCredie KB, Dicke KA: Human Leukocyte interferon preparation blocks granulopoietic differentiation. Blood 54: 1423, 1979.

Zarling JM, Eskra L, Borden EC, Horoszewicz JS, Carter WA: Activation of human natural killer cells cytoxicity for human leukemia cells by purified interferon. J Immunol 123: 63, 1979.

13th International Cancer Congress, Part E
Cancer Management, pages 327–336
© **1983 Alan R. Liss, Inc., 150 Fifth Avenue, New York, NY 10011**

THE STABILITY OF HUMAN FIBROBLAST INTERFERON (HuIFN-β)

Drs. Susan S. Leong, Ph.D., Julius S. Horoszewicz,
M.D., D.M.Sc. and Edwin A. Mirand, Ph.D., D.Sc.,
Department of Biological Resources
Roswell Park Memorial Institute
Buffalo, New York 14263

The stability of purified lyophilized HuIFN-β produced
at Roswell Park Memorial Institute, Buffalo, New York, USA
for clinical trials was determined after: a) storage for up
to 32 months; b) reconstitution and dilution in parenteral
solutions; and c) incubation in vitro with human blood,
plasma and serum. The potency of the purified lyophilized
HuIFN-β was preserved reliably after storage at 4°C for the
longest time after storage tested of 32 months. The activity
of this interferon was better retained after dilution into
the parenteral solution 5% glucose as compared with 0.9%
sodium chloride under the simulated conditions (as intravenous
infusion over a period of 1 to 3 hours at room temperature)
of interferon administration to patients. The short term
stability of HuIFN-α and HuIFN-β were found to be similar
in human whole blood, defibrinated blood, plasma and serum.
Thus, the likelihood of any significant depletion of these
two interferons by fibrin or cellular elements of blood is
reduced and confirms the relevance of measurements of the
levels of either interferon in serum.

INTRODUCTION

Human fibroblast interferon (HuIFN-β) and leukocyte
interferon (HuIFN-α) are natural products of corresponding
human cells stimulated with either synthetic or viral inducers. Both interferons are glycoproteins with a high
degree of species specificity in their action. Although
the amounts of interferon elaborated in vitro are minute
(less than 10^{-14} g per cell) the concentrations of interferon
capable of inducing measurable biological effects compare

favorably with the most potent polypeptide hormones. Human interferon molecules are carriers of antiviral, antiprolifera- tive and immunomodulatory activities. Each of these proper- ties suggests that interferon should find in the near future an appropriate place in our arsenal of therapeutic approaches to the management of viral and neoplastic diseases of man.

Clinical trials to determine efficacy of human inter- ferons in human diseases can only be conducted if large quantities of purified and stable interferon are available. This necessitates that the biological activity of the inter- ferons be stably retained during production, purification, processing, safety testing and the subsequent storage and shipment as well as during the period of clinical administra- tion. Although HuIFN-β and HuIFN-α have generally been considered to be stable molecules, especially at low pH (Fantes, 1973), it is now recognized that they can be readily inactivated by heat or mechanical stress during handling (Ng and Vilcek, 1972). A large-scale production facility for the purpose of obtaining sufficient quantities of puri- fied, safety-tested and stable human fibroblast interferon for clinical investigation has been in operation at Roswell Park Memorial Institute since 1976 (Horoszewicz et al., 1978; Murphy, 1981). The produced interferon is currently used in clinical trials locally (Horoszewicz et al., 1978; Dolen et al., 1979; Horoszewicz et al., 1980; Jacobs et al., 1981), nationally, under the sponsorship of the American Cancer Society (Borden et al., 1980; Hawkins et al., 1982) and internationally (Misset et al., 1981 and 1982). The stability of HuIFN-β produced at our facility during each step of the manufacturing process was extensively studied. We have previously reported that the stability of HuIFN-β is enhanced by the addition of human serum albumin (2.5 mg/ ml) and by storage of purified HuIFN-β at -90°C in 25 to 50% ethylene glycol in polypropylene or polystyrene con- tainers (Carter and Horoszewicz, 1979). This paper summar- izes the results of further studies on the stability of our purified lyophilized HuIFN-β produced for clinical trials after: a) storage for up to 32 months; b) reconstitution and dilution in parenteral solutions; and c) incubation in vitro with human blood, plasma and serum.

MATERIALS AND METHODS

Human fibroblast interferon was produced in our laboratory in human diploid fibroblasts by the superinduction

procedure and purified by sequential affinity chromatography
on Concanavalin A-agarose and phenyl-Sepharose CL-4B as
previously described (Horoszewicz et al., 1978; Leong and
Horoszewicz, 1981). After elution from phenyl-Sepharose,
HuIFN-β with a specific activity of 2 x 10^7 IU/mg protein
was obtained and human serum albumin (3 mg/ml) was added to
enhance stability. After dialysis against phosphate buffered
saline, the HuIFN-β was freeze-dried, stored at 4°C, and
safety tested (Horoszewicz et al., 1978; Leong et al., 1981).
Each vial of the lyophilized product contained HuIFN-β, 0.5
to 5 x 10$_6$ IU; 3 to 10 mg of normal human serum albumin; 3
to 9 mg of sodium chloride; 1 to 3 mg sodium phosphate and
0 to 0.1 mg of calcium chloride. This interferon was produced and used under an Investigational New Drug permit
(BB-IND 1325) issued by the Bureau of Biologics of the U.S.
Food and Drug Administration.

Human leukocyte interferon (specific activity 1 x 10^6
IU/mg protein) prepared at the Finnish Red Cross Blood
Collection Center and kindly provided by Dr. J. Gutterman
was used for the in vitro studies.

Interferon assays were performed in triplicate on
monolayers of human diploid fibroblasts (Strain BG-9) using
the modified colorimetric technique of Finter as previously
described (Finter, 1969). Bovine vesicular stomatitis
virus was used as the challenge virus. An internal lyophilized laboratory HuIFN-β standard, calibrated against the
international reference standard of human fibroblast
interferon (G-023-902-527, Research Resources Branch,
National Institutes of Health) was included in each assay,
and titers are expressed in international units (IU).

Six lots of HuIFN-β prepared for clinical use were
tested for stability after lyophilization and storage at
4°C for 5 to 32 months. Sample vials from each lot were
reconstituted to isotonicity with sterile water (1 ml) for
injection U.S.P. (Invenex) and the interferon content
assayed. The geometric mean potency of between 6 and 12
measurements of activity was determined and the standard
errors calculated.

To study the stability of HuIFN-β in parenteral
solutions, lyophilized HuIFN-β prepared for clinical use
was reconstituted to isotonicity with sterile water (1 ml)
for injection (Invenex) and then diluted with Elliott's B

solution (5 ml) (Division of Cancer Treatment, NCI), 0.9%
sodium chloride for injection U.S.P. (250 ml) (Travenol) or
5% glucose for injection U.S.P. (250 ml) (Travenol).
Elliott's B solution is an experimental diluent for chemotherapeutic drugs for intrathecal administration and has
electrolyte composition similar to that of human spinal
fluid. Each ml contains: 7.3 mg sodium chloride; 1.9 mg
sodium bicarbonate; 0.8 mg dextrose, hydrous; 0.3 mg
magnesium sulfate · 7 H_2O; 0.3 mg potassium chloride; 0.2
mg calcium chloride · 2 H_2O; 0.2 mg sodium phosphate
dibasic · 7 H_2O; and 0.1 mcg phenol-sulfonphthalein (pH
adjusted with carbon dioxide). The diluted interferon
solutions containing 12 µg/ml (0.9% sodium chloride and 5%
glucose solutions) and 600 µg/ml (Elliott's B solution)
of total protein were stored at room temperature for $3\frac{1}{2}$
hours and then at 4°C for the duration of the experiment.
Samples were taken from these solutions at time intervals
after reconstitution and the interferon content determined
by biological assay.

To assess the possible losses of HuIFN-β activity due
to the time and manipulation required for separating from
whole blood the serum used in interferon assays, aliquots
(100 µl) of stock HuIFN-β solution (in saline with 2 mg/ml
human albumin) were mixed with 4 ml of: (a) freshly drawn
uncoagulated blood, (b) blood defibrinated with glass
beads, (c) fresh plasma without anti-coagulants (collected
in plastic tubes), (d) fresh serum, and (e) fetal calf
serum. For comparison aliquots of HuIFN-α were used in
parallel experiments. The mixtures were incubated for
30 min at 37°C and 75 min at 4°C. After centrifugation
the serum was collected and immediately assayed for interferon content. The expected interferon concentrations in
serum were calculated from the hematocrit and from data
obtained in assaying the interferon stocks.

RESULTS

Accelerated storage tests (Jameson et al., 1979)
has predicted that for long term storage of interferon,
freeze-drying is the method of choice to preserve potency
reliably. However, little information is available on the
stability of lyophilized HuIFN-β under actual storage conditions after a period of 12 to 24 months. In our studies
we detected no significant loss of activity after storage
at 4°C of up to 32 months (the longest storage time tested)

for the lyophilized HuIFN-β prepared for clinical use
(Table I). Each sample was measured on 6 to 12 occasions.
The geometric mean potency was calculated and the standard
error was found to be well below 10%.

Table 1

STABILITY OF LYOPHILIZED HUMAN FIBROBLAST
INTERFERON DURING STORAGE AT +4°C

Sample #	Original Potency*) I U	Length of Storage Months	Potency After*) Storage I U $\pm$ SE	%
A	$10^{6 \cdot 176}$	5	$10^{6 \cdot 110} \pm 0 \cdot 122$	86%
B	$10^{6 \cdot 114}$	7	$10^{6 \cdot 179} \pm 0 \cdot 032$	116%
C	$10^{6 \cdot 481}$	11	$10^{6 \cdot 455} \pm 0 \cdot 022$	94%
D	$10^{6 \cdot 301}$	17	$10^{6 \cdot 294} \pm 0 \cdot 019$	98%
E	$10^{6 \cdot 010}$	27	$10^{6 \cdot 061} \pm 0 \cdot 084$	112%
F	$10^{5 \cdot 707}$	32	$10^{5 \cdot 629} \pm 0 \cdot 018$	84%

*) Geometric mean of between 6 and 12 measurements.

The stability of HuIFN-β in 0.9% saline and 5% glucose
solutions for injection were compared to determine if the
biological activity of interferon is preserved better in
one or the other parenteral solution during the usual
infusion period of 1 to 3 hours of intravenous administration to patients. No loss of activity was observed for up
to 3 1/4 hours when HuIFN-β was diluted in 5% glucose at
room temperature (Table 2). In contrast 40% of the biological activity was lost when HuIFN-β was diluted in 0.9%
saline. The stability of HuIFN-β in Elliott's B diluent
solution used for intrathecal administration was also tested. No loss of activity was observed for up to 2 1/2 hours
of the test period (Table 2).

Existing reports (Edy et al., 1978; Quesada et al.,
1982), as well as our own experience, indicated that only
trace or no detectable interferon activity was observed
after intramuscular or subcutaneous injections of HuIFN-β
(Merigan, 1977; Emodi et al., 1975). In contrast, injections of HuIFN-α produced readily measurable interferon

Table 2

STABILITY OF LYOPHILIZED PURIFIED HuIFN-β AFTER RECONSTITUTION AND DILUTION IN PARENTERAL SOLUTIONS

	Interferon Content					
	Elliott's B Solution		0.9% saline		5% glucose	
Time of storage	IU/ml	% recovery	IU/ml	% recovery	IU/ml	% recovery
immediately after reconstitution	2,700	100	1,400	100	1,400	100
1 1/4 hrs	3,000	111	1,600	114	1,400	100
2 1/2 hrs	3,100	115	820	59	1,100	79
3 1/4 hrs	–	–	850	61	1,400	100
8 days	–	–	280	20	880	63
15 days	–	–	270	19	800	57
24 days	–	–	98	7	633	45
5 months	–	–	105	8	410	29

Lyophilized HuIFN-β purified by Con-A and phenyl-sepharose column chromatography was reconstituted to isotonicity and diluted with Elliott's B solution, 0.9% saline and 5% glucose. Elliott's B solution is an experimental solution for intrathecal administration. The saline and glucose solutions are for intravenous administration. The diluted solutions were stored at room temperature for 3 1/2 hours and then at 4°C for the duration of the experiment. Samples were taken from these solutions at time intervals after reconstitutions and the interferon content determined by biological assay.

serum levels (Cesario et al., 1979). This prompted us to examine whether any selective loss of HuIFN-β vs. HuIFN-α activity could occur during the processing of human blood to obtain serum prior to interferon assays. Our findings indicated that the antiviral activity of both HuIFN-α and HuIFN-β, after mixing with human whole blood, remain essentially unchanged for at least 2 hours (Table 3). Thus, the likelihood of any significant depletion of HuIFN-β or HuIFN-α by fibrin or cellular elements of blood is reduced.

DISCUSSION

Although crude HuIFN-β preparations were found to be stable, no loss of activity when stored for many weeks at 4°C or at -70°C (Ng and Vilcek, 1972), purified HuIFN-β must be stabilized even for short periods of storage. Knight reported that purified poly I·poly C induced fibroblast interferon (specific activity 1 x 10[7] units/mg protein) was unstable losing 50 to 75% of its potency in 24 hours (4°C) when the total protein concentration was less than 10 μg/ml (Knight, 1976). In order to generate large quantities of purified, stable interferons for research and clinical use, considerable effort has been expended in the past few years toward establishing methods to prevent inactivation of human interferons during preparation, purification, processing, safety testing and storage. The addition

Table 3

STABILITY OF PURIFIED HuIFN-β AND HuIFN-α FOLLOWING
IN VITRO INCUBATION WITH HUMAN BLOOD, PLASMA AND SERUM

Patient	Diagnosis	Specimen	HuIFN-β		HuIFN-α	
			IU/ml added	% recovery in serum	IU/ml added	% recovery in serum
#1	breast Ca.	whole blood	350	99	550	65
#2	breast Ca.	whole blood	350	116	550	82
#3	melanoma	whole blood	350	105	550	120
#4	blastic CML	whole blood	350	98	550	139
#5	blastic CML	whole blood	875	11	N.D.*	
	blastic CML	serum	80	81	N.D.	
#6	normal	whole blood	350	92	550	105
	normal	defibrinated blood	350	82	550	93
	normal	plasma	350	81	N.D.	
	normal	serum	600	124	900	126
#7	normal	pool of human sera	600	119	900	134
#8	Pool of fetal calf sera		600	112	900	134

*N.D., not done.

of various proteins, i.e. bovine serum albumin (Davey et al., 1976) or cytochrome C (Anfinsen et al., 1974), rare earth salts of atomic numbers 57 to 71 (Sedmak and Grossberg, 1982) and the use of acid pH conditions (Fantes, 1973) were report- ed to be helpful. Some protection were also reported to be gained by the addition of chaotropic salts (Jariwalla et al., 1977) or sodium dodecyl sulfate (Knight, 1976). Although these techniques are useful because of their protective properties against both thermal and mechanical stress in- activation, the purification procedure developed in our laboratory have avoided the exposure of the HuIFN-β product to denaturing (partial or complete) condition which might affect the native conformational state of this glycoprotein. Thus, any exposure to (a) chaotropic salts (as thiocyanates), (b) detergents (as sodium dodecyl sulfate), or (c) extreme pH values of the solvent, has been carefully avoided through- out the purification of HuIFN-β. Exposure, even transient, to such denaturing agents carries the theoretical concern for irreversible alteration of the protein. Such alteration could result in unexpected biological effects, such as mod- ification of antigenicity on repeated administration, as well as undesirable biochemical changes such as molecular aggregation.

We have found that the activity of purified HuIFN-β is preserved during the manufacturing process by storage at -90°C in 25 to 50% ethylene glycol in polypropylene or polyethylene containers (Carter and Horoszewicz, 1979). The addition of human serum albumin (3 mg/ml) and freeze-drying of the purified interferon product resulted in preservation of the interferon potency reliably after storage at 4°C for 32 months (the longest time after storage tested).

We have determined the stability of HuIFN-β after dilution with parenteral solutions under the simulated conditions (as intravenous infusion over a period of 1 to 3 hours at room temperature) of interferon administration to patients. Our results indicated that the activity of purified HuIFN-β is better preserved at room temperature after 2 hours by 5% glucose as compared with 0.9% sodium chloride under conditions of low protein concentration (12 to 36 μg/ml).

We observed that the short term stabilities of HuIFN-α and HuIFN-β are similar in human whole blood, defibrinated blood, plasma and serum, therefore, the measurements of HuIFN-β level in sera reflected the actual concentrations of interferon circulating in vivo within the limits of the accuracy of the assay.

Anfinsen CB, Bose S, Corley L and Gurari-Rotman D (1974). Partial purification of human interferon by affinity chromatography. Proc. Natl. Acad. Sci. U.S.A. 71:3139-3442.

Borden E, Dao T, Holland J, Gutterman J and Merigan T (1980). Interferon in recurrent breast cancer: Preliminary report of the ACS clinical trials program. Proc. of AACR 21(3750):187.

Carter W and Horoszewicz J (1979). Production, purification and clinical application of human fibroblast interferon. Pharmac. Ther. 8:359-377.

Cesario T, Vaziri N, Slater L and Tilles J (1979). Inactivators of fibroblast interferon found in human serum. Infec. Immun. 24:851-855.

Davey MW, Sulkowski E and Carter WA (1976). Binding of human fibroblast interferon to Concanavalin A-agarose. Involvement of carbohydrate recognition and hydrophobic interaction. Biochem. 15:704-713.

Dolen J, Carter W, Horoszewicz J, Vladutiu A, Leibowitz A and Noan J (1979). Fibroblast interferon treatment of a patient with chronic active hepatitis. Am. J. Med. 67: 127-131.

Edy VG, Billiau A and DeSomer P (1978). Non-appearance of injected fibroblast interferon in circulation. The Lancet p. 451.

Emodi G, Just M, Hernadez P and Hirt HR (1975). Circulating interferon in man after administration of exogenous human leukocyte interferon. J. Nat. Cancer Inst. 54:1045-1049.

Fantes KH (1973). Purification and physico-chemical properties of interferons. In Finter NB (ed): "Interferons and interferon inducers," New York: North-Holland Publishing Co., p. 171-200.

Finter NB (1969). Dye uptake methods for assessing viral cytopathogenicity and their application to interferon assays. J. Gen. Virol. 5:419-429.

Hawkins MJ, Krown SE, Borden EC, Real F, Krim M, Cunningham-Rundles S, Oettgen H, Fox RW, Stock CC and Rauscher FJ (1982). ACS Phase I trial of human interferon beta (IFN-β). Proc. of AACR 23 (973):246.

Horoszewicz JS, Leong SS, Ito M, DiBerardino L and Carter WA (1978). Aging in vitro and large scale interferon production by 15 new strains of human diploid fibroblasts. Infec. Immun. 19:720-726.

Horoszewicz JS, Leong SS, Ito M, Mikulski AJ, Buffett RF, Karakousis C, Holyoke D, Job L, Dolen JG and Carter WA (1978). Human Fibroblast interferon in human neoplasia: Clinical and laboratory study. Cancer Treat. Reports 62: 1988.

Horoszewicz JS, Leong SS, Dolen J, Bucher M, Tebbi C, Freeman A, Aungst W and Mirand E (1980). Human fibroblast interferon as a potential anti-cancer drug-Phase I studies on intravenous and intrathecal administration. In Serrou B and Rosenfeld C (eds): "International Symposium on New Trends in Human Immunology and Cancer Immuno-therapy," France: Doin Editeurs, p. 908-919.

Jacobs L, O'Malley J, Freeman A and Ekes R (1981). Intrathecal interferon reduces exacerbations of multiple sclerosis. Science 214:1026-1028.

Jameson PD, Greiff D and Grossberg SE (1979). Thermal stability of freeze-dried mammalian interferons. Analysis of freeze-drying conditions and accelerated storage tests for murine interferon. Cryobiology 16:301.

Jariwalla RJ, Grossberg SE and Sedmak JJ (1977). Effect of chaotropic salts and protein denaturants on the thermal stability of mouse fibroblast interferon. J. Gen. Virol. 35: 45-52.

Knight E, Jr (1976). Interferon: Purification and initial characterization from human diploid cells. Proc. Natl. Acad. Sci. U.S.A. 73:520-523.

Leong SS and Horoszewicz JS (1981). Production and preparation of human fibroblast interferon for clinical trials. In Pestka S (ed): "Methods in Enzymology," Vol. 78 Interferon Part A, New York: Academic Press, p. 87-101.

Merigan TC (1977). Pharmacokinetics and side effects of interferon in man. Texas Reports on Biology and Med. 35:541-547.

Misset JL, Mathe G and Horoszewicz JS (1981). Intrathecal interferon in meningial leukemia. The New England J. Med., p. 1544.

Misset JL, Mathe G, Gastiaburu J, Goutner A, Dorval T, Gouveia J, Hayat M, Jasmin C, Schwarzenberg L, Machover D, Ribaud, De Vassal F and Horoszewicz JS (1982). Treatment of lymphoid neoplasia with interferon. I. Human fibroblastic interferon (beta) In Malignant Gammapathies Phase II Trial. Anticancer Research 2:63-69.

Murphy GP (1981). Current report on the interferon program at Roswell Park Memorial Institute. J. Surg. Oncol. 17: 99-111.

Ng MH and Vilcek J (1972). Interferons: physico-chemical properties and control of cellular synthesis. Advances in Protein Chemistry 26:173-239.

Quesada JR, Gutterman JU and Hersh EM (1982). Clinical and immunological study of beta interferon by intramuscular route in patients with metastatic breast cancer. J. of Interferon Res. 2:593-599.

Sedmak JJ and Grossberg SE (1982). Approaches to the stabilization of interferons. Texas Reports on Biology and Med. 41:274.

CONGRESS SYMPOSIA

THE ENVIRONMENT AND CANCER: RECENT EPIDEMILOGIC
DEVELOPMENTS Higginson, J., France, Chairman;
Graham, S., USA, Co-Chairman; Opera House

Some Thoughts on Preventive Oncology.
*Wynder, E. L., New York, NY USA.

Dietary Factors in Human Carcinogenesis.
*MacLennan, R., Brisbane, Australia.

Exposure to Polychlorinated Dibenzo-P-Dioxins and
Dibenzofurans in the Environment. *Hardell, L.,
Umea, Sweden.

Assessement of Low Level Risks. Land, C., USA.
(By Title Only)

Carcinogens and Anti-Carcinogens. *Ames, B. N.,
Berkeley, CA USA. (By Title Only)

Please note: Papers that are listed as "By Title
Only" were presented at the 13th International
Cancer Congress, but are not included in these
volumes.

13th International Cancer Congress, Part E
Cancer Management, pages 339–345
© **1983 Alan R. Liss, Inc., 150 Fifth Avenue, New York, NY 10011**

SOME THOUGHTS ON PREVENTIVE ONCOLOGY

Ernst L. Wynder, M.D., President

American Health Foundation
320 East 43rd Street
New York, NY 10017

The Evidence
Tobacco. Numerous studies have investigated the
influence of environmental factors on the development of
cancer in man. In general, they concluded that up to 80%
of all human cancers could be attributed to specific
environmental factors. Our evaluation indicates that
one-third of all male cancer deaths relate to smoking and
that the corresponding figure is 8% for women and is
rising. The effect of cigarette smoking principally is to
cancer of the lung, vocal cords, bladder and pancreas with
other types of smoking (cigar and pipe) also affecting the
risk for cancer of the oral cavity, extrinsic larynx and
esophagus. Tobacco chewing increases the risk for cancer
of the oral cavity as well, indicating that there are
carcinogens in raw tobacco itself.

The evidence that smoking is causatively related to
these cancers is so well established that it does not
demand to be repeated here. From an etiological point of
view, one of the few questions remaining is how quickly
does the risk of a tobacco-related cancer decline when one
stops smoking. The longer and heavier one smokes, the
longer it takes to observe a decline. In heavy, long-term
smokers, there is no decline for the first 3 years. After
12 to 15 years, levels are reached comparable to those
that have never smoked. Another important question
remains as to whether low-yield cigarettes are associated
with a lower rate of cancer risk. Data on lung and larynx
cancer indicate a small reduction in risk. This finding
may be due to the fact that non-filter cigarettes have

also been reduced in tar yield and that all filter cigarette smokers now in the cancer age began their smoking
career with a non-filter cigarette. It needs to be determined what the risk would be in individuals who begin
their smoking career with filter cigarettes and particularly, what the risk would be in those cases where only
cigarettes are smoked with very low tar yield (5 mg. per
cigarette or less). These studies still remain to be done
since cigarettes with such low tar yields have not been
smoked long enough for appropriate evaluation.

Alcohol. Like tobacco, data on alcohol is well
established in showing that for cancer of the oral cavity,
larynx (both intrinsic and extrinsic), as well as cancer
of the esophagus, alcohol is an important promoter or co-
carcinogen to cancer in these sites among smokers. We
emphasize the word "promotion" because there is little
evidence that alcohol can increase the risk by itself.
The data also suggest that it makes no difference what
type of alcohol one consumes. The key point is the total
amount of alcohol consumed. For this reason, it is not
surprising that in the United States, the risk is higher
among consumers of lard liquors compared to beer. Part of
the effect of alcoholism and cancer of the upper alimen-
tary tract relates to the fact that alcoholics often have
inadequate nutrition. It is not quite clear whether heavy
drinkers who eat well (particularly fresh fruits and
vegetables and a reasonably high intake of vitamin B) have
a lower risk than drinkers who eat less well. The effect
of nutrition deficiencies in alcohol-related cancers needs
to be explored further.

Weight. Caloric excesses as distinct from the
excesses of specific macronutrients as a risk factor for
cancer is principally limited to the endometrium and the
gall bladder. The data on cancer of the breast are relatively inconsistent. American data in particular, including our own, do not show a strong relationship of obesity
to cancer of the breast either in pre- or post-menopausal
age groups.

High-fat Diet. The effect of dietary fat, which has
been called causative by a Committee of the National Academy of Sciences, relates principally to cancer of the
breast, prostate and colon. The evidence rests on experimental data as well as on a variety of epidemiological

evidences including the correlation between dietary fat
intake and cancer in various populations and the rise of
these cancers as low-risk populations as the Japanese
migrate to a high-risk country like the United States.

The effect of fat, which can be mediated by a variety
of mechanisms can, as far as cancer of the colon is concerned, probably be reduced by high intake of dietary
fiber. Studies from Finland show that a high intake of
dietary fat, mostly saturated in this case, can be coun-
teracted by high intake of dietary fiber which results in
a greater stool bulk, thereby diluting bile acids.

Occupations. Occupations account for 5% or less of
male cancer deaths. The comparable percent for women is
less then 1%. Some of these occupations, such as asbestos
and uranium mining, work primarily synergistically with
tobacco smoking. One needs to carefully standardize data
for smoking before making claim for specific occupations
since blue collar workers smoke significantly more than
white collar workers. Industries that deal with expected
occupational hazards should keep life-long medical records
on all workers so as to better judge the effect of different occupational exposures on the development of human
cancer.

Miscellaneous Factors. Having outlined the role of
some of the major factors that relate to human cancer, our
data show no relationship to cancer of the bladder and
pancreas to consumption of coffee, nor could we confirm
the relationship of hair dye use to breast cancer, nor of
saccharin to cancer of the bladder. The effects of pro-
lactin, estrogen and viruses in the pathogenesis of select
cancer sites is well-established. Epidemiology has some
general problems when dealing with low order associations. It is not surprising, therefore, that in regard
to these variables there have been inconsistent reports in
the literature. Of course, the more carefully one asks
questions relative to such variables, the better one
selects cases and controls, the more fully one understands
confounders, the more reliable results will be. Weak
associations, such as passive inhalation of smoke to lung
cancer, a very important public health issue, remain to be
studied further.

In addition to careful epidemiology, one needs to examine the nature of the suspected carcinogen not only in terms of dose and potency, but also whether the component is genotoxic or epigenetic. If it is epigenetic, we have a reversible situation, and one where high doses are required to observe effects. Looking at the issue from this point alone, it was unlikely that saccharin, established to have promoting activity in the experimental setting, would increase bladder cancer in humans.

Preventive Approaches

Individual Prevention. Of key concern to society and science is, or at least should be, what to do about those factors that have been established to increase the risk of human cancer or of other diseases. What obstacles have prevented us from doing what we know we should have done in respect to smoking, alcoholism, obesity, excessive sunlight, poor genital hygiene, factors known for a long time to contribute to the development of cancer in humans.

These obstacles include human apathy to anything preventive. We tend to suffer from an illusion of immortality and believe that risk factors do not apply to us. If we add the relative disinterest of the medical profession, of the hospital system and the insurance companies' lack of support of prevention, it is clear that but few persons will get up every morning and say, "What can I do for disease prevention today?" It is obvious that the media give much more attention to acute health care than to prevention. Crisis always seems to motivate more people and sell more newspapers than prevention. If we survey the monuments in our cities we find them to represent heroes of wars rather than of men who kept us at peace. There are obvious inherent problems as to why preventive medicine will never be as exciting to society as cancer chemotherapy or coronary bypasses.

In addition to these obstacles, there are industries whichprofit from such goods as tobacco, alcohol and high-fat foods, that heavily advertise their wares. Thus, we have a dilemma where we have on the one hand human apathy, and on the other hand aggressive marketing. No wonder that we continue to be surrounded by risk factors and pay relatively little attention to them.

Nonetheless, we have been successful in certain areas. There has been a significant reduction of smoking habits, particularly in the United States, a reduction greatest in upper income males and particular physicians. We are learning from this that if we as a society frown upon a habit as being socially unacceptable, we are more likely to see change than on the basis of a factor being regarded as harmful. The same reasoning applies to weight, particularly of upper income group women. These women may not be so much concerned about ill health effects of obesity but rather that the fashionable dresses they see in magazines only come in certain sizes. By analogy, if we as a society would discredit alcohol abuse, we would see a greater reduction in alcoholism.

One point to make in a strategy of prevention is that we need to teach the public not only knowledge, we must change the attitude towards risk factors to change the public's behavior. The basic endpoint of health education is not more knowledge but improved health behavior. The governmental and voluntary health organizations, the medical profession, and the media should join forces in a continuous education of the public as to what constitutes good health behavior. We need to set a norm for others to follow not because this norm will help you, but because this norm is "the thing to do."

A proper strategy of health education should begin early in childhood. We should know from every dictator and every church leader that the way to persuade people is by teaching the children. At present there is no mandatory health education program in most school districts in the United States. The American Health Foundation has developed a Know Your Body School Health Education Program that is different from other programs in that it takes a health record of each child, gives each child a "Health Passport", and has developed a curriculum and corresponding teacher's guide from grades 1 to 8 designed to affect health knowledge, health attitude and health behavior. It measures these factors each year to determine what progress has been made. The schools have 40 hours per year to teach the program. Early results are satisfactory in showing, for example, a reduction in the use of skim milk, an increase in health knowledge, and, in one instance, the reduction of smoking habits among parents. Clearly, the parents need to be closely involved in this program. Our program is too new to have long-term results. The most successful results can be expected to occur when a six year old has been in the program through his entire school life. We strongly believe that if we are ever going to change the health behavior of the public, we must have a mandatory school-based health education program that is intensive, involves teachers, parents and the entire community as well as students, and is evaluated each year. Such a program can lead to better health knowledge, better health attitude, and better health behavior of children.

Product Modification. Another area of preventive medicine deals with product modification. We need to further reduce tar and nicotine levels of cigarettes. It remains to be determined at what level tar yields will be significantly less carcinogenic. Progress has been made not only in reducing tar yield to about 5 mg. per cigarette that gives a satisfying smoke, but there also has been selective reduction in tumorigenic agents in smoke. More progress can be made. It is likely that we can reduce the carcinogenesis of a cigarette before we are able to reduce its effect on the cardiovascular system. Seemingly, the threshold level to tumorigenic agents in tobacco smoke is quite higher than that of nicotine and its effect on the cardiovascular system and on epinephrine release.

In terms of nutrition, some progress must be made in reducing the fat content of the American diet and simultaneously increasing the intake of vegetable protein, complex carbohydrates, and fibers. The food industry can certainly contribute toward accomplishing such dietary goals by making meat leaner, by reducing the fat content of dairy products, by producing more tasteful vegetable proteins and complex carbohydrates and by helping to educate the public in the merits of such foods. At present, the public consumes too many calories and particularly too many fat calories in view of its low caloric expenditures. In terms of incentives, the insurance industry could provide economic incentives for individuals with proper health behavior as some countries have done for seat belt users.

Legislative Prevention. We must also consider legislative prevention. Ideas that come to mind include legislation to increase the drinking age, legislation regarding the maximum permissible tar and nicotine levels of cigarettes, and for the fat content in frankfurters and hamburgers. There is an obvious need for regulatory measures for occupational carcinogens. Political considerations are obvious limiting factors for legislative preventive strategies to be achieved.

Epilogue

Epidemiologists can obviously give further leads to the experimentalists to enhance understanding about mechanisms whereby environmental factors cause cancer. At the present time, a particular focus should be on applied epidemiology. Let us apply what we already know in prevention. We need to work toward modifying human behavior and changing the human environment. Thus, we hope to see the true endpoint of preventive medicine and of epidemiology, a reduction in the incidence of cancer in man. To accomplish this goal requires the commitment and the involvement of the entire oncological community and of society.

13th International Cancer Congress, Part E
Cancer Management, pages 347–355
© **1983 Alan R. Liss, Inc., 150 Fifth Avenue, New York, NY 10011**

DIETARY FACTORS IN HUMAN CARCINOGENESIS

Robert MacLennan MS MRCP FRACP

Principal Medical Research Fellow
Queensland Institute of Medical Research,
Bramston Terrace,
Brisbane, Qld 4006, Australia

Although there is, as yet, little direct evidence for
the current theory that diet is a major component of the
presumed environmental causation of cancer there is much
suggestive evidence. Geographical variation in cancer
incidence and the changes in cancer patterns following
migration, strongly suggest that environmental factors in
general are a necessary (but not sufficient) part of the
etiology in around 80 per cent of cancer. One third has
been attributed to diet, but although there is a high
correlation between dietary patterns and cancer incidence
rates (Armstrong & Doll 1975) the proportion attributed to
diet appears to have been estimated on the basis of
exclusion of specific causes (such as smoking, or
occupation) for which there is more compelling evidence.
Dietary factors become more credible in human carcinogenesis
where epidemiological data are consistent with possible
mechanisms of carcinogenesis. Although the latter are
poorly understood a more theoretical mechanistic approach,
instead of an empirical search for specific dietary
factors, could facilitate more effective prevention by
modification of mechanisms in addition, or as an
alternative, to reduction in exposure to dietary risk
factors. This hypothesis testing approach is needed to find
soluble problems for study in an extremely difficult area.
Human carcinogenesis is poorly understood, but it is assumed
that some dietary mechanisms may result in initiation and
others in promotion, with an interval of at least 20 to 30
years between the former and the clinical diagnosis of a
cancer. Further, measuring dietary factors retrospectively
is very difficult due to poor human memory and possible

changes in diet. Some of the theoretically possible ways in which diet may be related to human carcinogenesis are listed in table 1. Cancers of specific sites could be produced by a combination of these possible means.

Table 1. Possible ways in which diet may be related to human carcinogenesis*

Possible role of diet Example

Carcinogens or their immediate Aflatoxin
precursors in food and drink Methods of cooking

Endogenous formation Dietary substrates for
of carcinogens carcinogen formation
                  Dietary fat and
                  bile secretion

Modification of Cruciferous vegetables
metabolic activation or
inactivation

Concentration of Alcoholic beverages
carcinogens   Dietary fibre

Progression of epithelial Vitamin A
premalignant "states"

Other metabolic High energy intake
effects

* Based on MacLennan (1978).

CARCINOGENS IN FOOD AND DRINK

Although carcinogens may be frequently found in very low concentration in much of the food we eat and the intake of mutagens is very common, only relatively few preformed carcinogens have been found in what are believed to be active concentrations in human food. Chief among these are the mycotoxins, notably aflatoxin produced mainly by

Aspergillus flavus. Aflatoxin is a very powerful carcinogen
for the liver in animals and occurs commonly in human foods,
especially peanuts and maize. The geographical variation in
primary carcinoma of the liver has suggested an association
with contamination of food with aflatoxins, an hypothesis
which has been further strengthened by the studies of
Linsell and Peers (1977) in Africa. In Kenya, for example,
they measured aflatoxin in food prior to its preparation and
at the same time developed an ad hoc cancer registry for
primary liver cancer in the same population of Murang'a who
live over a considerable range of altitude. Both aflatoxin
and liver cancer were found to vary inversely with altitude.
Serological studies have shown that a very high proportion
of cases of primary liver cancer have persistent infection
with Hepatitis B virus (HBV). It is possible that
aflatoxins and HBV infection interact, with the latter
inducing hepatocellular necrosis and regeneration, thus
facilitating the carcinogenic action of aflatoxin. In New
Zealand primary liver cancer is fourfold higher in Maoris
than in non-Maoris (Foster 1976). Maoris have been reported
to have a much higher prevalence of HBV than Europeans in
New Zealand (Boveington & Stephens 1972), but relative
intake of aflatoxin is unknown.

Highly mutagenic amino acid pyrolysis products have
been found in charcoal broiled fish (Sugimura et al 1976).
It is possible that roasting and barbequing of foods
containing amino acids could produce similar products, which
in large quantities could produce human cancer. The latter
mechanism may explain the high rectal cancer rates in Dublin
brewery workers (Dean et al 1979). Geographical analysis
had shown a high correlation between national beer
consumption and mortality from cancers of the colon and
rectum (Breslow & Enstrom 1974). It was postulated that
groups with a known high beer consumption would have high
mortality from cancers of the colon and rectum. We found
increased mortality from rectal cancer in brewery workers in
general, and analysis of place of work within the brewery
showed a higher proportion of the rectal cancer deaths had
worked throughout their working lives in the brewhouse.
Surviving widows were interviewed in a survey described as
an inquiry into the leisure time activity of the deceased.
Among other things they were asked about drinking habits. A
higher intake of beer was reported by the spouses of men
dying from rectal cancer compared with other causes.

Samples of the beer have been tested and show strong
mutagenic activity. This is possibly due to the dark
roasted barley which is added to the malt during beer
production. This study suggests that dark beers may be
carcinogenic but that an effect is seen only with very high
consumption.

ENDOGENOUS FORMATION OF CARCINOGENS

Apart from the ingestion of carcinogens or their
immediate precursors it is possible that diet in man can
result in the endogenous formation of carcinogens. Sander
(1970) has induced tumours in various organs of rats by
feeding nitrites and alkylureas. Alkylnitrosoureas were
presumed to be formed in the stomach. In man a lunch
consisting of 310 g of spinach, 170 g cooked bacon, 200 g
tomato, 120 g bread and 460 g of beer resulted in increased
volatile nitrosamines in the blood (Fine et al 1977).

Gastric Cancer

Although the incidence of gastric cancer appears to be
decreasing in most countries, rates continue to be very high
in Japan and many areas of Latin America. Nitroso
compounds, one of the most powerful groups of experimental
carcinogens, could be involved in the etiology. Gastric
cancer has been associated with high nitrate in water in
several populations notably Narino in Colombia (Cuello et al
1976). Nitrate in the diet after ingestion could circulate,
be excreted in the saliva and bacterial action result in
reduction to nitrite; or, gastric nitrate may be reduced in
vivo in the stomach to gastric nitrite. Alternatively
ingestion of nitrites, as occurs with certain water
supplies, could result together with dietary amines and
either gastric acidity or appropriate bacteria, in the in
vivo formation of nitrosamines. This formation is thought
to be inhibited by ascorbic acid and protein. Vegetables
also contain catalysts (e.g. phenols) of nitrosation
reactions. Nitrosamines might result in gastric atrophy and
in intestinal metaplasia of the stomach, which are highly
prevalent in Narino. Both are known to increase the risk of
the intestinal type of gastric carcinoma. Case control
studies have indicated some protective effects for Western

vegetables such as tomatoes and lettuce which are eaten raw, among Japanese in Hawaii (Haenszel et al 1972). The studies of gastric cancer illustrate complex metabolic mechanisms which may relate dietary factors to cancer, with some dietary factors facilitating and others inhibiting endogenous carcinogen formation.

Colo-rectal Cancers

Current interest in the role of gut bacteria in carcinogenesis stems from work on the toxicity of cycasin whose possible toxic properties were investigated in relation to the extraordinary prevalence of amyotrophic lateral sclerosis in Guam. Cycasin unexpectedly produced tumours of the small intestine of normal but not in germ-free rats (Laqueur 1965). Hill et al (1971) have invoked bacterial metabolism to explain the geographical variation in colon cancer and its correlation with national consumption of fat and meat, which are postulated to increase the excretion of bile, a substrate for intestinal bacteria capable of metabolising biles salts to chemical structures resembling known carcinogens. In international metabolic studies they found a high correlation between colon cancer incidence and the concentration in the faeces of the bile acid metabolite dihydroxycholanic acid.

MODIFICATION OF METABOLIC ACTIVATION OR INACTIVATION

Many carcinogens require in vivo metabolism to their active forms, often by cellular enzymes such as the mixed function oidases in the intestine. The levels of these oxidases can be modified by the diet. Graham et al (1978) in a case contol study of colon cancer found a protective effect for cruciferous vegetables, a finding supported in Japan (Haenszel et al 1980).

CONCENTRATION OF CARCINOGENS

Alcholic Beverages

The concentration of carcinogens at their target sites could be increased by the diet. In North-western France a case-control study of oesophageal cancer showed that both increasing consumption of alcoholic beverages and of tobacco resulted in increased relative risks for oesophageal cancer but there was a much greater effect for alcohol and smoking combined (Tuyns et al 1977). There may thus be potentiation by alcohol (possibly acting as a solvent) of the carcinogenic action of tobacco tars.

Dietary Fibre

Risk factors for colo-rectal cancer have been investigated in many studies. No single dietary factor is likely to explain the variation in colo-rectal cancer and a complex multifactorial mechanism involving several dietary factors and endogenous metabolism is likely. From population studies in Denmark and Finland (IARC 1977) and some recent case control studies, it appears that dietary fibre could protect from the effects of an otherwise high-risk diet rich in fat or meat (MacLennan 1980). The mechanism whereby dietary fibre may exert an effect is uncertain, but it may be by reduction in the concentration of carcinogens in the large intestine (IARC 1977; Reddy et al 1978). There could be direct effects on metabolism and formation of carcinogens in the colon by lowering of pH.

PROGRESSION OF EPITHELIAL PREMALIGNANT "STATES"

Diet might halt or reverse the presumed early stages of malignant transformation. Evidence is accumulating that the intake of vitamin A and beta carotene can modify the effects of carcinogenic risk factors such as cigarette smoking. Several studies (e.g. Bjelke 1975, MacLennan et al 1977) have shown at least a two-fold protective effect against lung cancer of dietary intake of foods rich in vitamin A, and/or beta carotene, although the possibility remains that some other dietary factor present in such foods is responsible for the observed lower risk.

OTHER METABOLIC EFFECTS

There is experimental evidence that "low" energy intake decreases the tumour yield compared with "high" intake. Evidence in man is less convincing although in a follow-up of 750 000 men and women in the American Cancer Society prospective study (Lew & Garfinkel 1979) cancer mortality was elevated among persons 40% or more overweight. The sites of increased cancer were mainly colon and rectum in men; and endometrium, gall bladder and biliary passages, breast, cervix and ovary in women. A contrary trend was shown for lung cancer, but these data were not adjusted simultaneously for smoking.

CONCLUSION

Evidence is accumulating in colorectal and other cancers that diet may be a necessary, although not sufficient factor in causation. Clearly, preventive measures would be more feasible if high risk persons could be identified. This might be possible without a full understanding of the mechanisms of carcinogenesis, as is possible with skin cancer. There are now sufficient leads to justify a major research effort into diet, nutrition, and cancer involving many scientific disciplines. Research on modifiers of carcinogenesis appears to hold most promise and is based on the possibility that while exposure to carcinogens may be unavoidable, the subsequent development of cancer may be prevented. Dietary factors in developing countries are more likely to be naturally occurring carcinogens than in the West, where overnutrition is more likely. Strategies for prevention may therefore be different, but in any case must be based on a fuller understanding of dietary factors in human carcinogenesis.

REFERENCES

Armstrong B, Doll R (1975). Environmental factors and cancer incidence and mortality in different countries, with special reference to dietary practices. Int J Cancer 15:617.

Bjelke E (1975). Dietary vitamin A and human lung cancer. Int J Cancer 15:561.

Boveington CM, Stephens RG (1972). Australia antigen in New Zealand. Lancet 2:138.

Breslow NE, Enstrom JE (1974). Geographic correlations between cancer mortality rates and alcohol-tobacco consumption in the United States. J Natl Cancer Inst 53:631.

Cuello C, Correa P, Haenszel W, Gordillo G, Brown C, Archer M, Tannenbaum S (1976) Gastric cancer in Colombia. I Cancer risk and suspect environmental agents. J Natl Cancer Inst 57:1015.

Dean G, MacLennan R, McLoughlin H, Shelley E (1979). Causes of death of blue-collar workers at a Dublin brewery, 1954-1973. Br J Cancer 40:581.

Fine DH, Ross R, Rounbehler DP, Silvergleid A, Song L (1977). Formation in vitro of volatile N-nitrosamines in man after ingestion of cooked bacon and spinach. Nature 265:753.

Foster FH (1976). In Waterhouse J, Correa P, Muir C, Powell J. (Eds) Cancer Incidence in Five Continents, vol III. Lyon, International Agency for Research on Cancer.

Graham S, Dayal H, Swanson M, Mittelman A, Wilkinson G (1978). Diet in the epidemiology of cancer of the colon and rectum. J Natl Cancer Inst 61:709.

Haenszel W, Kurihara M, Segi M, Lee RKC (1972). Stomach cancer among Japanese in Hawaii. J Natl Cancer Inst 49:969.

Haenszel W, Locke FB, Segi M (1980). A case-control study of large bowel cancer in Japan. J Natl Cancer Inst 64:17.

Hill MJ, Crowther JS, Drasar BS, Hawksworth G, Aries V, Williams REO (1971). Bacteria and aetiology of cancer of the large bowel. Lancet 1:95.

IARC Intestinal Microecology Group (1977). Dietary fibre, transit-time, faecal bacteria, steroids and colon cancer in two Scandinavian populations Lancet 2:207.

Laqueur GL (1965). The induction of intestinal neoplasms in rats with the glycoside cycasin and its aglycone. Virchows Arch (Pathol Anat) 340:151.

Lew EA, Garfinkel L (1979). Variations in mortality by weight among 750,000 men and women. J Chron Dis 32:563.

Linsell CA, Peers FG (1977). Aflatoxin and liver cell cancer. Trans R Soc Trop Med Hyg 71:471.

MacLennan R, de Costa J, Day NE, Law CH, Ng YK, Shanmugaratnam K (1977). Risk factors for lung cancer in Singapore Chinese, a population with high female incidence rates. Int J Cancer 20:854.

MacLennan R (1978). Diet and human carcinogenesis with special reference to colon cancer. Marabou Symposium. Supplement nr 16 till Naringsforskning,argang 22, p29.

MacLennan R (1980). The incidence of colon carcinoma and dietary fibre intake. In Rottka H (Ed). Pflanzenfasern-Ballastoffe in der manschlichen Ernahrung, Stuttgart: Thieme.

Reddy BS, Hedges AR, Laakso K, Wynder EL (1978). Metabolic epidemiology of large bowel cancer. Fecal bulk and constituents of high-risk North American and low-risk Finnish population. Cancer 42:2832.

Sander J (1970). Induktion maligner Tumoren bei Ratten durch orale Gabe von N,N' - Dimethylharnstoff und Nitrit. Arzneimittelforschung 20:418.

Sugimura T, Nagao M, Kawachi T, Honda M, Yahagi T, Seino Y, Sato S, Matsukura N (1977). Mutagen-carcinogens in foods, with special reference to highly mutagenic, pyrolytic products in broiled foods. In Hiatt HH, Watson JD and Winsten JA (Eds.). Origins of Human Cancer. New York, Cold Spring Harbor Laboratory, p 1561.

Tuyns AJ, Pequignot G, Jensen OM (1977). Le cancer de l'oesophage en Ille-et-Vilaine en fonction des niveaux de consommation d'alcool et de tabac. Des risques qui se multiplient. Bull Cancer 64:45.

Acknowledgement

The assistance of the Queensland Cancer Fund in attending the 13th International Cancer Congress is gratefully acknowledged.

**13th International Cancer Congress, Part E
Cancer Management, pages 357–369
© 1983 Alan R. Liss, Inc., 150 Fifth Avenue, New York, NY 10011**

EXPOSURE TO POLYCHLORINATED DIBENZO–P–DIOXINS AND DIBENZO–
FURANS IN THE ENVIRONMENT.

Lennart Hardell, M.D.

Department of Oncology, University Hospital
S–901 85   Umeå
Sweden

Polychlorinated dibenzo–p–dioxins (PCDDs) and dibenzofurans
(PCDFs) are two series of tricyclic aromatic compounds with
similar chemical, physical and toxicological properties. In
all there are 75 PCDD and 135 PCDF isomers. The chemical and
environmental stability coupled with lipophility has resulted in their widespread detection throughout the global system. They have a potential for accumulation in food chains
and therefore they present a threat for man and the environment. Neither PCDDs nor PCDFs occur naturally and they have
never had any technical use but they are impurities in several commercial preparations. It is now evident that the
phenoxy herbicides 2,4,5-trichlorophenoxyacetic acid (2,4,5-
T) and 2,4-dichlorophenoxyacetic acid (2,4-D) are not the
only sources of PCDDs and PCDFs.

Table 1. Levels of 2,3,7,8-Tetra-CDD in 2,4,5-T Acid and
2,4,5-T Ester Formulatins (Rappe et al 1978, Norström et
al 1979).

Sample	Origin	2,3,7,8-TCDD µg/g
2,4,5-T acid	1952, Sweden	1.10
2,4,5-T ester	1960, Sweden	0.40
2,4,5-T ester	1962, Finland	0.95
2,4,5-T ester	1967, Finland	0.22
2,4,5-T acid	1964, USA	4.8
2,4,5-T acid	1969, USA	6.0
Herbicide Orange	unknown, USA	0.12
Herbicide Orange	unknown, USA	5.1

The major identified sources are associated with the use of
chlorophenols (CPs) in the wood industry.

Table 2. Levels of PCDDs and PCDFs in Commercial Chlorinated Phenols (μg/g/). (Rappe et al 1981).

	PCDDs	PCDFs
2,4,6-Trichlorophenol, Sweden	<3	60
2,4,6-Trichlorophenol, USA	0.3	4.6
2,3,4,6-Tetrachlorophenol, Finland	12	160
Pentachlorophenol, USA	2625	190
Pentachlorophenol, USA	1900	790
Pentachlorophenol, Germany	6.8	2.1

Also combustion of organic materials treated with CPs and
chemical dumps are sources of contamination. Pyrolysis of
commercial polychlorinated biphenyls (PCBs) generates PCDFs
whereas no PCDDs were identified (Buser el al 1978a).

Table 3. Levels of PCDFs in commercial PCBs (Bowes et al
1975).

Sample	Total μg/g
Aroclor 1248, 1969	2.0
Aroclor 1260, 1969	1.5
Clophen A 60	8.4
Phenoclor DP-6	13.6
Mitsubishi (used)[a]	10.0

a) Rappe and Buser, unpublished

Hexachlorophene (3,4,6-trichlorophenol) is another product
contaminated with PCDDs and PCDFs. Hexachlorophene has been
widely used as antiseptic and has been added to a wide
variety of over-the-counter products, including soaps,
shampoos, acne medications, deodorants, toothpastes, "vagi-
nal hygiene" preparations, and shaving creams (Martin-
Bouyer et al 1982).

CPs were first described in 1936 by the Dow Chemical Company under the trade name of Dowicide. Already in 1937
chloracne developed among workers manufacturing CPs (Butler
1937). PCDDs as being the responsible substances as inducers of chloracne were first described by Schulz in 1957.

Hexachlorophene was developed in 1939. The toxicity of
orally ingested hexachlorophene in animals was first described in 1939 and percutaneous hexachlorophene toxicity
in rabbits was described the same year (reports by Applied
Research Laboratories, Inc., to Givaudan Corporation, unpublished). Human percutaneous hexachlorophene poisoning
was first reported in 1959 (Herter 1959).

Sources:

In 1977 Olie et al reported on the occurrence of PCDDs and
PCDFs in fly ash of municipal incernators in the Netherlands. Also Buser et al have reported the same findings
(Buser et al 1978b). The variation of isomers of PCDDs
found in various samples of fly ash strongly suggests commercial CPs as the precursors. Regarding PCDF isomers identified in fly ash most of them are also formed in the pyrolysis of commercial PCBs (Aroclor 1254 and 1260) strongly
suggesting these commonly used products as the precursors
of the PCDFs in fly ash (Rappe, Buser 1981).

It has been suggested that PCDDs, including 2,3,7,8-TCDD,
can be generated by a pyrolytic de novo formation from carbon and chlorides (Bumb et al 1980). This "trace chemistries
of fire" hypothesis was orginally postulated by Dow
Chemical Company (Dow Chemical Co. 1978). However, the experimental data available strongly indicate that the domi-
nating part of the PCDDs found originate from chlorinated
aromatics used as industrial chemicals, the chlorinated
phenols being the major source (Rappe et al 1981). Moreover,
attempts to identify PCDDs in emmissions from coal-fired
power-plants have failed (Kimble, Gross 1980).

The estimated yearly input of PCDDs in the Canadian environment has been estimated to about 1500 kg, the major
source being CPs whereas the phenoxy herbicides and combustion sources were calculated to contribute only to a
minor degree (NRCC 1981).

Persistence in the Environment:

PCDDs appear to be resistant to photolysis except in the
presence of a hydrogen donor. In pure water and on soil
surfaces very little photolysis occurs (Dobbs, Grant 1979).

In fact, photoformation of PCDDs from pentachlorophenol
(PCP) can occur in very low yields (Lamparski et al 1980).
The PCDDs tend to be rapidly and strongly absorbed to most
soils. Migration of TCDD deep into soils have been reported
around Seveso in Italy (Cavallaro et al 1979). The PCDDs
are, however, relatively insoluble in water (Crummett,
Stehl 1973). PCDDs are considered highly persistent with a
reported half-life in biologically active soils and sedi-
ments of 1-2 years (Ward, Matsumara 1978) and possibly up
to 10 years (DiDomenico et al 1980).

Exposure:

PCDDs are present in various matrices including food.
Primary dermal contact is difficult to assess but exposure
to pesticides has shown an about 10% uptake when such
chemicals are spilled on the forearm (TGOEP 1974). No estimates have been made of the exposure through secondary
dermal contact, i.e. contact with treated vegetation, wood
etc. PCDDs have been reported in some samples of beef fat
(US), fish (Lake Ontario), chicken livers (Canada) and
gelatin (US) (NRCC 1981).

Table 4. PCDD residues associated with food.

| | Number | | PCDD (ng/kg) | Comments | Ref |
	Sampl	Pos	Range de-tected		
Cattle fat	85	2	20-60	2,4,5-T treated and untreated rangeland	a)
milk	10	9	59-7900	Seveso 1976	b)
Chicken liver	19	9	100-1420	PCP impregn.	c)
Fish many species	12	8	20-170	Locations around Midland	d)
	12	3	20-102	Lake Ontario	e)
Gelatin	15	10	80-1290	Associated with PCP residues	f)

References to table 4:
a) Harless et al (1980)
b) Fanelli et al (1980)
c) Ryan, Pilon (1981)
d) Dow Chemical Co (1978)
e) McLeod (1981)
f) Firestone (1977)

PCDDs can enter the diet by different routes (NRCC 1981):
1. Accumulation in the aquatic systems like PCBs and DDT.
2. Accidental spillage of contaminated fluids into foods or feeds during processing etc.
3. Use of CPs treated wood products or by-products in agriculture or gardens.
4. Use of treated wood waste in the pulp industry and use of potentially contaminated products in the food industry.
5. Use of herbicides contaminated with PCDDs.

Groups among the general population who may be exposed to PCDDs through inhalation are those who use wood treated with CPs and those who live within houses whose interior surfaces are treated with CP-based products. Another possibility is the contribution of incineration of CPs-treated wood. Workers in wood treatment plants, tanneries, pulp and paper mills are at occupational risk to be exposed to PCDDs and PCDFs (Klemmer et al 1980, EPA 1978). Sawmill-workers, tannery-workers, textile impregnators and seamstresses sewing treated fabric all have elevated PCP urine levels (Rappe et al 1981). In almost all cases the exposure would also include PCDDs and PCDFs. A large part results thus from extensive use of CPs, in particular PCP as a preservative. Additions are use or manufacture of phenoxy herbicides, chlorobenzenes and hexachlorophene. It is thus necessary to consider the use of products contaminated with PCDDs such as wood preservatives, as herbicides but also contaminated materials as treated lumber, mouthwashes, cleansers, etc. Also recycling of contaminated products must be considered such as contaminated wood chips for pulp or burning, inadequate disposal practices, accidents, dumping of contaminated chemicals etc. Regarding exposure to PCDFs factories manufacturing or reparing transformers or capacitors containing PCBs should be considered.

Toxicology:

Most of the data available refer to PCDDs of which 2,3,7,8-TCDD has been most investigated due to its extreme acute toxicity. However, the same toxicological pattern seems to attribute to PCDFs as to PCDDs. The highest human tissue concentration of TCDD has been found in fat whereas the highest accumulation of PCDFs is in the liver.

Table 5. Human tissue concentrations of 2,3,7,8-T CDD (after Facchetti et al 1980).

Tissue	2,3,7,8-T CDD/wet tissue (ng.kg^{-1})
Fat	1840
Pancreas	1040
Liver	150
Thyroid	85
Brain	60
Lung	60
Kidney	40
Blood	6

A variety of signs and symptoms have been reported in human populations following accidental exposure to PCDDs and relaed compounds. These have included (NRCC 1981):

- skin lesions, including chloracne, hyperpigmentation and thickening of the skin

- hair loss and hirsutism

- porphyria cutanea tarda

- central and peripheral nervous disorders

- liver, kidney and gastrointestinal disturbances

- neurasthenia, including lack of drive and vigor, sleep disturbances, emotional instability and altered basic frame of mind

- respiratory and cardiac disorders

- hypothyroidism

TCDD has been shown to be a potent inducer of the hepatic enzymes aryl hydrocarbon hydroxylase (AHH) (Poland et al 1979), 5-amino levulinic acid synthetase (ALAS) (Poland and Glover 1980) and glutathine transferase (S-GT) (Kirsch et al 1975). ALAS activity is associated with defect hepatic porphyria synthesis causing porphyria cutanea tarda. The bulk of the data suggest that PCDDs are not mutagenic. Immunosuppressive effects have been demonstrated (Vos, Moore 1974). Regarding teratogenic effects cleft palate and kidney abnormalitites predominate in mice. (Smith et al 1976).

Carcinogenicity:

During the past few years exposure to phenoxy acids or chlorophenols has attached an increasing interest as a possible cause of malignant disorders. Thus Swedish rail-road workers were found to have an increased incidence of tumour mortality related to both amitrole and phenoxy acid preparations (Axelson et al 1980). Case reports on soft-tissue sarcomas (Hardell 1977) and malignant lymphomas (Hardell 1979) as possibly related to exposure to phenoxy acids, have strengthened the suspicion that these substances are carcinogenic. These clinical observations initiated two subsequent case-referent studies of soft-tissue sarcoma which demonstrated a roughly 6-fold increase in the risk after exposure to phenoxy acids or chlorophenols (Hardell, Sandström 1979, Eriksson et al 1981). A similar matched case-referent study of malignant lymphoma (both Hodgkin's disease and non-Hodgkin lymphoma) indicated an association also between that disease and exposure to phenoxy acids or chlorophenols but also to organic solvents (Hardell et al 1981).

In a cohort study of mortality among workers exposed to TCDD in a 1949 trichlorophenol (TCP) accident a suspicious increase of lymphatic and hematopoetic malignancies was observed, i.e. 3 deaths as compared to 0.88 expected (Zack, Suskind 1980). In a British plant manufacturing pentachlorophenol 2 men with NHL of the scalp have been reported versus 0.28 NHL expected (Bishop, Jones 1981). Also a study by Cantor (1982) is in agreement with the Swedish study showing an elevated risk among younger farmers for histiocytic lymphoma in counties high in summary measures of general agricultural activity (OR = 3.2), of rural grain acreage and acres treated with insecticides (OR = 6.6), and of wheat acreage (OR = 4.4). Several studies have revealed an increased incidence of Hodgkin's disease in lumberjacks and woodworkers (Milham, Hesser 1967, Grufferman et al 1976, Greene et al 1978).

In four separate studies of cohorts of workers occupationally exposed to 2,4,5-T or to trichlorophenol a total of 3 deaths (2,9%) from soft-tissue sarcoma were observed versus 0.07% expected (Honchar, Halperin 1981). A fourth case of soft-tissue sarcoma has been reported in one of these groups of men (Cook 1981). Another employee exposed to 2,4,5-T in one of the firms concerned in these studies has recently died of neurogenic sarcoma (Moses, Selikoff 1981). Three thoracic soft-tissue sarcomas have lately been reported among Vietnam war veterans exposed to the mixture of phenoxy acids known as agent-orange, but it is not clear whether or not these cases represent an excess (Sarma, Jacobs 1982). In Vietnam an increase in the number of persons with primary liver cancer in proportion to the number of all cancers in North Vietnam during the period when herbicides were used in South Vietnam was reported (Tung 1973).

Regarding animal testing, groups of mice administered 2,7-DCDD showed increased incidence of leuchemias and lymphomas, hemangiosarcomas and hemangiomas and of hepatocellular carcinoma (NCI 1979). In a study by Van Miller et al (1977) feeding rats with TCDD various tumour types were induced among them different soft-tissue sarcomas. A NCI study (1980[a]) studying the carcinogenicity of TCDD showed in mice a significant increase in hepatocellular carcinoma but also of fibrosarcoma, histiocytic lymphoma, thyroid follicular cell adenoma and adrenal cortical adenoma. Fibrosarcoma in the integumentary system was found in female mice treated dermally with 2,3,7,8-TCDD (NCI 1980 [b]). In summary these data demonstrate that 2,3,7,8-TCDD is carcinogenic in rats and mice. Whether 2,3,7,8-TCDD acts as a promotor as suggested by Pitot et al (1980), as an initiator or as both a promotor and initiator is unclear, however.

Exposure to PCDDs and PCDFs occurs thus occupationally in different types of work. Industrial accidents may give high grade of exposure. The bioaccumulation and spreading of PCDDs and PCDFs in the ecological system result in large groups of populations being at risk of exposure. Moreover products contaminated by PCDDs and PCDFs contribute to such exposure. Local exposure of the general population occurs where chemicals have been dumped in soil or in water as in Love Canal (USA), Tecomatorp (Sweden) or through industrial accidents as near Seveso in 1976. In the presence of the carcinogenic and toxicological data of PCDDs and PCDFs it is necessary to limit the exposure of the populations to those compounds to an absolute minimum.

References:

Axelson O, Sundell L, Andersson K, Edling C, Hogstedt C, Kling H (1980). Herbicide exposure and tumour mortality; an updated epidemiological investigation on Swedish railroad workers. Scand J Work Environ Hlth 6: 73-79.

Bishop CM, Jones AH (1981). Non-Hodgkin's lymphoma of the scalp in workers exposed to dioxins. Lancet ii: 369.

Bowes GW, Mulvihill MY, Simoneit BRT, Burlingame AL, Risebrough RW (1975). Identification of chlorinated dibenzofurans in American polychlorinated biphenyls. Nature 256: 305-307.

Bumb RR, Crummett WB, Cutie SS, Gledhill JR, Hummel RII, Kage RO, Lamparski LL, Luoma EV, Miller DL, Nestrick TJ, Shadoff LA, Stehl RH, Woods JS (1980).
Trace chemistries of fire; a source of chlorinated dioxins. Science 210: 385-390.

Butler MG (1937). Arch Derm Syph 35:251.

Buser HR, Bosshardt HP, Rappe C, Lindahl R (1978a). Identification of polychlorinated dibenzofuran isomers in fly ash and PCB pyrolysis. Chemosphere 7: 419-429.

Buser HR, Bosshardt H, Rappe C (1978b). Identification of polychlorinated dibenzo-p-dioxin isomers found in fly ash. Chemosphere 7: 165-172.

Cantor KP (1982). Farming and mortality from non-Hodgkin's lymphoma; a case-control study. Int J Cancer 29: 239-247.

Cavallaro A, Tebaldi G, DeFelice G, Colli G, Gualdi R (1979). Indagine sperimentale sulla penetrazione di TCDD nella zona A di Seveso. Boll Chim d'Unione Ital Lab Prov Sci 5: 489-541.

Crummett WB, Stehl RH (1973). Determination of chlorinated dibenzo-p-dioxins and dibenzofurans in various materials. Environ Health Persp 5: 15-25.

DiDomenico A, Silano V, Viviano G, Zapponi G (1980). Accidental release of 2,3,7,8-tetrachlorodibenzo-p-dioxin (TCDD) at Seveso, Italy. V. Environmental persistence of TCDD in soil. Ecotoxicol Environ Safety 4: 339-345.

Dobbs AJ, Grant C (1979). Photolysis of highly chlorinated dibenzo-p-dioxins by sunlight. Nature 278: 163–165.

Dow Chemical Co (1978). The trace chemistries of fire – a source of and routes for entry of chlorinated dioxins into the environment. The Chlorinated Dioxin Task Force. Dow Chemical Co, Midland, Michigan: p 46 plus Appendices.

EPA (1978). Pesticide programs. Rebuttable presumption against registration and continued registration of pesticide products containing pentachlorophenol. Fed Regist 43(202): 48443–48617.

Eriksson M, Hardell L, Berg NO, Möller T, Axelson O (1981). Soft tissue sarcomas and exposure to chemical substances; a case-referent study. Br J Indust Med 38: 27–33.

Facchetti S, Fornari A, Montagna M (1980). Distribution of 2,3,7,8-tetrachlorodibenzo-p-dioxin in the tissues of a person exposed to the toxic cloud at Seveso. Adv Mass Spectrom 8B: 1405–1414.

Fanelli R, Bertoni MP, Bonfanti M, Castelli MG, Chiabrando C, Martelli GP, Noe MA, Noseda A, Garrattini S, Binaghi C, Marazza V, Pezza F, Pozzoll D, Cicognetti G (1980). 2,3,7, 8-Tetrachlorodibenzo-p-dioxin levels in cow's milk from the contaminated area of Seveso, Italy. Bull Environ Contam Toxicol 24: 634–639.

Firestone D (1977). Determination of polychlorodibenzo-p-dioxins and polychlorodibenzofurans in commercial gelatins by bas-liquid chromatography. J Agric Food Chem 25: 1274–1280.

Greene MH, Brinton LA, Fraumeni JF, D'Amico R (1978). Familial and sporadic Hodgkin's disease associated with occupational wood exposure. Lancet ii: 626–627.

Grufferman S, Duong T, Cole P (1976). Occupation and Hodgkin's disease. J Nat Cancer Inst 57: 1193–1195.

Hardell L (1977). Soft tissue sarcomas and exposure to phenoxy acids; a clinical observation. Läkartidningen 74: 2753–2754.

Hardell L (1979). Malignant lymphoma of histiocytic type and exposure to phenoxyacetic acids or chlorophenols. Lancet i: 55–56.

Hardell L, Sandström A (1979). Case-control study: soft tissue sarcomas and exposure to phenoxyacetic acids or chlorophenols. Br J Cancer 39: 711–717.

Hardell L, Eriksson M, Lenner P, Lundgren E (1981). Malignant lymphoma and exposure to chemicals, especially organic solvents, chlorophenols and phenoxy acids; a case-control study. Br J Cancer 43: 169–176.

Harless RL, Oswald EO, Wilkinson MK, Dupuy AE Jr, McDaniel DD, Han Tai (1980). Sample preparation and gas chromatography-mass spectrometry determination of 2,3,7,8-tetrachlorodibenzo-p-dioxin. Anal Chem 52: 1239-1245.

Herter WB (1959). Hexachlorophene poisoning. Kaiser Fnd Med Bull 7: 228-230.

Honchar PA, Halperin WE (1981). 2,4,5-T, trichlorophenol and soft tissue sarcomas. Lancet i: 268-269.

Kirsch R, Fleischer G, Kamisaka K, Arias JM (1975). Structural and functional studies of ligandin, a major renal organic anion binding protein. J Clin Invest 55: 1009-1019.

Klemmer HW, Wong L, Sato MM, Reichert EL, Korsak RJ, Rashad MN (1980). Clinical findings in workers exposed to pentachlorophenol. Arch Environ Contam Toxicol 9: 715-725.

Lamparski LL, Stehl RH, Johnson RL (1980). Photolysis of pentachlorophenol-treated wood. Chlorinated dibenzo-p-dioxin formation. Environ Sci Technol 14: 196-200.

Martin-Boyer G, Lebreton G, Toga M, Stolley PD, Lockhart J (1982). Outbreak of accidental hexachlorophene poisoning in France. Lancet i: 91-95.

McLeod HA (1981). Personal Communication to MJ Boddington. Health Protection Branch, Health and Welfare Canada.

Milham S, Hesser JE (1967). Hodgkin's disease in woodworkers. Lancet ii: 136-137.

Moses M, Selikoff IJ (1981). Soft tissue sarcomas, phenoxy herbicides and chlorinated phenols. Lancet i: 1370.

NCI (1979). Bioassay of 2,7-dichlorodibenzo-p-dioxin (DCDD) for possible carcinogenicity. Carcinogenesis Testing Program, National Cancer Institute. Tech Rpt Ser #123. NTIS Dept Comm PB290570.

NCI (1980a). Bioassay of 2,3,7,8-tetrachlorodibenxo-p-dioxin (gavage study). Carcinogenesis Testing Program, National Cancer Institute. DHHS Publ # (NIH) 80-1765. (original unseen).

NCI (1980b). Bioassay of 2,3,7,8-tetrachlorodibenzo-p-dioxin for possible carcinogenicity. Carcinogenesis Testing Program, National Cancer Institute. Tech Rpt 201. DHHS Publ # (NIH) 80-1757. (original unseen).

NRCC (1981). Polychlorinated dibenzo-p-dioxins; criteria for their effects on man and his environment. Ottawa, Canada: pp 23-165.

Olie K, Vermeulen PL, Hutzinger O (1977). Chlorodibenzo-p-dioxins and chlorodibenzofurans are trace components of fly ash and flue gas of some municipal incinerators in the Netherlands. Chemosphere 6: 455-459.

Pitot HC, Goldsworthy T, Poland H (1980). Promotion by 2,3,7,8-tetrachlorodibenzo-p-dioxin of hepatocarcinogenesis from diethylnitrosamine. Cancer Res 40: 3616-3620.

Poland A, Glover E (1980). 2,3,7,8-Tetrachlorodibenzo-p-dioxin; studies on the mechanism in action. In The Scientific bases of toxicity assessment. Edited by H Witschi: pp 223-239.

Poland A, Greenlee WF, Kende AS (1979). Studies on the mechanism of action of the chlorinated dibenzo-p-dioxins and related compounds. Ann N.Y. Acad Sci 320: 214-230.

Rappe C, Buser HR (1981). Occupational exposure to polychlorinated dioxins and dibenzofurans. Am Chem Soc Symp Ser 149: 319-342.

Rappe C, Buser HR, Bosshardt HP (1978). Identification and quantitation of polychlorinated dibenzo-p-dioxins (PCDDs) and dibenzofurans (PCDFs) in 2,4,5,-T-ester formulations and Herbicide Orange. Chemosphere 7: 431-438.

Rappe C, Garå A, Buser HR (1978). Identification of polychlorinated dibenzofurans (PCDFs) in commercial chlorophenol formulations. Chemosphere 7: 981-991.

Rappe C, Nygren M, Buser HR, Kauppinen T (1981). Occupational exposure to polychlorinated dioxins and dibenzofurans. In Impact of chlorinated dioxins and related compounds on the environment. Edited by O Hutzinger, RW Frei, E Merian, F Pocchiari. Pergamon Press, Oxford: pp 495-513.

Ryan JJ, Pilon JC (1981). Chlorinated-dibenzodioxins and dibenzofurans in chicken liver and litter arising from pentachlorophenol contamination of wood shavings. In Impact of chlorinated dioxins and related compounds on the environment. Edited by O Hutzinger, RW Frei, E Merian and F Pocchiari. Pergamon Press, Oxford: pp 183-189. (In press).

Sarma PR, Jacobs J (1982). Thoracic soft tissue sarcoma in Vietnam veterans exposed to agent orange. N Engl J Med 306: 1109.

Schultz KH (1957). Arch Klin Exp Derm.

Smith FA, Schwetz BA, Nitschke KD (1976). Teratogenicity of 2,3,7,8-tetrachlorodibenzo-p-dioxin in CF-1 mice. Toxicol Appl Pharmacol 38: 517-523.

TGOEP (1974). Occupational exposure to pesticides. Rpt to Federal Working Group or Pest Management from the Task Group on Occupational Exposure to Pesticides. NTIS, US Dept Commerce #PB-244259: p 154.

Tung TT (1973). Le cancer primaire du foie du Viet-Nam. Chirurgie 99: 427-436.

Van Miller JP, Lalich JJ, Allen JR (1977). Increased incidence of neoplasms in rats exposed to low levels of 2,3, 7,8-tetrachlorodibenzo-p-dioxin. Chemosphere 10: 625-632.

Vos JG, Moore JA, Zinkl JG (1974). Toxicity of 2,3,7,8-tetrachlorodibenzo-p-dioxin in C57B1/6 mice. Toxicol Appl Pharmacol 29: 229-241.

Ward CT, Matsumura F (1978). Fate of 2,3,7,8-tetrachloro-dibenzo-p-dioxin (TCDD) in a model aquatic environment. Arch Environ Contam Toxicol 7: 349-357.

Zack JA, Suskind RR (1980). The mortality experience of workers exposed to tetrachlorodibenzo-p-dioxin in a tri-chlorophenol process accident. J Occup Med 22: 11-14.

CONGRESS SYMPOSIA

ECONOMICS OF CANCER CARE Einhorn, J., Sweden, Chairman; Monaco, G., USA, Co-Chairman; Opera House

Economic Cost of Cancer in the United States, 1980. *Hodgson, T. A., Hyattsville, MD USA.

Issues of Payment for Cancer Care. *Hoffman, R. W., Seattle, WA USA.

Economics as a Significant Contributor to Family Stress in Childhood Cancer. *Monaco, G., Washington, DC USA.

The Economics of Cancer Care in Canada. *Lentle, B. C., Edmonton, Alberta, Canada.

Cancer Care Cost in Japan. *Maeda, N., Tokyo, Japan.

Please note: Papers that are listed as "By Title Only" were presented at the 13th International Cancer Congress, but are not included in these volumes.

13th International Cancer Congress, Part E
Cancer Management, pages 373–382

ECONOMIC COST OF CANCER IN THE UNITED STATES, 1980

Thomas A. Hodgson, Ph.D.

Chief Economist
National Center for Health Statistics
Hyattsville, Maryland   20782

INTRODUCTION

It is estimated that about 1.25 million persons were
diagnosed as having cancer in 1980 in the United States,
including 400,000 new cases of nonmelonoma skin cancer
(American Cancer Society 1980), and 414,320 persons died of
the disease (National Center for Health Statistics 1981).
The social and economic implications of cancer for victims
and the society at large are pain, suffering, disability,
and death; millions of years of life lost; vast amounts of
human and economic resources devoted to detection, diagnosis, treatment, and rehabilitation; and billions of
dollars of economic output forgone annually because of lost
human resources.

Direct economic costs are those connected with the use
of medical care in the prevention, diagnosis and treatment
of illness and disease, and for the continuing care, rehabilitation, and terminal care of patients. These costs
include expenditures for hospitalization; outpatient clinical care; nursing home care; home health care; services of
primary physicians and specialists, and other health practitioners; drugs and drug sundries; and rehabilitation
counseling and other rehabilitation costs, such as for
prostheses, appliances, and speech devices related to overcoming impairments resulting from illness or disease.

In this paper we give estimates of the medical care
expenditures associated with the prevalence of cancer in
1980 according to age, sex and cancer site, and compare the

costs of cancer with expenditures for heart disease, stroke, injury and poisoning. In conclusion, we briefly discuss indirect costs, or lost output, in 1977.

EXPENDITURES FOR PERSONAL HEALTH CARE

The Health Care Financing Administration estimates annual expenditures for health care. In 1980, spending for personal health care amounted to $219 billion (Gibson, Waldo 1981). Of this total, figure 1 shows that 46 percent ($100 billion) was for hospital care, 21 percent ($47 billion) for physicians' services, 9 percent ($21 billion) for nursing home care, and 24 percent ($51 billion) for other health services, including drugs. These expenditures can be distributed by diagnosis, sex, and age according to the number of services used and the unit prices or charges for these services. For example, expenditures in community hospitals are allocated to a disease category in proportion to the number of days of care attributable to the diagnosis weighted by the cost per patient day. Similar procedures are applied where possible to other types of health care to distribute the total among diagnoses. By this method,

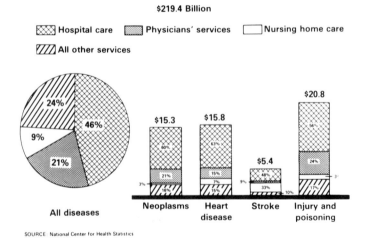

Fig. 1. Medical care expenditures, 1980.

neoplasms accounted for $15.3 billion in medical care expend-
itures, 7 percent of the total. By comparison, injuries
and poisoning required almost $21 billion worth of services,
nearly $16 billion was spent for heart disease, and expen-
ditures for stroke were $5.4 billion. In each case, hospi-
tal care accounted for the largest proportion of spending,
from 48 percent of the cost of stroke to 63 percent of the
cost of heart disease. Although expenditures were much
less for physicians' services than for hospital care, they
were the next largest component for neoplasms (21 percent),
heart disease (15 percent), and injuries and poisoning (24
percent). For these three categories of disease relatively
small amounts were spent for nursing home care. For stroke,
however, nursing home care accounted for one-third of the
total spent, while physicians' services represented only 9
percent of expenditures.

Of the $15.3 billion spent for neoplasms, $12.1 billion
(79 percent) resulted from malignant neoplasms or cancers
and $3.2 billion was due to benign neoplasms (figure 2).
More was spent for hospital care ($9.1 billion) than for all
other services combined. Women used more medical services

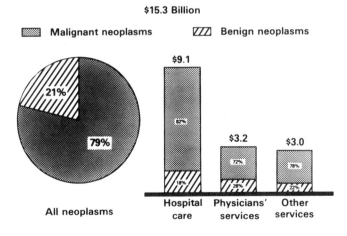

Fig. 2. Medical care expenditures for neoplasms by type of
care, 1980.

than men, $8.9 versus $6.3 billion, and persons under 65
years of age required $9.7 billion worth of medical care
compared to $5.6 billion for those age 65 years and over
(figure 3). Figure 4 shows that $11.7 billion was spent on
cancer for hospital care, physicians' services and all
other services, excluding nursing home care. The amount
spent varied according to the cancer site. For the sites
shown in figure 4, malignant neoplasms of the digestive
organs and peritoneum required the largest expenditures
($2.3 billion), while the least amount was spent for
cancers of bone, connective tissue, and skin ($0.9
billion). The proportions spent for hospital care and
physicians' services also varied with site. For cancers of
the trachea, lung, and bronchus, hospital care accounted
for 70 percent of expenditures and physicians' services 13
percent. For malignant neoplasms of bone, connective,
tissue, and skin, on the other hand, 52 percent of the
total was spent for hospital care and 31 percent for
physicians' services. For the sites shown, all other services represented a relatively constant share of expenditures, varying from 15 to 17 percent of the total for each
site.

The prevalence-based costs discussed above provide an
estimate of the direct economic costs incurred in the year
1980 (the base period) as a result of the prevalence of
disease during this same base period. Included are the
costs of the base year manifestations or sequelae of
disease which may have had its onset in the base year or
any time prior to the base year. Prevalence costs measure
the value of resources used during the specified period of
time, regardless of the time of disease onset. In addition
to prevalence costs, it may be important to know the costs
associated with the incidence of disease. For a specific
case these include the medical care expenditures from onset
until cure or death, a period that can extend over many
years. Incidence costs represent the lifetime costs
resulting from the disease or illness. In the aggregate,
incidence costs in a given base year refer to the total
lifetime costs of all cases with onset of disease in the
base year. Incidence costs measure savings, or benefits,
of reducing the incidence of disease or preventing new
cases, or of successful intervention during the course of
the disease. Both the prevalence and incidence approaches
measure expenditures for medical care. The difference
between the two methods is in terms of which cases occuring

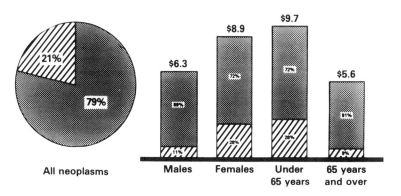

Fig. 3. Medical care expenditures for neoplasms by sex and age, 1980.

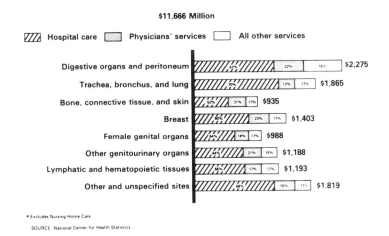

Fig. 4. Medical care expenditures for malignant neoplasms by site, 1980.

in the base period are included in the analysis, and the time period that determines the costs to be counted.

To determine the reduction in health costs that would result from changes in the incidence of disease, as might result from incremental changes in environmental conditions or new prevention initiatives, it is not only necessary to calculate the costs of particular health conditions during the recent past (prevalence costs), but also to predict the consequences of various types of changes in the incidence and natural history of these conditions on the future utilization of health services. Incidence costs are difficult to estimate since they require knowledge of the likely course of a disease and its duration, including survival rates by time since onset, medical care that will be used, and its cost during the length of the disease. These factors vary greatly, even within a specific diesease category, and for a disease such as cancer will depend on organ site, histological type of cellular change, and stage of disease development when treatment commences. Relatively few incidence based studies exist, but the current state of the art is illustrated by Hartunian, Smart, and Thompson (1980; 1981) who estimate the costs of cancer, coronary heart disease, stroke, and motor vehicle injuries, and Policy Analysis, Inc. (1981) who examine the costs of breast cancer, diabetes mellitus, rheumatoid arthritis, stroke, and acute lymphocytic leukemia. Both studies demonstrate that incidence based costs are methodologically feasible, but attempts to estimate incidence costs still suffer from limitations of data and knowledge.

In addition to medical care expenses, other costs may be incurred by patients and family. These include costs resulting from special diets and clothing, dwelling modifications, homemaker care (household help for cleaning, laundering, cooking and babysitting), vocational, social and family counselling services, transportation to medical care providers, out of area living by those individuals who travel, for example, to medical centers and live there while undergoing treatment, relocation of place of residence, lost earnings or salaries and wages of family members who have to give up work or work part-time in order to care for a patient in the home, forced liquidation of tangible assets (interest lost on withdrawal of savings to pay expenses), and other financial costs such as interest charges on funds borrowed to pay for illness-related expenses, including

interest on personal loans, mortgages, and loans against
the cash value of life insurance. Unfortunately, we have
no way of knowing the magnitudes of these costs since the
necessary studies have not been done.

LOSSES IN OUTPUT

Illness and disease may result in the cessation or
reduction of productive activities due to morbidity,
mortality, and disability. Illness may prevent persons
from leading their accustomed productive lives in terms of
working and keeping house. They may lose time from their
activities, be forced out of their jobs or become institutionalized, or die prematurely. The resulting losses are
called indirect costs. The measure of output loss is earnings and the imputed market value of unperformed housekeep-
ing services. The value of other nonmarket activities,
both work and leisure, is also an indirect cost but lack of
data and conceptual difficulties prevent calculating the
monetary loss when these activities are curtailed.

The year 1977 is the latest for which estimates of
indirect costs are available. In 1977, 38.2 million
productive person-years were lost (figure 5). Of this
total, 84 percent (32.1 million person-years) resulted from
premature mortality and 16 percent (6.1 million person-
years) were due to morbidity among persons currently
employed, those unable to work because of chronic illness
or disability, and women unable to keep house. Not
included in this figure, however, is the morbidity loss
among the institutionalized population. Neoplasms
accounted for 6.5 million person-years, or 17 percent,
heart disease 9.3 million person-years, accidents 4.2
million person-years, and stroke 2.2 million person-years.
The 38.2 million person-years represented a total of $176
billion lost to the economy in 1977 (figure 6). Neoplasms
accounted for $26.3 billion, or 15 percent of the total,
while $33.6 billion were lost to heart disease, $26.5
billion to accidents, and $6.6 billion to stroke.

When the medical care expenditures are combined with
the annual morbidity costs and life-time mortality losses,
the total economic costs in 1977 were $325 billion based on
a 6 percent discount rate for estimated mortality losses
(figure 7). Medical care expenses accounted for 46 percent

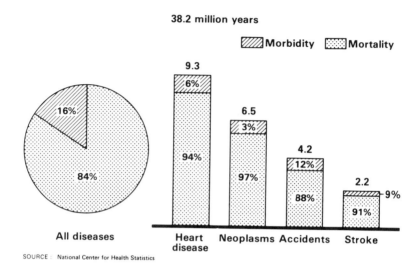

Fig. 5. Person-years lost to illness and disease, 1977.

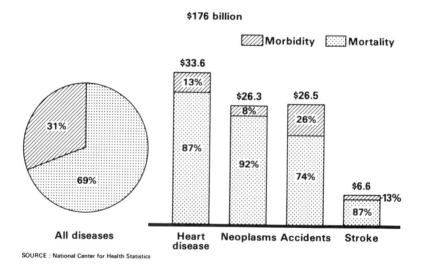

Fig. 6. Earnings lost to illness and disease, 1977.

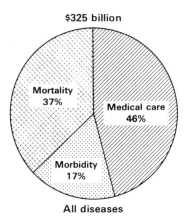

$325 billion

All diseases

SOURCE : National Center for Health Statistics

Fig. 7. Economic costs of disease, 1977.

of the total costs, mortality losses for 37 percent, and morbidity for 17 percent. Indirect costs of morbidity and mortality have not yet been estimated for 1980. But if the relationships in 1980 approximate those in 1977, the $219.4 billion in medical care expenditures in 1980 were accompanied by about $256 billion of indirect costs of morbidity and mortality, for a total economic cost in 1980 of about $475 billion.

American Cancer Society (1980). "1981 Cancer Facts and Figures," New York: American Cancer Society.
Gibson RM, Waldo DR (1981). National health expenditures, 1980. Health Care Fin Rev 3:1.
Hartunian NS, Smart CN, Thompson MS (1980). The incidence and economic costs of cancer, motor vehicle injuries, coronary heart disease, and stroke: a comparative analysis. Amer J Pub Health 70:1249.
Hartunian NS, Smart CN, Thompson MS (1981). "The Incidence and Economic Costs of Major Health Impairments." Lexington, Mass.: Lexington Books.

National Center for Health Statistics (1981). Annual summary of births, deaths, marriages, and divorces: United States, 1980. Monthly Vital Statistics Report No. 13, 29:20.

Policy Analysis, Inc (1981). Evaluation of cost of illness ascertainment methodology: part II applications of methodology to ascertain lifetime economic costs of illness in an incidence cohort. Final report, DHHS contract no. 233-79-2048.

13th International Cancer Congress, Part E
Cancer Management, pages 383–386
© 1983 Alan R. Liss, Inc., 150 Fifth Avenue, New York, NY 10011

ISSUES OF PAYMENT FOR CANCER CARE

Robert W. Hoffman, M.D.

Medical Director
King County Medical Blue Shield
Seattle, Washington 98101

I am the Medical Director of a Blue Shield plan here
in Washington State. We are a rather typical third party
health insurance carrier and the problems and concerns of
my company are common to the health care insurance industry
in the United States. My thoughts and a few suggestions,
however, may well be at variance with others in my position.

The health insurance industry in the United States is
not completely well. The cost of providing medical/surgical
coverage is escalating at a much more rapid rate than most
other essential goods and services and shows no real indication of an easing of its climb. Rapid increases in the
fixed costs of clinics and hospitals, growing numbers of
physicians and para-professional providers, our aging
population,new and effective, but costly diagnostic and
therapeutic techniques are all central to these rising costs.
There are also less apparent pressures such as shifting of
responsibility to the medical profession of problems previously left to the family or the community.

Health insurance carriers are now hard-pressed to
provide coverage for all the things that can and are being
done for patients at a premium which the average American
can afford to pay.

As a society we regard illness or disability as unacceptable, and death as someone's failure. The American
health care system invests enormous resources in the treatment of patients who, as it turns out, are in the final
weeks or months of their life.

The time may come when this country will have to make some decisions about the cost of treatment as it relates to age and prognosis. But I believe that for now our professions and the American people are unwilling to consider a system of health care that makes the cost of treatment its primary concern rather than the extension of life and improvement in its quality.

People want and expect to have access to all of what contemporary medicine has to offer; and this I fully understand. But it also must be understood that someone must somehow pay the bills. For the foreseeable future private and public health insurance programs will continue to be the most practical method of supporting our health care system. But under our present arrangement or some future alternative system of financing, American people must be prepared to budget a larger portion of our wealth to health services.

The progress being made in the understanding and treatment of malignant disease is a major contribution to the well being of all people and can only be applauded. But narrowly viewed, it extends and expands the obligation of health insurance carriers to provide new and often costly benefits, and at a time when similar advancements and demands are coming from almost every field of medicine.

Health insurance premiums in the United States are increasing at 30% or more each year, and are approaching that level which the purchaser of coverage, be it an individual, and employer or a government agency will be unable or unwilling to pay.

Various restraints on the utilization of medical services and their costs such as larger deductibles, co-payment, HMO's, and peer review functions are of some small help, but they do not significantly address the large expenditures required for the care of the kinds of high cost illness with which you people and this Congress are concerned.

The health care insurance industry in this country, and I include both private and public funded carriers, does not know with any accuracy at all what portion of its premium dollar is used in the care of cancer patients. We relate the cost of diagnosis and of much actual treatment to the body system involved and not to the basic underlying disease. An electrocardiogram for a patient with an as yet undiagnosed carcinoma of the pancreas will appear in our statistics on cardiovascular disease. Long range studies on significant numbers of patients with a specific carcinoma are required to give any credibility to estimates on the cost of care. Our actuaries calculate premiums on age and sex distribution, occupations, and our, or some other carrier's previous experience with a specific subscriber pool. Knowing the average cost of care for every important disease entity would be an expensive refinement for which we would have little real use.

Agencies providing broad coverage health care insurance must find the means of meeting their increasing responsibilities. There are important lessons for us in such a Congress as this.

If we agree that the least costly cancer is the one which does not exist then we must give more than lip-service to recognized cancer prevention programs and look to your discipline for focused direction.

Because of much more effective therapy, the early detection of cancer can reduce the cost of care. In the past the health insurance industry has not been convinced that large scale screening programs are cost effective. Perhaps we are wrong and should be listening more to you.

Providing benefits for the palliative and supportive care of the terminally ill patient consumes large numbers of dollars, mainly for hospital services. Attractive and cost effective alternatives to traditional hospital care exist, but because of lack of support are in short supply. My industry must do more to enhance the hospice concept, skilled nursing facilities and care at home.

I would like to say a few words about the role of insurance carriers in the financing of research. The requirements of quality clinical study can add, and at times substantially, to the cost of treatment. Supporting clinical investigation

is an anathema to some health insurance companies and a part
of corporate policy for others. The lack of uniformity in
third party coverage of new technology delays the availability
of your contributions to many patients and sometimes leads to
non-factual billing in an effort to obtain third party reim-
bursement.

Bunker, Fowles, and Schaffarizick in the New England
Journal of Medicine propose the formation of an independent institute for the evaluation of new medical technology.
A multi-disciplinary panel would, among other things serve
as a reference point for the health insurance industry as it
considers coverage for recent advances in medicine. Uniformity and a more timely acceptance of new medical technology
should follow, and I believe this is an objective we can all
support.

The rapid escalation in the costs of medical care will
continue to burden the American people and their health
insurance programs.

We must look to prevention, early detection, and less
costly care environments if we are to continue to have the
quality of care we need and want.

13th International Cancer Congress, Part E
Cancer Management, pages 387–394

ECONOMICS AS A SIGNIFICANT CONTRIBUTOR TO FAMILY STRESS
IN CHILDHOOD CANCER

Grace Powers Monaco, J.D.
Law Firm of White, Fine & Verville
1156 15th Street, N.W.
Washington, D.C. 20005

INTRODUCTION

A 1979 Candlelighters study of 268 families reveals that
even when insurance pays most medical expenses, the cost of
childhood cancer is a significant factor in family stress.
The treatment time factor -- years of in and out patient
services -- poses major time management and employment
condition hardships.

Employed mothers took from 51 or more days (9%) off from
work to accompany their child to the treatment center.
Time away from work related directly to their child's
therapy status. A majority of mothers employed prior to
their child's illness quit or took indefinite leave.
Fathers took between 1-10 days (21%) from work over a
period of 1-6 months (18%). Days taken were deducted from
parents' personal, sick or vacation times; days in excess
of these allotments were "without pay."

The cost of paid child care for siblings was $101 or
more (57%) over a minimum time span of 1-10 days (21%) and
cost from $25.00 to $9,000.00. For 95% of these families
there was no financial assistance for paid child care.

One to 25 miles (35%) was the distance to the treatment
center with the car (82%) the principal mode of transport.
Cost was between $101.00 and $300.00 (18%) with $1.00 to
$5.00 per day for parking and tolls. Temporary housing at
the treatment center used by 27% accounted for out of
pocket expenses as well as for the average cost at the
treatment center of $1,584.21.

Although cancer is the second leading cause of death for
our children and the most common disease cause of death for
children between 3 and 14 in the United States, children
account for only 1% of the population affected by cancer in
this country. This is significant. The size of the population treated for pediatric cancer means that specialized

cancer care facilities to provide skilled treatment are not
right around the corner as they may be for the adult cancer
population. The corollary of this is that even if a family
has medical insurance or resources to pay all of its direct
medical expenses, the indirect medical expenses -- of
transportation costs to a far facility, board, lodging,
child care for other children remaining at home, loss of
work time, the requirement often of quitting work for the
mother -- that must be borne by the family are usually
staggering.

In 1980, the Candlelighters Foundation, an international
organization for parents of children with cancer affiliated
on a national basis with the American Cancer Society,
published the results of an analysis of 268 families in
Candlelighters parents groups to determine the financial
impact on families of children with cancer. A profile on
family structure was the starting point for the analysis:

FAMILY STRUCTURE

	MOTHER		FATHER	
AGE	31-35	29%	31-36	26%
EDUCATION	H.S. Grad.	33%	Some College	22%
EMPLOYMENT STATUS	Unemployed	39%	Employed	90%
MARITAL STATUS	............Married............87%			
INCOME	........$15,000 to 24,000 ......30%			
FAMILY SIZE	........2 children (1 boy, 1 girl)..			

An initial examination supported general expectations about
family composition. Families of children with cancer are
as "typical" as other families when compared to national
statistics in the 1977 Statistical Abstract of the United
States. More specifically, the comparison showed that the
survey family was younger in age than the national average
(44 years, men, 38 years, women), average in education
(12.6 years of school), comparable in employment status
(1.86 wage earners per family), above age for marital
status (78%), within the national income range ($19,480),
and, slightly above the norm for number of children (1.17
per family).

The study confirmed that a seriously ill child presented
a wide range of psychological, emotional, and physical
problems that directly resulted in family instability. The
most severely affected relationships were husband-wife,
parent-children, ill child-healthy child and family-friend.
Family priorities were reassessed; the ill child's medical

and personal needs came first and other family concerns
received secondary considerations. To the majority of
respondents, this was most difficult to handle and a
paramount concern.

Financial hardship due to the child's illness added to
the pressures of the family unit. Concern was expressed
not only over family instability, but also over financial
instability. Some families said they had been faced with
the decision of stopping treatment because of financial
demands. Skepticism was expressed over the family's
ability to ever again achieve financial parity and mobility.
Many families depleted their savings, stocks and bonds, and
personal credit to offset the financial burden.

The study presented the following profile on patient
history:

	PATIENT HISTORY	
DIAGNOSIS	ALL	35%
AGE AT DIAGNOSIS	1-3 years	29%
SEX	Male	63%
STATUS	alive	84%
THERAPY STATUS	on therapy	54%
TIME SPAN FOR THOSE STILL ON THERAPY	13-18 months	19%
TOTAL NUMBER OF IN-PATIENT CARE DAYS	11-20	16%
LONGEST STAY AS IN-PATIENT	1-10 days	19%
SHORTEST STAY AS IN-PATIENT	1-10 days	61%

The question regarding diagnosis produced data reflecting
44 different forms of cancer among the patients responding.
After the majority of response of ALL (acute lymphocytic
leukemia), the three most frequently reported forms of
cancer were non-Hodgkins lymphoma, osteogenic sarcoma and
Ewings sarcoma. Ages ranged from under 1 year of age (6%),
to over 20 years (1%), with the 11-15 (19%) bracket having
the next highest total.

The majority of patients were male; female patients
accounted for 35% of the responses. Only 15% of the survey
group had lost their child to cancer. Twenty three percent
of the patients had discontinued therapy and had been off
chemotherapeutic drugs on an average of 15 months. For
those patients on continuing therapy, the time span was as
short as 1-6 months (16%) and as long as four (4) years or
more (7%). The time span studies was from date of diagnosis

to December 1979.

The data confirm that cancer is a pervasive disease
requiring extensive treatment procedures that extend over
periods of years through both in-patient and out-patient
services. This treatment time factor poses significant
hardship in relation to finances, time management, and
employment conditions. The nature and extent of the cancer
has a strong correlation to the degree of the hardship
endured by patient and family. Prolonged treatment adversely
affects financial considerations because of the time and
costs of health care.

The majority of patients were accompanied to treatment
center by either one (50%) or both (40%) parents. Two
related aspects were examined: time taken from the job, and
child care provision for the remaining child. Those
mothers who were employed took from 51 or more days off
from work to accompany their child to the treatment center.
The time employed mothers spent away from work was directly
related to the child's therapy status, 13-18 months. A
majority of the mothers employed prior to their child's
illness either quit their job or took an indefinite leave
of absence. Fathers took between 1-10 days (21%P from work
over a period of 1-6 months (18%)). Days taken from work
were generally deducted by employers from the parents'
personal time, sick time or vacation time; days taken off
in excess of these allotments were "without pay".

Fifty nine (59%) percent found it necessary to secure
child care for the remaining child through either relatives
(47%), friends (34%), or paid help (17%). The cost of paid
help was $101.00 or more (57%) over a minimum time span of
1-10 days (21%). The range of cost for paid child care
services was from less than $25.00 to $9,000.00. Ninety-
five (95%) percent of these families did not receive any
financial assistance for paid help they retained.

Having secured time from the job and child care services,
the family next faced the expenses of travel to the
treatment center. One to 25 miles (35%) was the distance
of travel with the car (82%) being the principal mode of
transportation. The cost of transportation was between
$101.00 and $300.00 (18%) on average. The distances, modes
of transportation and costs are arrayed below:

DISTANCE FROM MEDICAL CENTER (MILES)		MODE OF TRAVEL TO CENTER		COST OF TRANSPORTATION TO CENTER	
1-25	35%	Car	82%	$1-100	10%
26-50	20%	Bus	6%	$101-300	18%
51-75	9%	Plane	7%	$301-650	13%
76-100	9%	Other	4%	$651-1,000	12%
101-125	1%	No response	1%	$1,001-2,000	10%
126-150	3%			$2,001-4,000	6%
151-175	1%			$4,001-8,000	1%
176-200	2%			Over $8,000	1%
over 200	13%			No response	27%
no response	7%				

The detailed added comments enclosed with most of the questionnaires provide flesh to the bones of the transportation impact. One telling financial impact is the plane fare needed to transport families from states like Nevada, where there are no facilities for the treatment of cancer in children to California, where they receive treatment. These costs may be about $6,000 to $8,000 per year per family. However in other states such as Arkansas, New Mexico and Washington, families may have to drive 240 to 500 miles for treatment. Gas, car upkeep, meals away from home can gut a family's cash on hand resources.

For the parents who could stay with their child in his/her room or travel to and from the center as required (37%), temporary housing facilities at the treatment center were not an important consideration. However, twenty seven percent (27%) did utilize temporary housing. These families reported that 45% of this available temporary housing was without cooking facilities, 44% was without laundry facilities. The survey did not consider the availability of housing such as the McDonald's houses that are now available for families in most pediatric cancer treatment settings. At the time the questionnaires were administered (1978) the McDonald's houses and similar houses were just beginning to open and operate, and a later survey will consider the impact of these facilities.

There follows a general expense profile. Because most respondents reported costs after insurance coverage it is not a true indication of total costs of illness but rather more of a profile of costs that the family must bear alone:

EXPENSES

MEDICAL

COST OF ILLNESS	AVERAGE	$28,633.37

NON-MEDICAL

COST AT CENTER (food, lodging, etc.)	HIGH	25,000.00
	LOW	18.00
	AVERAGE	1,584.21

TRANSPORTATION	18%	$101--$300

PER DAY OUT OF POCKET

Food	17%	$6-$10
Laundry	9%	$1-$5
Transport	14%	$1-$5
Lodging	4%	$31

PAID CHILD CARE	4%	$101 and up

From the 79% of families providing complete financial responses, the collective cost of illness (200 families) irrespective of insurance coverage was $5,704,010.00. The majority reported that they had 80% insurance coverage. Assistance from outside agencies such as the State Crippled Childrens Program was negligible with 68% reporting no assistance, only 3% reported assistance from this source.

The written comment addenda again permit to graphically depict the plight of families from the overall costs of cancer treatment. A mid-west teenager with a cancerous bone in her right leg was advised that the only alternative to amputation was to travel to a cancer center in New York that had developed a procedure that might save her leg. Her mother had to quit her job in order to accompany the child to New York for treatment and to care for her. The mother's living expenses in New York, travel bills, and caring for five other children left at home completely depleted the family's savings. Thus, even though the family's insurance covered most of the teenager's medical bills and the State Crippled Childrens program paid remaining medical expenses, the family was in effect destitute. This same scenario repeats itself regularly in families that travel to obtain bone marrow transplants for their children at the 7 major centers of excellence for this treatment in children in the United States.

A further complication lies with state rehabilitation agencies who are often reluctant to provide necessary prosthetic and rehabilitation services for children unless they can be assured that the child is going to be a survivor of his or her bout with cancer.

The Foundation's response to the data obtained from this survey is to propose a laundry list of items that we feel would relieve substantially the financial burdens on families and at the same time enhance the quality of care and outcome for our children.

* Any Catastrophic insurance plan advocated through the federal government must include transportation costs as an insured, reimbursable expense for pediatric and adolescent cancer patients.
* The network for the care of pediatric and adolescent cancer patients should contain sufficient pediatric and adolescent hematology/oncology specialists to permit the day to day care of children/adolescents to be accomplished at a local level BUT each child should be linked through her/his hometown pediatric/ adolescent oncology specialists to a cancer center or clinical cooperative group and entered into a protocol. The center/group would perform the initial staging of treatment and periodically as needed evaluate and suggest changes in the course of treatment. All specialized surgery and chemotherapy would be conducted through the center.

Under this plan 90-95% of all treatment could be conducted at home with quality of life and cost savings. However, no child's opportunity for cure would be compromised. It would permit the centers and groups to concentrate more on tertiary care, research and innovative treatment problems and leave routine care to the front line physical members of the team.

A large step forward in this direction is evidenced by the new NCI CCOPS programs and by some of the outreach programs in place at major treatment centers.

* Pediatric oncology nurse and social worker expertise which means so much to quality of care and life should be extended beyond the treatment center into the community through liaison with home town social workers and nurses that form the community care part of the treatment team.
* A cadre of volunteers to provide home care, babysitting, meal preparation, and tutoring needs to be obtained to reduce parent out of pocket costs.
* Home care of the dying child should be reimbursed in lieu of hospital care where the teams to support

it are in place.
* Employers should be encouraged to permit co-workers
to volunteer their sick leave, personal leave time
to other co-workers and to stand their shifts for
them to reduce the financial impact on families.

If we can implement the common sense suggestions set
forth above, we will have achieved the financial health of
families and enhanced the opportunities of them to emerge
from a personal experience with cancer in a child or
adolescent with not only their child in tact but also their
financial resources.

13th International Cancer Congress, Part E
Cancer Management, pages 395–401
© 1983 Alan R. Liss, Inc., 150 Fifth Avenue, New York, NY 10011

THE ECONOMICS OF CANCER CARE IN CANADA

Brian C. Lentle

Alberta Cancer Board
Edmonton, Alberta   T6K 2A9

Let me say at the outset that I am a physician and not an economist. There can be no other professional group, taken as a whole, any member of which can discuss economics with less expectation of credibility.

No discussion of the financing of cancer care in Canada would be complete without recognizing the social, geographical and historical context within which cancer care is delivered.

Canada has enjoyed a standard of living this century second only to the United States. However, according to a United Nations classification of nations reflecting the portion of gross national product which is finished goods as distinct from raw materials, Canada ranks as only a semi-industrialized nation.

In geopolitical terms the conventional map of Canada differs from the demographic map to an exceptional degree. Despite the agricultural industry Canada's population is largely to be found in urban areas while the true north, such a conspicuous feature of Canada's geography, is largely empty of people, or indeed the developed capacity to support them.

For most people Canada is probabaly defined by its geography and climate as much as by any reconizable national identity. A Quebecois chanteuse has said "my land is not a country, it is winter". Thus despite its great beauty and strength Canada does not lend itself to generalizations. It is a country of marked regional differences, reflected in a comment by Peter Newman that "the search for a Canadian identity has become the Canadian identity". This introspection has unduly hurt a country rich in human and material resources so that our economy is in great trouble at present with a Canadian dollar worth less than 80¢ U.S.. The provision of health care has to recognize the implications of this fact, particularly as nearly all of our high technology equipment is supplied from outside the country. The weakness of the Canadian dollar compounds the adverse effects of the present rates of inflation from which we all suffer to some degree.

*   *   *

Meilicke and Storch (1980) have divided Canadian health care up into five periods and I will use their analysis here.

The first era dates from before Confederation which was the birth of the modern Canadian state. During this time social security programs were minimal and amounted to local parochial responsibilities except for quarantine regulations and institutional care.

Between 1867 and the mid 1940s there was little real change except for some clarification of federal and provincial responsibilities. That issue haunts Canada still, and not only in Quebec.

Between the mid 1940's and 1960s several important federal programs were introduced. These included national health grants including provision for cancer control. These cancer control agencies thus often antedated the introduction of universal medical insurance which followed during this era and was in place in every province by 1972.

Although not directly related to cancer another important milestone in the provision of health care in Canada occurred in 1974 with the publication of "A New Perspective in the Health of Canadians" (Lalonde), a working document more widely known as the "Lalonde white paper", after the cabinet minister chiefly responsible for it. Lalonde clearly articulated a political position, the substance of which was that the economics of care had reached a new plateau in which the marginal social (or personal) value of further gains in life expectancy from traditional medical strategies were disproportionately small in comparison to the mariginal social or personal cost of achieving them.

Since that time, and exacerbated by other adverse changes in the economy, there has been a great reluctance by Canadian provincial governments to commit additional funds to any aspect of health care. The "lifestyle" recommendations of the Lalonde document have found an echo in the "Participaction" movement which has swept a nation otherwise as physically indolent as its southern neighbor.

However, government restraints in Canada come at a time when my country's health care expenditure, at a little over 7% of gross national product (GNP), is above that of the U.K. (5.8%) but below France, Holland, Sweden, the U.S. and West Germany where expenditures are between 8.0% and 9.5% of GNP.

In the political climate following the Lalonde paper it is difficult to justify a greater share of the GNP without some event to radically change the slope of the "Lalonde plateau" or alter the equation such that marginal social value does indeed exceed marginal social cost.

I have pointed out that health care in Canada is a provincial responsibility with the federal government using fiscal strategies to influence provincial policies. Such a strategy is the federal-provincial cost sharing program. For a province to benefit from this program it must provide a universal and portable insurance scheme.

Thus at present, apart from in Quebec, comprehensive cancer care is a provincial responsibility administered, in effect, by a crown corporation. That is a British Commonwealth strategy to allow for an organization which is government funded but enjoys a great deal of autonomy. If I may use my home Province of Alberta as an example the result is that a Board, appointed by Government, administers goverment funds through a provincial administration to provide care at two major cancer centres and, through them, a number of outreach programs of varying degrees of sophistication. Systems in other provinces are similar but not identical.

In Table 1 a comparison is presented of the levels of program support available in selected Provinces across Canada. I must emphasize that because of regional differences this comparison is only of limited validity as the operational costs involve differing expenses and cover different programs in each Province across the country.

Table I.

Provincial Cancer Program Operating Budgets+
(For 1981 or the fiscal year ending therein)

Province	Population $X10^6$	OperatingBudget ForCancerCare $\$X10^6$	Local Research Funding $\$X10^6$
British Columbia	2.6	19.0	0.03
Alberta	2.1	16.0	3.6*
Saskatchewan	1.0	9.0	0.3*
Ontario	8.7	51.0°	0.7
Nova Scotia	0.9	2.5	0.0

$Canadian 1981
*largely (90%) or entirely coming from Provincial Governments.
°excludes some professional fees coming from this budget
  item in other provinces.
+It must be emphasized that this comparison is only of limited
  validity as different components make up the operating budget
  in each province.

The Ontario program is similar to that in Alberta but size
determines that it is more multi-facetted. In addition, the Princess
Margaret Hospital in Toronto acts as a flagship of cancer care in
Ontario and has a somewhat privileged status. Quebec, which to
outsiders must consistently seem to exist in a state of imminent
separation from the remainder of the nation, but which is in fact a
profoundly civilizing influence on Canada, is again an exception. In
Quebec until recently no distinction has been made between the
care of cancer patients and patients with other diseases. Equally,
cancer care and, particulary, the facilities for radiation treatment
are not centralized in the way that they tend to be elsewhere in the
country.

To return to the more usual pattern of cancer care, there are
some very distinct advantages to the Canadian strategy. The chief
one is that patients all tend to be seen by a central referral centre
so that entry of patients into clinical trials is considerable and
oncologists have the opportunity to see as many patients as possible
in their community with a given disease. Thus patient flow is highly
structured in Canada.

A further advantage is that epidemiological studies and
professional audit are greatly facilitated by the lack of
fragmentation of care. This is made even more true by cancer being
a reportable disease in Alberta so that we do not just think that our
experience is as broad as possible - we can know it.

The centralization of programs in the major part of Canada has obvious advantages in providing comprehensive cancer care as it is usually defined. Close university links allow many cancer centres such as those in Alberta to function also as the focus for a division or department of oncology in the faculties of medicine and other professional interactions.

No description of cancer care in Canada would be complete without reference to the educational dimension. Training programs for residents in radiation oncology exist in several centres but staffing is a problem in respect of manpower. The higher salaries to be earned in the private practice of this specialty in the U.S.A. compared with the Canadian system, which in most provinces is in whole or in part government funded and staffed by salaried physicials, somewhat compounds this problem. On the other hand there is as yet no formal specialty of medical oncology so that cancer centres in Canada have not graduated medical specialists to compete for patients. This has ensured a monopolistic position for most cancer centres in terms of patient referrals. Thus the slight economic disadvantage for our physicians is offset by the greater research opportunities and wide multidisciplinary clinical experience available at a typical cancer centre in Canada.

Thus in northern Alberta 70% of all patients with cancer (exclusive of in-situ lesions of the cervix or basal skin cancers) are referred to the Cross Cancer Institute. This figure rises to 100% for cancers for which we believe a multi-disciplinary diagnostic and treatment service to be essential, for example cancers in children, Hodgkins disease and testicular cancer.

The funding of cancer research in Canada is a mixture of local endowments, andprivate and public money. However, the main support derives from monies collected in money raising campaigns by provincial divisions of the Canadian Cancer Society. Each provincial Division keeps about one-third of these monies for local purposes —chiefly public education and the provision of patient services, but specifically not for research support. The remaining proportion of the monies is administered by the National Cancer Institute of Canada and goes to provide research support by peer review in a number of traditional ways. This fact is reflected in Table 2.

Table 2.

NATIONAL CANCER INSTITUTE OF CANADA
FINANCIAL ACTIVITIES IN THE YEAR
ENDED MARCH 1981
$Canadian $X10^3$, to nearest 1,000

Receipts		Disbursements	
Canadian Cancer society	15,980	Research	15,801
Marathon of Hope	18,925	Professional	
Breast Cancer screening		Education	42
Federal & Prov. grants	2,432	Meetings and	
Interest	2,432	travel	32
Donations and		Administration	241
contributions	17		
Total	$37,773		$16,116
	Net increase in resources		$21,656

Canada has also been fortunate in having had, in the person of Terry Fox, a young man who, while dying of metastatic osteogenic sarcoma lived a life of purpose and courage with a maturity far beyond his years. His example and his "marathon of hope" has yielded what is, in Canadian terms, a large sum to support new initiatives in cancer research. This enables the award of larger sums of money over a longer time than is usually possible to be awarded to particularly able investigators across the country. It is this "marathon of hope which has caused the financial picture of the NCI of Canada to look so favorable.

Against this picture, which has many good aspects, must be set some sober facts. As a nation we spend 0.9% of our gross national product on research and development (R & D) compared with 1.8% in France, 2.0% in West Germany and the U.K., 2.2% in the U.S. and 2.4% in Japan. Thus Canada appears to lack the will or the intent to effect a transition to full industrialization. This lack of R & D support spills over into medicine.

Despite the size of Canada it has a small population of less than 10% that in the U.S. As a result Canada has an inadequate population base to suppport any truly autonomous pharmaceutical manufacturing companies or makers of high technology equipment, with the notable exception of Atomic Energy of Canada Ltd.. The result is that value for dollar spent is less than might be the case, further compounding the difficulties caused by limited levels of spending, the "weak" Canadian dollar, and inflation.

Fortunately, in much of Canada cancer as a disease is

privileged in the support it commands. Anyone looking at our programs is unlikely to sense dire need. Indeed, in Alberta the greatest problem is that of enough space to house clinical care, and a successful and imaginative group of clinical scientists and researchers.

That we in Edmonton can have our government studying with us the building of a heavy ion accelerator for cancer treatment (among other applications) at a cost of $200,000,000 reflects not only the happy chance by which oil deposits are distributed around this globe, but also the enormous discrepancies within Canadian national borders. Quebec is not the only province to march to the beat of its own drummer.

To secure national equity, to consolidate a good but troubled national system, and to plan to build for the future are dilemmas not only for cancer care in particular and health care in general, but also the substance of the challenge my country faces in every aspect of its social fabric for some time to come. I suspect, however, that our problems are trivial on a global scale.

Acknowledgements:
I wish to acknowledge that Dr. Neil MacDonald has, in discussion, helped to develop some of the observations made here.
I am grateful to Mrs. Doreen McGonigle for secretarial help.

Lalonde M. A new perspective on the health of Canadians. Ottawa Government of Canada, p 31-34.
Mielicke CA, Storch JL (1980). Introduction: on historical framework. In Meilicke CA, Storch JL (eds): "Perspectives on Canadian Health and Social Services Policy: History and Emerging Trends," Ann Arbor, Michigan: Health Administration Press, pp 3-34.

13th International Cancer Congress, Part E
Cancer Management, pages 403–410
© **1983 Alan R. Liss, Inc., 150 Fifth Avenue, New York, NY 10011**

CANCER CARE COST IN JAPAN

Nobuo Maeda, Dr Med Sci.

Head, Section of Social Security
Institute of Public Health
4-6-1 Shirokanedai
Minato-ku, Tokyo, Japan 108

Ministry of Health and Welfare estimated 577 billion yen ($3 billion) for cancer care in 1979 and 650.9 billion yen in 1980. Significant annual increase of cancer care cost was observed as 25.8% in 1978, and still now total expenditure is increasing by the rate of over 10% more than the previous year. The proportion of total cancer cost in total medical expenditure in Japan is minor between four to five percent, but this proportion is also steadily growing (Table 1).

Table 1. Total Cancer Care Cost in Japan   ¥1 Billion

Year	A. Total Cancer Care Cost	B. Total Medical Care Cost	Proportion % of A in B	Annual Increase
1977	376.9	8 568.6	4.4	
1978	508.1	10 004.2	5.1	+ 25.9%
1979	577.4	10 951.0	5.3	+ 12.0%
1980	650.9	11 980.5	5.4	+ 11.3%

Table 2. Cancer Care Cost by Site   ¥1 Billion

Year	Stomach	Trachea Bronchus Lung	Breast	Uterus	Others	Total
1979	135.3	39.3	37.1	28.2	337.5	577.4
	(23.4)	(6.8)	(6.4)	(4.9)	(58.5)	(100.0)
1980	140.8	41.3	41.9	29.4	397.5	650.9
	(21.6)	(6.4)	(6.4)	(4.5)	(61.1)	(100.0)

Ministry of H.& Welfare, ¥1 Billion=US$4 Million   (1980)

Stomach cancer care cost is almost 20% in total cost and other sites cancers are spending 60% (Table 2).

Age groups over 45 years incurred most of cancer cost. Recently, older patients over 65 years became the major age group contributing to costs of medical care for cancer (Table 3). It is interesting to note the gradual tendency toward ambulatory care from hospital care. Outpatient care with chemotherapy and radiotherapy is growing and is costly. But, hospital care remains as a core component for cancer patients. We are able to recognize the specific situation of cancer care by comparing the cost of hospitalization and outpatient care among cancer, heart disease and stroke. One day charge for cancer patients is averageing ¥20.6 thousand for hospitalization. But the charge of other disease represents only ¥14 thousand for one day charge including medical care (Table 4).

Table 3. Total Cancer Care Cost in Japan by Age Groups

¥1 Billion

Year	Total Cancer Cost	Age Groups 0-14	15-44	45-64	65ys-	Hospital Care	Other Care
1977	376.9	5.4	56.1	161.9	153.5	304.0	72.9
(%)	(100.0)	(1.4)	(14.9)	(43.0)	(40.7)	(80.7)	(19.3)
1980	650.9	11.3	85.6	264.6	289.3	465.5	185.4
(%)	(100.0)	(1.7)	(13.2)	(40.7)	(44.4)	(71.5)	(28.5)

Ministry of Health & Welfare, Japan

Table 4. One Day Charge for Insured Patients under Health Insurance -1980,4-

¥ 1000

Diseases		Hospitalization	Outpatient Care
Cancer	(9-15)*	20.6	13.0
Heart	(43)*	14.1	4.5
Stroke	(45-47)*	14.6	4.0

Ministry of Health & Welfare, Survey of Medical Care Benefit, 1980. * I.C.D. Number. ¥10 thous.=$40

Because of tremendous economic burden of cancer care and other costly diseases to the small group of health insurance, National Federation of Health Insurance Societies introduced the special fund system for reallocation of benefits to help economically unbalanced group by the high cost payment. I picked up five highest cost patients from the case report on the high cost illness (Table 5). A most expensive bill amounted to 3 205 thousand yen ($10 thousand) in 1975 for the care of Leukaemia lady of 50 years during only one month. The cost of same category grew up every year toward 8 million yen level in 1980. Acute Myeloid Leukaemia was most popular diagnosis in this higher ranking of high cost illness. We could not see breast and uteri cancer and cancer of male genitals in these high cost bills.

Table 5. Ranking of Highest Costs of Five Cancers among One Month Bills, in Japan, by Sex & Age, Health Insurance Report of N.F.H.I.S.   ¥ 1000

Year	1st	2nd	3rd	4th	5th
1975	Monocytic Leukaemia	Stomack	Cardia	A.Myeloid Leukaemia	Stomach
	F 50ys	F 77ys	M 59ys	F 34ys	M 46ys
	3 205	3 038	2 900	2 861	2 860
1976	Malignant Lymphoma	A.Myeloid Leukaemia	Stomach	Stomach	A.Myeloid Leukaemia
	M 33ys	M 43ys	F 69ys	M 58ys	M 28ys
	5 324	5 273	4 568	4 631	4 431
1977	Leukaemia	A.Myeloid Leukaemia	Lung	Cardia	A.Myeloid Leukaemia
	F 3lys	M 49ys	M 58ys	M 63ys	M 32ys
	8 063	4 963	4 497	4 460	4 436
1978	Leukaemia	Leukaemia	Chronic Leukaemia	Leukaemia	A.Myeloid Leukaemia
	F 16ys	M 17ys	F 36ys	M 75ys	M 28ys
	7 246	6 586	6 396	6 166	5 754
1979	Acute Leukaemia	A.Myeloid Leukaemia	Liver	Leukaemia	Stomach
	F 19ys	M 35ys	M 5lys	M 67ys	F 64ys
	7 547	7 447	7 328	6 595	6 465
1980	A.Myeloid Leukaemia	A.Promyeloid L.	A.Myeloid Leukaemia	Stomach	A.Promyeloid L.
	M 4lys	M 15ys	M 4lys	M 64ys	F 3lys
	8 543	7 517	7 330	6 924	6 866

Ca. ¥1000=$3.30 in 1975, $4.00 in 1977. $4.50 in 1978. $4.00 in 1980. *27million population under N.F.H.I.S.

Fukushima and Fujii studied the hospitalization cost in the National Cancer Center of Tokyo on the data from 1979 until 1981, by breaking down to the components of care. I put similar hospitalization cost of rural area with 12 948 population on table 6. We can know average cost for a hospitalized patient through these data. The range of average charges was from ¥147 thousand to ¥914 thousand (ca. $4000). Even though the charges in rural area was lower than in National Cancer Center, the level of charge for one cancer inpatient on table 6 is greatly below the higher group of table 5 which showed in national level. The amount of charges varies greatly according to the stage of cancer, malignant site, age and technical level of hospital. The proportionate charges to consultation, medication and others differ significantly among different diagnosis. Hospitalization cost amounted around 50% in total charge among breast and cervix uteri, but stomach patient paid 41% of cost for injection. For lung cancer patients, laboratory test was major component of care in terms of payment.

Table 6. One Hospitalized Patient's Charge & Components of Care by one episode   ¥ 1000

| | N.C.C. Hospital *1979-81 | | | | Rural 1980** | |
	Stomach 3 cases	Breast 5	Cervix.U. 9	Lung 4	Stomach 1	Cervix.U 1
Charge	723	384	914	851	147	199
Total	100.0	100.0	100.0	100.0	100.0	100.0
Consultaion	0.2	0.1	-	-	0.4	0.5
Medication	3.6	1.2	5.6	3.7	1.4	3.9
Injection & Blood	18.0	8.3	17.5	13.3	41.2	14.0
Operation & Treat.	17.0	26.6	9.7	16.7	15.3	22.4
Lab.Test	21.2	12.0	11.0	33.8	9.3	8.9
X-Ray	3.3	1.1	1.9	4.4	3.4	0.3
Hospitalization	36.7	50.5	49.6	27.8	28.9	50.0
Other	0.1	0.2	4.8	0.4	0.0	-
Hosp. Days	45	25	68	39	65	34

* Stage II only, from Fukushima & Fujii.

I mentioned the stomach patient cost and lung patient cost on Table 7 and 8 by showing the charge per one episode found the malignant after January 1980 until November 1981. Roughly speaking, the level of charges related to the length of stay in hospital, however, the cost of each case differs greatly among lung cancer group. Longer stay in hospital is very significant in most of hospitals not only for cancer patients but also all of other patients. I can't conclude definit factors influenced to the level of charge by the current data without much more detail data. Yet, I am very sure that the high cost of lung patient care and stage IV stomach cancer care will be dominant in many municipalities without planned programs for preventation, early detection and appropriate curative efforts.

Table 7. Stomach Cancer Care Costs per One Episode & Length of Hospitalization in Three Towns of Northern Japan (Rural)

Case Number	Length of Stay in Hospital	Age	Charge (thous.yen)
1*	387	57	4 964
2*	267	49	1 801
3	111	75	4 083
4*	83	69	2 205
5*	82	65	2 305
6	69	64	1 207
7	61	59	3 236
8	55	54	3 166
9	55	49	2 175
10	52	42	1 800
Average	122.2	58.3	2 698.7

1980.1-1981.11. Under N.H. Insurance. *died
Total population of three towns is 12 948.

Table 8. Lung Cancer Care Cost per One Episode & Length of Hospitalization in Three Towns of Northern Japan (Rural)

Case Number	Length of Stay in Hospital	Age	Charge (thous,yen)
1*	378	59	9 316
2	55	60	1 137
3*	45	64	2 354
4*	21	45	375
Average	124.7	57	

1980.1-1981.11 *died

Finally, we estimated total economic costs due to cancer of 1979 including direct cost and indirect cost (Table 9). Beside of direct cost of ¥577.4 billion, the income loss due to death, as the indirect cost of mortality was ¥812.8 billion in Japan. The economic loss by hospitalization as the morbidity cost was ¥98.5 which shows underestimate figures. If we will get new reliable data on ambulatory care which can clarify how many days patients stopped their jobs, we might add further income loss. Mortality cost was calculated like table 10 according to Hishinuma's table on the present value of lifetime earnings which is taken by similar to Dublin and Lotka. Total estimated cost of cancer in Japan was ¥1 488.7 billion ($6 767 million).

Table 9. Estimated Economic Costs due to Cancer in Japan

	1979	
	Yen amount in billions	Dollar amount in millions*
1. Total Medical Costs of Cancer Care (Direct Costs)	577.4	2 624
2. Total Income Loss due to Hospitalization of Cancer (Indirect Costs)	98.5	448
3. Total Income Loss due to Death by Cancer (Indirect Costs)	812.8	3 695
Grand Total	1 488.7	6 767

* $1.00=¥220

Table 10. Income Loss due to Deaths by Cancer in Japan

Age Group	A.Number of Deaths by Cancer (1979)	B.Present Value of Lifetime Earnings* in Thousands Yen (1979)	C.Income Loss due to Deaths by Cancer in Millions Yen (A x B)
0- 4	513	4 053	2 079
5- 9	472	8 336	3 935
10-14	352	14 404	5 070
15-19	441	22 725	10 022
20-24	552	29 100	16 063
25-29	1 067	31 599	33 716
30-34	1 944	31 389	61 020
35-39	3 204	29 288	93 839
40-44	4 871	25 339	123 426
45-49	8 459	19 805	168 243
50-54	12 094	13 244	160 173
55-59	12 289	6 485	92 664
60-64	17 673	2 407	42 539
65-69	23 723	-	-
70-	66 970	-	-
Total	156 660		812 784

* by Hishinuma, Discount Rate=5%

We can easily expect cancer will keep the first position among major killers in Japan until next century. This
means that we have to pay not only medical cost of 6 or 8%
in total medical cost but also much more money for income
loss by untimely malignant deaths. Ministry of Health and
Welfare expended 16.7 billion yen for the national programs
against cancer including the building of hospitals, training
of experts, cancer research and mass screening programs like
table 11. Most amount of budget in these programs was
granted for the construction and operation of regional
cancer centers and hospitals in Japan. We have to find most
effective and efficient strategy in the preventive programs
and the early detection at the community level by using
limited budget. This strategy shall contribute to reduce
and contain the sky-rocketing increase of cancer care cost
in Japan. In order to defind the programs, the data and
analysis on the economic costs due to cancer is primary
requisite for all of experts in this area.

Table 11. National Grants for Cancer Care Programs

Million yen

	1970	1975	1979	1981
Total	3 367	10 045	15 187	16 779
Construction*	2 729	7 738	11 998	13 125
Training	7	15	6	6
Research	298	1 250	1 520	1 600
Prevention**	311	749	1 087	1 155

* including equipments ** mainly for mass screening
  cars and programs

References

1. Fukushima M., Fujii M,, Statistical observations on
   medical care for cancer patients. in Cancer Report
   of 1979, Ministry of H.& W. Japan. pp.243-248 (in
   Japanese)

2. Hartunian N.S., Smart C.N., Thompson M.S., (1981).
   The incidence and economic costs of major health
   impairments. D.C. Health and Company. P.417

3. Ministry of Health and Welfare, Japan, Public Health
   Bureau (1980). Future Cancer Prevention Measures in
   Japan. P.108 (Draft)

4. Maeda, N, (1979). Health Economics. Tokyo University
   Press. P.175 (in Japanese)

5. U.S. Department of Health and Human Services, National
   Center for Health Statistics (1981). Social and
   economic implications of cancer in the United States.
   DHHS Pub. No.(PHS) 81-1404. P.43

CONGRESS SYMPOSIA

CANCER NURSING: AN INTERNATIONAL PERSPECTIVE
Joyson, G., Australia, Chairman; Hilkemeyer, R.,
USA, Co-Chairman; Opera House

Cancer Nursing an International Perspective:
Developing of Cancer Nursing in the United
States. *Hilkemeyer, R., Houston, TX USA.

Problems Encountered in an Intensive Care Medical
Oncology Unit in Paris. *Adonis, C., Bobigny,
France.

Cancer Nursing in the Netherlands. *Strak,
E. M. K., Rotterdam, The Netherlands.

The Development of Oncology Nursing in the
United Kingdom. *Tiffany, R., London, England.

Cancer Nursing in a Comprehensive Cancer Center.
*Park, R. N., New York, NY USA.

Please note: Papers that are listed as "By Title
Only" were presented at the 13th International
Cancer Congress, but are not included in these
volumes.

13th International Cancer Congress, Part E
Cancer Management, pages 413–422
© 1983 Alan R. Liss, Inc., 150 Fifth Avenue, New York, NY 10011

CANCER NURSING AN INTERNATIONAL PERSPECTIVE: DEVELOPMENT OF
CANCER NURSING IN THE UNITED STATES

Renilda Hilkemeyer, R.N., B.S.

Staff Asst. to President, Prof. Oncology (Nursing)
The University of Texas System Cancer Center
6723 Bertner, Houston, Texas 77030 U.S.A.

Modern cancer "oncology" nursing practice, education, and
research developed into a vibrant, expanding, specialty field
over the past two decades. Nurses historically cared for cancer patients, but the care was often basic and given by nurses
who had learned by experience. There were no physician specialists in oncology as today. Preventive, diagnostic, therapeutic, and rehabilitation programs were not comparable to the
present. Nurses in cancer institutions had more opportunities
to gain knowledge and experience in cancer nursing. We were
often the "experts". We opened our doors to registered nurses
from here and abroad, students and faculty, to provide opportunities for clinical practice, cancer information, special
education programs, or individual assistance with specific patient care needs, policies, and development of similar programs.
We actively promoted "cancer nursing" as a desirable clinical
practice field through every possible means using the spoken
and written word. It was not easy, because many nurses feared
cancer and felt it was a hopeless disease, just as the public
and patient did. This was understandable; the nurses' knowledge, the opportunities to see patients who survived were
limited, and survival rates were poor compared to the present.
Those nurses who had been involved in Cancer Nursing, whether
practice, education, or research, had the vision, courage, and
determination to move forward; initiate changes and revise approaches through use of the nursing process to provide care
for clients/patients; define roles and collaborate with other
health care professionals; provide academic and continuing
education programs to meet the needs of the practitioner; and
initiate nursing research.

Nurses in cancer institutions, the American Cancer Society Nursing Consultant and nurses serving on various National and Division Committees of ACS, and a few faculty members interested in cancer nursing developed an informal network for helping each other. As more nurses became involved in cancer nursing, the need for a formal organization became apparent. The Oncology Nursing Society was organized in 1975. It has grown to 4,100 members and 23 local chapters. The International Union Against Cancer is to be commended for establishing a Nursing Committee, and Congress participation.

Many factors and trends have influenced the growth and development of oncology nursing including: changes in the nursing profession, practice, and education; medical, scientific, and technological advances in the field of cancer; changes in societal health care attitudes, needs and health care delivery systems; and legislation. The nursing profession has been undergoing major changes in practice roles, goals, education, and research.

Many expanded roles have emerged for oncology nurses since the late 1960s. In retrospect, as Director of Nursing at U.T.M.D. Anderson Hospital (MDA), we were in the forefront defining and implementing new and expanded roles for oncology nurses as: in clinical trials, for patients in germ free environments including the Laminar Flow Unit, Clinical Research Units, intravenous hyperalimentation teams, patient and family education, prevention and detection programs. I was successful in developing proposals and securing funds from the National Cancer Institute to support additional nurses for some of these expanded roles, and for continuing education programs for nurses in institutions, health agencies, and academic institutions. (Hilkemeyer, 1982).

Today, oncology nurses practice as generalists, clinical specialists, and nurse practitioners. They may be involved in primary care, including independent practice, or be responsible for specific patient populations as is the physician, such as the pediatric nurse practitioner or the nurse concerned with adult leukemia patients. Clinical nurse specialists and practitioners may have dual roles in screening and detection programs, general hospitals, visiting nurse association, public health and home health agencies, and nursing homes where their focus is on the cancer client/patient, education of staff, and as a resource person to health care professionals. Some studies on the effectiveness of these roles are being conducted.

Standards for practice, patient care and audit are a professional expectation for quality care. Standards for Cancer Nursing Practice (Oncology Nursing Society, American Nurses Association, 1979) provide guidelines for nursing intervention. Publications using the Standards provide assistance to nurses.

The National Cancer Act of 1971, revised in 1974, has as a major goal the reduction in incidence, morbidity, and mortality of cancer in human beings. The Act provided impetus to the development of cancer control programs; including prevention, detection, diagnosis, treatment, rehabilitation, and the education of professionals and the public. The Act provided many opportunities for expansion of oncology nursing practice, education, and research. Diffusion and transfer of knowledge was considered essential, since 80% of cancer patients receive treatment in community hospitals and clinics. The three major cancer institutions were designated as the first Comprehensive Cancer Centers, which now total 22. In addition, clinical research centers and oncology units in general hospitals have developed.

Every nurse has a responsibility in prevention and early detection of cancer regardless of the area of practice. This includes identification of high risk individuals, conduct of systematic screening, and educational programs. Linda White, MDA, was a pioneer in this area. She began the first structured, institutional, continuing education program to teach nurses prevention and early detection. Over 700 nurses in the U.S. and other countries have completed the program. It has served as a model for programs initiated and conducted by nurses in institutions, clinics, academic institutions, and industry. The original program was three weeks but there are also now one-week specific site modules. Many materials and teaching aids have been developed and are available at minimal cost. After the program had been in operation one year, a field evaluator was employed to evaluate the graduates, their screening practices, and to determine acceptance and utilization. Physicians reported positive acceptance of the program. The evaluator identified practice areas needing improvement. (Alvardo, Drean, Kean, 1979). As a result of this program, a Colposcopy Clinic was developed at MDA, which the cancer detection nurses conduct, providing service to patients and education for nurses and physicians. MDA also provides a free health screening clinic and education program for asyptomatic employee, conducted by the cancer detection nurses.

In 1973, a 5-year Breast Cancer Detection Demonstration
program was sponsored by NCI and ACS. The purpose of this
program was to disseminate the techniques of early detection
of breast cancer to both the public and the medical profession.
Nurses were involved in this program. Results of this study
(Baker 1982) demonstrated the value and effectiveness of a
public and medical education, recruitment of women including
high risk groups into the program, the use of mammography to
detect early breast cancer, and the saving of lives. Teaching
breast self examination was an important part of the program;
80.9% of the women indicated they practiced BSE prior to entry;
35.9% on regular basis. Many studies have been done on why
women do not practice BSE. With breast cancer still the leading cause of female deaths from cancer, nurses in all areas
of practice need to continue their efforts in this area of
prevention and early detection.

The development of clinical trials with investigational
and other antineoplastic agents in the 1960s had a significant
impact on the expanded role of the nurse. Not only did it affect nurses, but also physician investigators, particularly
the medical oncologist, pharmacists, and other support services. Nurses at MDA became actively involved in the conduct
of clinical trials, collaborated with principal investigators
to learn and plan together in order to provide necessary intervention, and evaluate the delivery of care to patients. As
Director of Nursing, I believed that nurses could contribute
to and understand protocols, aid in patient selection, administer investigational drugs, assess patients and determine necessary intervention, coordinate multiple services provided by
other disciplines, interpret and monitor laboratory findings,
observe patients for possible known and unknown side effects,
provide emotional support to patients and families, teach patients and families and develop instructions and teaching aids,
provide adequate documentation; collect and interpret data,
and contribute to the literature. Some of my colleagues ques-
tioned this practice. As clinical trials became more complex
with combination and adjuvant therapy and new blood components
and antibiotics became available, nurses provided more complex
intervention. As the need for psychosocial support for patients and families was intensified, nurses identified new
approaches as support groups, together with individualized as-
sitance to patients and families. Research and studies were
done to improve the quality of care for clients/patients and
to aid other nurses.

Changes in attitude of health professionals and the consumer together with legislation has resulted in more open communication with patients. Legislation was enacted in 1974 for the Protection of Human Subjects of Biomedical and Behavorial Research including the concept of informed consent. Nurses should be members of Institutional Review Boards, and Research Committees since they can contribute from their expertise, will be closely involved in execution of protocols, and can often serve as a patient advocate.

The initiation and expansion of comprehensive cancer centers, clinical centers, community programs, clinical trials, and supportive therapy has had a major impact on the increase in ambulatory care. When I came to MDA in 1955, there were six clinics with about 200 patients daily. They were open 8-5 Monday through Friday, since there was little need for services after those hours. Now there are approximately 1,100 patients seen in some 25 specialized clinics. We designed one clinic section for all patients who receive intravenous chemotherapy, blood component therapy, have long-line catheters, are on portable pumps, or have emergency needs after the clinics close. In 1975, I set up 24-hour nurse coverage for this area. There is an adjacent sattelite pharmacy and pharmacists responsible for preparation of all antineoplastic agents and other parenteral admixtures.

Another major impact of antineoplastic drugs and the clinical trials has been the need to develop delivery systems for administration. Nurses have been very involved in this aspect as they identified needs and problems of patients receiving intravenous therapy over long periods; concerns were preserving the integrity of the patients venous access, providing simplicity for self care management, comfort and ease of ambulation so patients could continue their daily activities, and providing savings in hospital costs. Physicians and nurses at MDA collaborated with Alza Corporation on one of the first delivery systems for chemotherapy. All of use were excited about future possibilities; at the same time we often had as much anxiety as the patient did over his ability to self-administer the drug and maintain the system. There are now patients on portable pumps on current or intermittent therapy outside treatment centers. At MDA this program has greatly expanded. Twenty-four hour access to the nurse and other health professionals are readily available, sometime by phone, to answer questions, resolve a problem, or provide support.

Millie Lawson, MDA, was a pioneer in expanding the role of nurses in infusion therapy. She identified needs and problems, and systematically established her own or collaborative research with physicians to improve the quality of patient care. She collaborated in the development of the long-line indwelling, silicone elastometer peripheral, central venous catheter and has nurses with special training insert the catheter, suture it in place, and verify placement by xray. She has also aided in research on the use of the shorter subclavian central venous catheter using a percutaneous overwire technique. She has established procedures tor heparinization, conducted collaborative research in the use of fibrinolytic drugs as declotting agents, and developed techniques to maintain sterility of the system. Other nurses also have identified needs and problem, combined research and practice to influence the development of new technology, as in home I.V.H. and Stoma Care.

Historically, health care professionals included patient education as an integral part of the health care program. There has been a major change in concepts and methods. Now, patient education programs provide for: client/patient needs assessment, systematic design and structure, teaching plans with identified responsibility for health care professionals, outcome criteria and documentation and evaluation. MDA was the first Comprehensive Cancer Center to establish an institution-wide, coordinated patient education program in 1979, with the employment of a director and health educator. Patient education materials developed are available, at minimal cost.

The first center for rehabilitation of the cancer patient was established at MDA in 1972. A multidisciplinary team was established for planning and establishing concepts for delivery of care, with consideration for maintenance of maximum levels of physiological, psychosocial, and vocational functioning. I established an expanded role for screening nurses at MDA who were responsible for patient assessment, based on a care level index developed. They determined eligibility for admission. The program and screening nurse plan still exist, with modification. Focus on rehabilitation and quality of life for the cancer patient began with legislation in 1965. The NCI in 1974 provided impetus through funds for development of institutional and home care programs using the multidisciplinary approach, and educational programs to train enterostomal therapists. I received a contract to develop a program which is still in

operation, and has trained E.T's from here and abroad. Sexual
rehabilitation of the cancer patient, spouse, or significant
other has been addressed only within the past two decades.
Prior to that time the major focus was on eradication of the
cancer. At MDA in 1982 a Sexual Rehabilitation Section was
established in the Urology Department with a urologist, a
chief enterostomal therapist, and a psychologist. They provide individual and group counseling.

While there has always been concern for the terminal cancer patient, the concept of the Hospice program was not initiated in the U.S. until 1978. The first pilot program was
modeled after St. Christopher's in England. The movement has
spread rapidly. There are in-patient hospital-based programs,
home care programs, and free-standing hospice programs. Recent legislation will make it possible for patients on Hospice
programs to have insurance (Medicare) coverage for home care.

The development of multidisciplinary teams has occurred
in the past 20 years. Quality patient care is better attainable through utilization of this concept. If you are still
struggling, take heart; it takes time and perserverance.

Major emphasis has been directed to the "care giver", the
oncology nurse, during the past decade. Stress and "burn-out"
have been recognized as a reality in this highly specialized
field. Attention has been directed to personal, institutional,
educational, and professional awareness and causes. Preventive and intervention programs have been initiated. Administrative recognition of the problem, changes in work schedules
and assignments, participatory management, clinical career
ladders, recognition, and caring atmosphere, peer support
groups,opportunities for "feeling rap" sessions, orientation
and continuing education programs, use of counselors for both
professional and personal problems, and courses in identification and management of stress have been suggested and used.

Nursing Education has changed dramatically in the U.S. in
the last 30 years. Prior to that time most of the programs
were diploma-based in hospital settings. The major thrust now
is baccalaureate degree programs in senior colleges and associate degree programs in junior colleges. In addition, the
number of nurses prepared at Masters and Doctoral levels has
increased.

In cancer nursing, much of the early detection was spon-

sored by the ACS and consisted of short 1- or 2- day programs.
Some cancer institutions and several universities offered
short courses. These early programs focused primarily on providing basic cancer information and nursing care of the cancer patient in the hospital and home. The first graduate program was offered in 1945 by Katharine Nelson at Columbia Uni-
veristy, N.Y. She had a faculty appointment while employed
as educational director at Memorial Hospital. Students had
clinical practice there and it was the first collaborative
effort for students in a cancer institution. Since the focus
in nursing at that time was on preparation of the "generalist"
rather than the specialist, only one class of students completed the program. There are now 3 Doctoral, 3 post-masters
and 30 schools offering a Masters program with cancer nursing
focus.

In 1954, the Nursing Section Chief, NCI, USPHS, secured
federal funds that were given to four baccalaureate schools of
nursing to integrate cancer nursing into the curriculum. Faculty developed curricula, a knowledge test, and evaluation
tools.

In 1978, ACS invited a distinguished group of nurses to a
workshop on curriculum construction and role definition to
clarify the role and academic preparation necessary in cancer
nursing. Guidelines for the masters degree with a speciality
in cancer nursing were developed and subsequently published.
Since 1981, the ACS has offered scholarships to nurses at a
Masters level in oncology nursing. While there are some common threads, curricula content, clinical practicum, and research as a component varied. A Task Force of ONS is working
on the development of standards for graduate education in oncology nursing. In 1982, ONS published "Outcome Standards for
Oncology Nursing at the Fundamental Level".

In 1980, ACS approved a proposal for the development of
clinical professors in oncology nursing; to date none have
been appointed. The aim was to have nurses at an Associate
Professor or Professor in academic institutions, to assist
faculty, nursing service, conduct research, and collaborate
with other health professionals.

Continuing education programs in oncology nursing have
increased, but most have no provision for clinical practice.
MDA now offers an oncology nurse clinician program of one
year or less for specific modules. It is open to outside

nurses. Whereas in some of your countries curriculum and continuing education programs are approved only to be given in
certain institutions, such as oncology nursing at the Royal
Marsden, London, in the U.S. academic institutions, hospitals
or specialty groups organize and conduct a variety of continuing education programs. Program approval and awarding of continuing education units to participants are based on meeting
established criteria.

Oncology nurses in practice, education, and research are
now contributing extensively to the literature. Two journals,
Oncology Nursing Forum and Cancer Nursing: an International
Journal for Cancer are excellent resources.

Research is essential in order to advance the knowledge
and science of oncology nursing. It is necessary to develop
a theoretical knowledge base for oncology nursing practice in
order for nurses to function effectively in dealing with cancer clients/patients, and for educators who prepare nurses.

Research in Cancer Nursing, while still in its infancy,
has made progress compared to general nursing research. The
American Nurses Association Commission on Nursing Research
identified practice priorities as a major area for research.
A study (Oberst 1973) determined priorities for research in
cancer nursing related to patients needs, practice, support
for practitioner, education and communication. Nurse researchers are addressing some of these problems. Oncology
nurses have and continue to do research in psychosocial aspects; the patient's perception; compliance, and the effects
of nursing intervention in prevention, detection, diagnosis,
treatment, rehabilitation, and pain control; and home care of
the terminal ill child and adult. Research includes not only
the client/patient but the family or significant other. These
research efforts have implications for nursing practice and
educational programs.

Nurses have had representation on the NCI Cancer Control
Grant Review Committee since 1970. Ruth McCorkle and I are
presently members. The committee reviews proposals submitted
for scientific and technical merit. I believe we have another
important responsibility in interpreting and supporting oncology nurses and nursing. Nurses have representation on
other NCI Committees related to Cancer Control and INtervention
Activities.

ONS has a Research Committee, and publishes a Research article and a Question-Answer column in each issue of their Journal. Individual members of the committee have offered assistance to their colleagues. At the 1982 meeting of ONS, the Research Committee sponsored a resolution supported by the Membership. The resolution supported voluntary collaboration in nursing and medical research, and the nurses' right to do nursing research independently. It was hoped that this would assist some nurses who now need to have a physician collaborator identified to do research. At the same ONS meeting, I initiated a resolution which was also supported by the membership to encourage and support·NCI funding of nurse principal investigators in cancer nursing research. Recent development may make this a reality.

Summary: As I have discussed, oncology nurses and cancer nursing have made great strides in the past two decades. Where do we want to be in the next two decades? Questions need to be raised, goals set, and a course of action determined. As Derdarian (1981) states, "Cancer Nursing as a specialty of nursing profession, can create a prototype- a model- for practice, curriculum development, and research." Cancer Nursing is now a colossus inspite of its fragile beginning. It developed and was built on caring, sharing, and daring. We must plan and build for the future while keeping pace with the present. I have been in this field for 32 years, and knowing and working with oncology nurses, the challenges will be met and resolved.

Alvardo E, Drean D, Kean T, (1980). Follow-up evaluation cancer control program for nurses, M.D.A.
Baker L, (1982). Breast cancer detection demonstration project: five year summary report, CA-J for Phys. 1, 194.
Hilkemeyer R, (1982). A Historical Perspective in Cancer Nursing. Onc Nurs Forum 9,47.
Oberst M, Priorities in Cancer Nursing, CA Nsg, 3, 281.
Onc Nurs Soc ANA, (1979). Standards for cancer nursing practice. Kansas City, Mo.
Vredevoe D,Deridarian A, Sarna L, (1981). Concepts of oncology nursing practice, Prentice Hall, New Jersey.

13th International Cancer Congress, Part E
Cancer Management, pages 423–426
© **1983 Alan R. Liss, Inc., 150 Fifth Avenue, New York, NY 10011**

PROBLEMS ENCOUNTERED IN AN INTENSIVE CARE MEDICAL ONCOLOGY
UNIT IN PARIS.

Catherine ADONIS

Oncology Division. CHU Avicenne

Bobigny. 93000. France

Oncology in France is in a very special situation.
20 large cancer centers are semi-private and receive about
25 % of the cancer patients, 75 % are treated either by
doctors in private practice or in public hospitals but
generally by radiotherapists or general surgeons and medical specialists of the various organs involved. In University hospitals, there are almost no oncology divisions, and
oncology is not yet considered as a speciality. That is the
reason why, as head nurse of a medical oncology unit in a
University hospital in Paris, I live a still very exclusive
experience, and I choosed to talk about it rather than
giving you a general view of cancer nursing in France
because I think this experience might be of interest for
several countries.

In my hospital in Bobigny, a suburb of Paris, the
medical oncology unit was created, 6 years ago, by Lucien
ISRAEL in a semi-clandestine way. Patients from all parts
of the country, started immediately to come to us, referred
by themselves, or other patients or private doctors, but
not by other services of the hospital or other hospitals in
the vicinity, and the situation has changed only slightly
since the beginning.

This may explain why 80 % of the cases we see are
relapses. Cancer is treated by organ specialists who generally do not seek advise from an oncologist and advise
against any systemic treatment or specialised surveillance.

This results in the fact that we are in the necessity of trying to rescue most of the patients that come to us in very advanced state, and that we have had some trouble in the beginning with young nurses that were discouraged. This situation also results in the fact that we have been obliged to design some therapies difficult to apply, or even unconventional, such as combination of local hyperthermia, plasmaexchange and intraarterial chemotherapy, together with heavy schedules of systemic chemotherapy involving continuous infusions for several days every 3 to 4 weeks.

The policy of the service being to give a chance to every patient who asks for it, except when it looks totally unreasonable. We have had to meet several challenges.

1. We have had to deal with an ever growing population of patients with only 34 beds for hospitalisation and 10 beds for out patients.

Patients that live outside the Paris area are hospitalized for their treatments, and come back every 3 to 4 weeks for 1 week, with all work-ups and tests performed as out patients. We are in touch with them and their doctor by phone. Soon we will need a computer for bed reservation only for our unit. I personnally spend two hours a day answering phone calls and managing appointments.

Most of the patients, after the first course, are treated as out-patients. We see about 50 patients a day in such conditions. Drugs that should be delivered in a continuous schedule are given every 6 or 8 hours, part in our out-patients unit, part at home by their family physician and the home nursing assistance service. Blood transfusions when needed are performed in this out-patient unit. Usually these patients are asked to consult once a week between therapy courses.

2. Another challenge has been to learn how to master situations such as repeated plasmaexchange, collection of very large amounts of white cells from normal donors that are injected in unresectable tumors, care of patients that may a white cell count between 100 and 500 for several days.

Moreover to treat patients whose veins are in a very bad state after one or two years of chemotherapy, arterio-veinous shunts with prosthetic material are currently perf rmed and sometimes I.V. infusions have to be elevated 2 and one-half meters higher than the infusion point at counter arterial pressure.

3. Perhaps the most interesting problem and the most demanding, has been to learn how to cope with patients that in many instances have been rejected by other centers, because they were told their disease was incurable, and they come to us with a mixture of great hope and great anguish. In some cases the patients had to fight their family and their physician. Of course we are far from succeeding in every case, but curiously most of these patients tell us they are grateful just because we accepted to try. And fortunately, in more and more cases the treat-ments are relatively successful, giving two years to a person who was given two months to live, or even three to five years, during which some surgery may be done that was impossible at the beginning, and or some radiation therapy, etc...

What our patients fear most is not intensive treatment, nor side effects ; it is to be abandoned. They do not ask us - unlike some family members - to be necessarily success-ful. They ask us to offer them an ultimate chance, as fellow humans, to show that we care for them, that we are prepared to try as long as possible, and that they are not only numbers in a protocol list.

This is not to say that no protocols are performed in our unit. However most protocols are phase II protocols of combined modalities designed for helping patients in advan-ced states, for improving second or third line regimens, for regaining control of disseminated disease, inflammatory carcinomas, unresectable tumors that do not respond to radiotherapy, etc...

In such a situation most people on the staff, nurses and doctors alike, feel like a "commando unit", living in a state of urgency, which may be sometimes exhausting. All of us resent intensely our failures, especially of course in young patients that are more and more numerous, although we treat only solid tumors. However all of us share a sense of victory when patients that were sent to us with multiple injections of morphin per day enter into complets regression and leave the hospital to go to the out-patient unit.

It has become clear to us that in a majority of our cases more intense and earlier treatment could have given the patient more chance. I do not dare to correlate the percentage of patients receiving from the beginning the optimal treatment, but it is far below 50 %, at least in France and probably in many other well developped countries. It seems to me very likely that without any major discovery, but just by giving every patient the proper treatment from the beginning the general results could be largely improved. However this is not My subject.

Now I will try to draw from my experience, a few general conclusions regarding cancer nursing.

Firstly, cancer nursing is a very difficult task that requires technical skill and we should try to recruit the best of our young colleagues, and devote a great deal of time to increasing their technical capabilities.

Secondly, it is diff cult, in the field of oncology to distinguish between routine tasks and research. All cancer nurses should receive detailed information and training concerning technical and ethical aspects of research.

Thirdly, as cancer is a very severe disease of uncertain outcome, it represents a situation in which patients need the assistance of special kind of human being, well balanced personalities with empathy and love, conscious of what life represents, able to understand things that will never be said, to forgive weaknesses, to give strenght, time, and be concerned. Just to show the goals and to delineate the directions, is a great challenge for the whole international community of cancer nurses.

13th International Cancer Congress, Part E
Cancer Management, pages 427–433
© **1983 Alan R. Liss, Inc., 150 Fifth Avenue, New York, NY 10011**

CANCER NURSING IN THE NETHERLANDS

Ellen M.K. Strak, S.R.N.
Director of Nursing Services
Dr. Daniël den Hoed Kliniek
Rotterdamsch Radio-Therapeutisch Instituut
P.O.B. 5201, 3008 AE Rotterdam

"Cancer nursing" is a generally accepted expression, although I myself do not like the term that much. I think "nursing of cancer patients" or "nursing patients with cancer" would be better. It reminds me of the time as a student nurse when we were forbidden to talk about "the stomach in room three" or "the broken hip in room seven".

The heightened efforts in the last decade have led to progressive improvements in the treatment of cancer. The time, when the only way to treat a tumour was surgery or radio-therapy is far behind us. The change in medical treatment, with its emphasis on chemotherapy, hormonal therapy and the refinements in surgery and radiation, the planning of treatment modalities, all taking place in multidisciplinary teams, has had a tremendous influence, also in my country, on the medical as well as the nursing profession. The U.S.A. took the lead, in 1971, with the acceptance by congress of the National Cancer Act. It resulted in the establishment of 20 comprehensive cancer centres. The Netherlands followed: 5 years ago the first comprehensive cancer centre was set up, and at the moment there are seven. These cover a greater part of the country. Comprehensive cancer centres in the Netherlands are financed through the hospitals in the area by raising slightly the hospital charges. That means that all patients, including those only operated on for varicose veins, or maternity cases, help to pay for better cancer care. Basic and clinical research is financed partly by the government (which is tightening the strings of the purse harder and harder) and partly by the Queen Wilhelmina Fund, which is dependent on gifts from the dutch people.

At the same time as the developments within the medical
profession, nurses in the Netherlands began to realize that
they needed to improve their knowledge and skills in cancer
nursing. Both cancer hospitals, in Amsterdam and Rotterdam,
have been organizing courses in cancer nursing for many
years. Primarily these courses were given in order to attract
nurses to work in this special field. A great stimulus for
nurses in general was the First International Cancer Nursing
Conference in London, in 1978, which was attended by several
dutch nurses. The next conference, 2 years later, was
attended by many more. This second conference has led, as a
consequence, to the establishment in the Netherlands of a
Foundation to promote cancer nursing. This Foundation wants
to improve the quality of cancer nursing by way of:
1. to inform hospital and community nurses about developments
   in cancer nursing
2. to promote discussions about these subjects
3. to organize a yearly conference
4. to stimulate attendance at congresses in the Netherlands
   or elsewhere
5. to give general information.
In the meantime the Foundation has organized 2 conferences.
The interest in these was immense, both times the hall was
filled to capacity, and many were disappointed. Last year a
specialist course in stoma-care was started, for nurses
working in hospitals and nursing homes as well as for
community nurses. Some hospitals have set up a stoma-clinic.
When one of the visitors of the First International Cancer
Nursing Conference realized that so many nursing textbooks
had been written relating to cancer care, but none of them in
the dutch language, which made them accessible to only some
of our nurses, he decided to write one himself. Last year it
was published.

All these events are a sign that also in my country nurses
are trying to become more professionalized. They feel
activated to become experts in their chosen field.

Let us go back to the comprehensive cancer centres. Although
the approach and the activities differ slightly, their
functions are:
1. The organization of consultation services in regional
   medical centres.
2. The organization of specific tumour working parties.
3. To organize the registration and documentation of cancer
   incidence and prevalence.
4. Education, training and postgraduate courses for health
   professionals in the region.

5. Providing information for health professionals, patients and the general public.
6. Providing psychosocial care and support for cancer patients.
7. Clinical and basic research.

As you can see: at point 4, 5 and 6 nurses are involved in:
- education, training and postgraduate courses
- providing information
- providing psychosocial care and support.

One can question if point 1: consultation services and part of point 7: clinical research, should be considered as tasks of a cancer nurse. In some centres we see a beginning of these activities.

Education and training

Comprehensive cancer centres must see it as a duty to stimulate and improve the nursing care for cancer patients. All our 7 comprehensive cancer centres include university hospitals; on top of that Amsterdam and Rotterdam each have a hospital specializing in cancer. As well as the courses in these hospitals, which I already mentioned, some university hospitals have also begun specialized education and training in cancer nursing. Others are considering it. Although it can not always be realized, the most ideal situation is to give these courses as in-service training. In this way it is possible to integrate theory and practice as well as to acquire a special attitude. During the courses the students are being taught the pathophysiology of malignant processes, the different modalities of cancer treatment and supportive management, such as nutrition, pain control and infection control. At the same time the implications for nursing practice are taught. Rehabilitation and psychosocial care and support are of course not forgotten.

Bedside teaching is in this matter very important. Students have not only to learn, but also in some ways to unlearn. Let me give you an example: As a nurse one has learned that patients must be rehabilitated as quickly as possible, everything they can do themselves, they must do. In our hospital we teach nurses to observe the patients very carefully. If they have little energy left, the patients should have the freedom to opt for whatever they want to use their energy for; if bathing themselves takes all their strength, the nurse should offer to help them with their bath, so that they can engage themselves later in the day with something more enjoyable. Cancer patients, who undergo an exhausting treatment, a treatment which takes very often years of their lives, have during that time very little choice. And is the possibility to choose not a very important part in each of our own lives?

From education and training now I come to
Postgraduate courses.
The improvements of modalities in treatment of cancer have to be followed carefully, both by physicians and nurses working in the field. Especially by staff nurses working in a cancer centre, in cancer wards or cancer clinics. New modalities have implications for nursing care. And as new modalities are preceded in cancer centres by pilot studies and clinical trials, the nursing staff should master the ins and outs of the procedures and should know what the aims are.

In my hospital one of the head nurses took it upon herself to create weekly discussions on various topics between nursing staff and physicians, who alternate in order to expose what is going on in their special field and report the outcome of studies they have performed in which nurses often participated. The Comprehensive Cancer Centre in Rotterdam organizes regularly symposia about different subjects. Although these meetings are mainly for members of the medical profession, nurses are gladly admitted. During these gatherings future developments are being discussed and in this way nurses are able to anticipate complementing nursing care.

Another group which must not be forgotten is the public health or community nurses. They come in contact with all sorts of people, healthy or ill, and only some of their patients suffer from cancer. As these patients need sophisticated care, the community nurse can seek advice from her colleagues in the hospital where the patient is treated, or still better: hospital nurses should encourage the community nurse to visit the hospital beforehand. But as more and more patients are hospitalized only on and off during their illness, and the contact between the community nurse and her patient becomes very frequent, patients tend to get information about their disease from her as well. Therefore comprehensive cancer centres are beginning to organize study programmes especially for this group.

That brings me to the next function of a comprehensive cancer centre:
Providing information.
For the general public the outlook on cancer is bleak. To talk about it, is one of the still existing taboos. A well known womens magazine in the Netherlands did an

investigation: it found out there were three taboo-subjects, which, when put on the cover, did raise the sale of copies considerably: they were Downs' syndrome, sex and cancer. I wonder if these taboos still exist among some members of the medical and nursing profession?

The physician, of course, will explain to his patient what sort of treatment he has in mind, but this explanation often takes place in an emotional situation. Booklets and folders can be a help but have to be accompanied by further interpretation and encouragement to come forward with questions.

It is my opinion that, exclusively by education and training, nurses can gather knowledge in order to inform the patient about his disease and the treatment he needs. By doing this they can help to motivate him to undergo and endure an often exhausting therapy.

Last year the Queen Wilhelmina Fund opened up an information centre. In this centre one finds experts, among them a nurse. They provide the general public with information about cancer. Visitors to this centre are not only patients themselves or relatives of patients, but also nurses from general hospitals and community nurses. Just like the American Cancer Society has been doing for years, the Queen Wilhelmina Fund publishes booklets about different kinds of cancer. They also pass on information about patients who have formed groups to give emotional and practical support to each other.

Psychosocial care and support
Nursing care and psychosocial support go hand in hand. The one can not be without the other. How do we master the latter subject? We can invite experts to teach us. Discussions with colleagues and sharing their experience are a help, or we can read what others have to say. Whole libraries can be filled with books on psychosocial care and emotional support of cancer patients! Of course, the diagnosis of cancer is a shattering experience for the patient and his family, and not all patients can be given hope of a cure. This brings about a feeling of helplesness. However, our own uncertainties should never be compensated by overdoing our emotional support with cancerpatients. By doing this we stigmatize them.

Psychosocial support is showing humanity. This is part of the nature of every human being. Let us not forget that in the end the patient himself chooses the person who he wants to support him. And this person is not necessarily a professional.

Listening to patients can be a revelation. In the chemotherapy department of our hospital we have group discussions. Once a week all patients are invited to join, though of course, it is not compulsory. The head nurse and the psychologist are always in attendance, the other nurses if time allows. The patients themselves choose the subject they want to discuss. Mostly they wish to talk about their disease, their therapy and its side effects. It is striking how well patients listen to each other and how freely they discuss their feelings and their experiences, inside and outside the hospital. The nurses were surprised to find that patients with whom it was very difficult to make any personal contact, because they stayed in their rooms, suddenly opened up in these group discussions. After this, in most cases, their openness mostly continued.

Besides that, the nurses were trying to activate their patients. The puzzles and games which they bought for them were hardly touched, records stayed in their covers. The patients' lethargy was especially evident in the morning when they were still waiting to receive their chemotherapy, and not feeling nauseous. After discussions with the physicians it was decided to give physiotherapy. Now all chemotherapy patients are recommended to go to the physiotherapy department in order to do some exercises each morning. Although especially new patients go under protest, afterwards they recognize these exercises as a help to overcome their feeling of weakness.

Nursing of cancer patients can be a heavy strain, because not only the patients but also their relatives have to be considered. Therefore an open relationship between all the people who work in a cancer ward is of the greatest importance. Support from colleagues, superiors and others, such as family and friends is needed, in order to enable nurses to keep their emotional strength.

I wish to end this paper by quoting Bob Tiffany. In his introduction to "Cancer Nursing Update" he wrote: "From a beginning of rather insular, in-service training programmes, based on maintaining standards of care, cancer nursing has now developed into an outgoing, internationally orientated, professionally aware group, eager to share information and ideas to achieve optimal care and support for patients with cancer."

Cleton FJ (1982). Integrale kankercentra. Tijdschrift voor Ziekenverpleging 10:319.

Leer JWH (1982). Patiënten met kanker in kliniek en polikliniek. In: Begeleiding van patiënten met kanker :20. Stafleu's wetenschappelijke uitgeversmaatschappij B.V. Alphen a/d Rijn.

American Cancer Society (1981). A cancer source book for nurses, reviced edition. Professional Education Publication.

Tiffany R (1981). Cancer nursing Update. Baillière Tindall, London.

13th International Cancer Congress, Part E
Cancer Management, pages 435–440
© 1983 Alan R. Liss, Inc., 150 Fifth Avenue, New York, NY 10011

THE DEVELOPMENT OF ONCOLOGY NURSING IN THE UNITED KINGDOM

Robert Tiffany, S.R.N., R.C.N.T., D.N.

Chief Nurse
The Royal Marsden Hospital,
London SW3 6JJ

When one looks at developments in the United Kingdom that have occurred within our speciality over recent years, it is difficult to realise that so much has been achieved in such a short time.

Nursing of cancer patients is not new; it has been in existence within my own institution for over a century, and looking back at some of the earliest nursing records makes fascinating reading. Many of the problems that we often think are new are easily identified as existing before the turn of the century, and as we think of the dramatic advances in nursing being made today, one can imagine the fire of enthusiasm that these early oncology nurses must have experienced during the 'Nightingale' era.

These early pioneers became oncology nurses not by education but by experience. The knowledge base of cancer nursing was experimental and not formalised for application outside their own institution. Despite the importance of lessons learned during ten decades, and the excellence attained by individuals and groups of nurses, the published literature on cancer nursing was sparse and often contributed by doctors rather than nurses. Thus, until recently there was no formal education programme for cancer nursing, no literature on which to base such a programme, no definition of the role of a cancer nurse and no formalised identity for the nurse except through the institution in which she worked.

Nurses were not alone in these early years in their lack of a formal approach to the cancer problem. There were no physician specialties devoted to cancer care. Radiotherapy, then in the kilovoltage era, was practised by individuals trained primarily in diagnostic radiology, and training in general surgery was often considered adequate for the delivery of complete cancer care.

Perhaps it is significant that our growth occurred at the same time as developments within the medical profession. The complex nature of the disease and the recognition that cancer is often systemic at the time of diagnosis has led to a collaborative approach between diagnosticians, surgeons, radiotherapists and physicians. Planning of treatment now takes place in multidisciplinary teams, using various forms of treatment at specific times in the overall management of a particular tumour. Coupled with this development has been the growing awareness, particularly as prognostic factors improve, of the need to provide adequate planned caring and support systems in conjunction with curative and palliative treatments.

These developments have led, in many centres, to a truly interdependent functioning between health care professionals to provide individualised comprehensive care plans for each patient.

Perhaps the most significant development in the United Kingdom was in 1973 when, following developments at the Royal Marsden Hospital and other cancer centres, the Joint Board of Clinical Nursing Studies recognised the need to establish a national curriculum for post basic training in oncology nursing. This development led to a recognition that post basic education in this speciality could no longer be considered a luxury for the privileged few but a necessary prerequisite for clinical practice if nursing was to continue to make a major contribution in cancer care. From 1974, when the first Joint Board of Clinical Nursing Studies Course was approved at the Royal Marsden Hospital, to the present time, over 2,000 nurses have successfully completed training.

The effects of the introduction of this programme of training have been quite dramatic. From a desert of literature on the subject of cancer nursing has blossomed a whole range of nursing textbooks on cancer care, and there is hardly an issue of our current nursing journals that does not contain a contribution from nurses on some aspect of cancer care. What is particularly significant is that these textbooks are being written by nurses for nurses, bringing greater credibility to the concept of nursing as a profession in its own right.

The 1970's saw another milestone in the development of cancer nursing. Recognition that there was a need for a learned body to advise the profession on cancer care led the Royal College of Nursing to establish the Oncology Nursing Society, which, whilst still in its infancy, has already made a major contribution to the development of an identifiable body of knowledge through the exchange of information and generation of interest in cancer nursing. This search for knowledge led to greater international cooperation, and in 1978 'Cancer Nursing', an international journal for cancer care, was launched and already has over 8,000 subscribers worldwide. The International Union Against Cancer recognised the unique contribution that nurses made and established their first nursing committee, and later in that year held their first nursing workshop at their 12th International Congress in Buenos Aires. For me personally, the event that had the greatest impact that year was the First International Conference on Cancer Nursing, held in London and sponsored by Nursing Mirror. At this event, over 1,200 nurses from 25 countries participated in a most remarkable week in which nurses addressed the problems faced by our patients, and provided many exciting and innovative approaches to finding solutions.

The Second International Conference in 1980 was also well attended with participants from over 30 countries, and commitment has now been made to continue these conferences on a two-yearly cycle, following the 1984 Conference in Melbourne, Australia.

Regarding international cooperation, it must be recognised, of course, that cancer nursing - unlike cancer medicine - cannot be internationally defined and specified except in general terms. The medical approach to cancer does not change dramatically from one country to another. The surgical procedure, radiotherapeutic technique or chemotherapy protocol remains basically the same and although there may be varying degress of sophistication in therapy, there are clear parameters that can be easily defined. Nursing, however, is concerned with the daily living

activities of people, the promotion of independent
functioning, providing physical and emotional support for
patients and their families to cope with their disease and/
or its treatment.

How this can best be achieved will, to a large extent,
depend on local environmental, social and cultural factors.
Even those aspects of care which are in support of our
medical colleagues' work are greatly influenced by local
differences and the degree of health care sophistication.
For example, enterostomal surgery may be the same procedure
in the United Kingdom and a rural Asian community. However,
methods of caring for and supporting this patient will differ
greatly. In one setting there may well be disposable aids
and appliances, expensive skin creams, disposal collection
services etc. In the other setting, lack of resources may
present innovative challenges to the nurse who will have to
develop a different type of care and support system.

During the past few years this momentum has been
maintained. The development of clinical nurse specialists
in a variety of areas, the creation of international oncology
nursing exchange programmes and the introduction of nursing
research programmes into cancer care have all helped to
generate a more dynamic and creative professional awareness.

At the present time we can observe three distinct but
linked areas of development in cancer nursing. Firstly, in
clinical practice we are developing more creative roles to
deal with the daily living problems of patients that arise
as a result of their disease and/or its treatment. Significant is the insistence that nursing is more than a collection
of skilled and semi-skilled tasks; it is a professional
discipline in its own right, underpinned by a particular
approach to patient care that is different from any other.
Nursing should not be viewed only as a back-up to medical
care or even as some kind of paramedical service. This
does not mean that we reject a collaborative role with other
professionals. On the contrary, one of the valuable roles
that nurses perform is to continue the prescribed therapy of
the doctor, physiotherapist, social worker, dietitian etc.
in their absence, and also to report the effects of this
prescribed therapy. However, this supplementary role of
nursing should not overshadow its unique complementary role.
Virginia Henderson amplifies this aspect of the nurse's role
when she portrays these challenging demands:-

'The nurse is temporarily the consciousness of the unconscious, the love of life of the suicide, the leg of the amputee, the eyes of the newly blind, the mouthpiece of those too weak to speak.'

Jean McFarlane at the First International Conference on Cancer Nursing outlined how we could develop this unique role by moving from a reactive to a scientific approach, from institutionalised to individualised care, from the routinised to the creative, and from the dependent to accountable functioning.

Coupled with this general development has been the concurrent progress in developing specialist nursing roles. In my opinion, this small group of nurses have achieved quite remarkable success and the results of their endeavours in improved patient care I would have thought were quite obvious to anyone who has worked with them or had the opportunity of observing them at work. However, it must be said that this is not a universal opinion. There is still some scepticism and, indeed, some opposition from within and outside the profession.

However, I would agree with the American philosopher, Oliver Wendell Holmes, who remarked 'I know no teachers so powerful as the little army of specialists. They carry no banners, they beat no drums, but where they are men learn that bustle and push are not the equals of quiet genious and serene mastery'.

The second development is in the field of nursing research, which is providing the stimulus to question and examine existing practices, and generating enquiry into alternative methods of care. No profession can continue indefinitely, least of all in a contemporary setting, to base its practices on the collected folklore and customs of its predecessors. If nursing is to continue to make an effective contribution to patient care it must evolve as an applied scientific discipline in a similar way to medicine. It is only by undertaking research that nursing can continue to develop as a profession, justify its own existence and, most of all, give patients the care they need.

However, we must remove some confusion. Research is not nursing research because it is done by nurses. Nurses who collect data for investigators from other disciplines are not 'nurse researchers' although they often like to style themselves by this title. They are data collectors and, valuable though their work may be, we must be careful not to confuse nurses working in research with research into nursing.

A number of major cancer centres now have nursing research units established and valuable information is being obtained.

Thirdly, there is the development in nursing education. I mentioned earlier the development of Joint Board Courses. In the United Kingdom it was considered a priority in cancer nursing education to prepare clinical nurses who were currently delivering care, to function effectively. This pattern was followed in a number of countries. However, others followed a different route, notably the United States. Here, Masters' programmes in cancer nursing were developed to produce leaders of the profession, academically prepared to take senior positions in nursing management and education related to cancer care, and to provide a core of clinical nurse consultants in a variety of sub-specialities. These two views are not necessarily opposing and, in my opinion, are complementary. In the United States, consideration is now being given to the establishment of courses similar to those available in the United Kingdom. Perhaps we should now be considering developing more advanced courses in cancer nursing similar to those established in North America. These would be a natural development for people with ability, who had undertaken our first line course and wished to pursue a career in cancer nursing at a senior level.

In conclusion, the last ten years have seen more developments in cancer nursing than the previous ten decades. Never has there been such an opportunity for nursing to exercise its influence in promoting optimal standards of care, and in assisting patients to overcome the problems of their disease and its treatment.

The future holds for us many exciting possibilities. If a collaborative approach can be fostered within our own profession, and with other professions, a nursing renaissance can occur over the next ten years.

****

13th International Cancer Congress, Part E
Cancer Management, pages 441–447
© 1983 Alan R. Liss, Inc., 150 Fifth Avenue, New York, NY 10011

CANCER NURSING IN A COMPREHENSIVE CANCER CENTER

Donna Park, R.N., MA
Memorial Sloan-Kettering Cancer Center

The nursing care of patients with cancer can be both physically and emotionally demanding, yet filled with many challenging and rewarding experiences. Nowhere is this more evident than in a Comprehensive Cancer Center where nurses respond to the needs of patients on a continuum from the prevention of cancer to supportive care in terminal stages of disease. Each nurse working in a Comprehensive Cancer Center is a member of a highly specialized multi-disciplinary team, and makes a unique contribution to the practice, education and research efforts of the Center. I would like to take you through Memorial Sloan-Kettering Cancer Center located in New York City and describe to you some of its many nursing practice roles.

Patients come to Memorial Hospital because of the specialized treatment available. A nurse, the Patient Service Coordinator, facilitates entry into the health care system by processing requests for treatment and making referrals to alternate health care facilities.

Many patients are initially evaluated by a Family Nurse Practitioner who uses knowledge and expert skills in the area of cancer prevention and detection to determine the presence or absence of a malignancy. Based on her findings, patients may be referred to medical or surgical oncologists or counseled regarding health status, personal risk factors and the importance of routine health care measures.

In the ambulatory care setting, the trend toward giving more intensive treatment on an outpatient basis requires that nurses function in a wide spectrum of oncology nursing practice. During the patient's first visit to the oncologist, the ambulatory care nurse establishes a relationship with the patient and family and begins to develop an individualized plan of care. On subsequent visits, each patient is assessed to ascertain any changes that have occurred since the last visit. Anticipating the need for additional health care and/or community resources is an important part of this assessment.

In each outpatient area, nurses design interventions to meet the special needs of their patient populations. For example, an important aspect of administering chemotherapy is reinforcing patient understanding of drug side effects and their management. In Ambulatory Surgery, efforts are focused on supporting the patient and family during the diagnostic period. In the Hematology Clinic, nurses perform bone marrow aspirations and biopsies. Their skill and understanding help allay patients' fears regarding this procedure. In fact, some patients will allow only nurses to perform their bone marrow aspirations. In Breast Clinic, post-mastectomy patients are seen after discharge from the hospital. Here, wound healing is assessed, hand and arm care reviewed and the importance of performing monthly breast self-examination is stressed. Working in the Transfusion Room offers the unique opportunity to meet the emotional and physical needs of patients who require frequent blood and/or platelet transfusions. As the outpatient treatment of cancer has intensified the development of complications at home has increased. Patients presenting to the emergency facility are evaluated initially by nurses. Being alert to the subtle signs of the medical emergencies associated with cancer, such as hypercalcemia or sepsis, requires a broad knowledge of cancer pathophysiology and current treatment modalities.

Specialization of cancer diagnosis, treatment and rehabilitation are reflected on each of the inpatient units. Here the nurses develop specialized expertise in responding to the multiplicity of problems brought about by the numerous treatment modalities for cancer. Because of the research efforts of the institution, patients with rare malignancies are frequently referred for treatment. It is the impact of these research efforts which pose the greatest challenge for nursing. For example, over the past year, Memorial has treated an increasing number of patients with Acquired Immune Deficiency with Kaposis Sarcoma. These patients are usually on Enteric and Hepatitis Precautions, and strict isolation for Herpes Zoster. In addition to managing the physical care and administering the multiple antibiotics and parenteral infusions, these patients require constant emotional support to enable them to cope with the stress of isolation, and to understand what is happening to them and why.

Nurses at Memorial have the opportunity to develop competency and to receive recognition for clinical expertise through a Clinical Career Ladder concept. When a new graduate is employed at Memorial Hospital the job title is Clinical Nurse I. At the end of an evaluation period, her performance should progress to the level of a Clinical Nurse II. The Clinical Nurse II has special knowledge and skills necessary to assist patients and families in adjusting to physiologic changes from cancer treatment and the resulting psychological impact of these alterations. For example, on the Thoracic Unit, the Clinical Nurse II conducts a preoperative teaching class to explain the importance of deep breathing and coughing post-thoracotomy. In all areas the nurse must create and maintain an atmosphere of support for the patient and family in which physical and emotional needs can be shared and discussed.

The third level of the Clinical Career Ladder is the Clinical Nurse III position. This level requires development of significant expertise in clinical nursing practice. Functioning as a resource for staff, the Clinical Nurse III assists in the design of specialized plans of care for specific patient populations. The final level of the Ladder is an advanced practice role – that of Nurse Clinician. This role provides an opportunity to demonstrate a high degree of professional competence in a selected specialty. Some Nurse Clinicians function in joint practice roles with physicians. For example, on the Hematology Service, the Nurse Clinician follows a caseload of patients on an inpatient and outpatient basis, and collaborates with a physician in management of care. A Psychiatric Nurse Clinician, in a consultant role assists with the integration of psychiatric/psychosocial elements into nursing practice. Referrals are made to the Psychiatric Nurse Clinician by the nursing staff regarding management problems of patients and/or families. In order to improve the staff's knowledge and skills, the Nurse Clinician assesses the problem and recommends interventions in the context of an educational process. Subsequent review, evaluation and support are provided during the implementation of the care plan. The Psychiatric Nurse Clinician also conducts support groups to assist staff in communicating thoughts and feelings regarding professional conflict situations. In an effort to maintain patients at home, a Supportive Care Program has been established. Two (2) Nurse Clinicians function as primary care providers in helping patients and families in managing pain and dealing with cancer. They provide assistance to families in negotiating the health care system and in mobilizing community resources.

All the Nurse Clinicians routinely meet as a Nurse
Practice Council to direct development of standards for
clinical nursing practice utilizing the conceptual framework
of nursing diagnosis. These standards serve as a resource
to staff in the development of individual patient care
plans. Examples include: Alterations In Immune Response
And Alterations In Comfort Related to Nausea And Vomiting.

In response to the needs of the highly complex treatment
programs, many specialized nursing roles have evolved. For
example, because the majority of surgical procedures
performed in a Comprehensive Cancer Center are more extensive
than in other facilities, operating room nurses make pre-
and postoperative visits to patients to assess needs and
answer questions. From these visits the need was recognized
for a liaison between the patient's family and physician
during the operative procedure. As a result the unique
nursing role of Surgical Nurse Coordinator was created.
The nurses in this role make rounds between the Operating
Room, Recovery Room and waiting area for families. They
obtain information on the progress of surgery thus enabling
them to provide needed support to family members.

Specialized roles also exist in other areas. Nurse
Practitioners function as members of the Clinical Nutrition
Team in order to provide optimum therapy for patients
requiring nutritional support. They assess the clinical
status and nutritional needs of patients and develop
nutritional therapy plans in collaboration with the other
members of the team. The nurses on the Intravenous Therapy
Team evaluate the effects of parenteral treatment on the
vascular system, and develop new techniques in an effort to
conserve the integrity of each patient's veins. The nurses
who fill the role of Enterostomal Therapist have specialized
clinical expertise in the care of ostomy patients. They
work with the staff in the preoperative and postoperative
management of patients with ostomies. In addition, they
provide classroom instruction to new staff as well as
bedside consultation for management problems such as
multiple abdominal fistulae. The Treatment Room nurses
assist with diagnostic and minor surgical procedures such
as the management of acute stomatitis, surgical wound
defects and cancer lesions. The nurses working in Diagnostic
Radiology perform special procedures such as lymphangiograms.
Their skill and understanding personalizes diagnostic
procedures, with the result that the patient undergoing
such procedures perceives an individualization of his care.
In the Radiation Therapy Department, nurses conduct orienta-

tion classes for patients about to receive therapy, and provide emotional and physical support during each treatment.

Pediatric oncology nursing is a specialized area of practice which requires an understanding of the complexities of childhood cancer and the impact of the disease and its treatment on the growth and development of the child. Most of the treatment is provided in the ambulatory care setting using a multidisciplinary family centered approach in an effort to help the family maintain as normal a life style as possible. In the Pediatric Outpatient Department, Nurse Practitioners, in collaboration with physicians, follow a caseload of patients who have a particular malignancy. During each visit the Practitioner performs a physical examination, and any necessary procedures such as bone marrow aspirations, lumbar punctures, and administration of chemotherapy. The development of the Pediatric Day Hospital has reduced the need for hospitalization. In the Day Hospital, nurses administer intensive chemotherapy requiring close monitoring of delicate fluid balances. Before discharge from the area the patient is given detailed instructions for management of the child's care at home. For children who are hospitalized, the nurses provide Play Therapy as a therapeutic outlet for the pediatric patient's anxiety. In an attempt to respond to the unique needs of the terminally ill child and his family, a Pediatric Home Care Project has recently been instituted. Designed as a research study, this project will focus on identifying the problems associated with establishing a home care program in an urban setting.

The Bone Marrow Transplant Unit is an area which presents many unique challenges for the nurse who chooses to work there. Caring for patients with Severe Combined Immuno-deficiency Disease, Leukemia and Aplastic Anemia requires intensive nursing intervention in controlling hemorrhage, infection and graft versus host disease during the post transplant period. It is the nursing care that sustains patients and their families throughout the long-term hospitalization required for this treatment modality. Maintaining a sterile environment requires that meticulous attention be paid to every detail. Yet the reward of watching a child receive his first kiss from his mother is something a nurse will never forget and makes every effort worthwhile.

Many nurses work in a variety of roles as members of Biomedical Research Teams. They collaborate with physicians and researchers on investigational studies. In addition to

functioning as the liaison between the nursing staff and
the research team, they are responsible for certain aspects
of direct patient care and for the collection of clinical
data. The following are examples of these roles. The
nurses on the Analgesia Team study the dynamics of pain,
the effectiveness of various medication schedules, and the
efficacy of new drugs. The Antiemetic Research nurses are
active in the study of new antiemetics, such as metoclo-
pramide, in an effort to alleviate the discomfort of nausea
and vomiting from cancer treatment. Chemotherapy Research
nurses are part of the team involved in the investigation
of new chemotherapeutic agents. These nurses administer
investigational drug protocols and observe for manifestations
of unknown adverse reactions anticipated with administration
of new agents. Immunology nurses monitor patient response
to treatment with immunotherapy. All nurses on Biomedical
Research Teams provide support to the patient and family
during what may be a frightening treatment course. They
are able to answer questions and reinforce or clarify
information given by the physician regarding specific
studies.

In order to provide for continuity of care when patients
are discharged, a Coordinator of Discharge Planning works
with the health care team in assessing and planning for
discharge needs. Multidisciplinary rounds are held weekly
on each unit and in the outpatient department to discuss
plans for the patient's discharge and reintegration into
the community. To help home health agencies deal with the
complex health care needs of the oncology patient, educational opportunities and materials are provided by the
Discharge Planning Coordinator.

The role of the Clinical Instructor is essential in
maintaining the level of expertise necessary to administer
to the needs of the cancer patient. Specialized orientation
of the new employee and ongoing staff development are
necessary components in the delivery of cancer nursing care
to patients and family. The Clinical Instructor has the
responsibility of maintaining and improving the quality
patient care through assessing the learning needs of the
staff and designing educational programs to those needs.
The nurse in this role has specialized clinical expertise,
leadership ability and knowledge of teaching methods.

Nurses working in the Department of Nursing Research
work both independently and collaboratively with staff on
clinical and administrative research problems. A clinical
nursing research program has been beneficial in developing

new approaches in the care of the cancer patient. One study in progress is identifying patterns of crisis and coping techniques in cancer patients post discharge. The results of this study will be useful in developing discharge planning programs and follow-up care.

In addition to their responsibilities within the institution, nurses in a Comprehensive Cancer Center have responsibility to share their knowledge of oncology nursing with other professional nurses in the community. At Memorial Sloan-Kettering Cancer Center an ongoing program of Continuing Education in Oncology Nursing is offered to nurses outside the institution. In addition, under a grant from the National Cancer Institute, a course on Cancer Prevention For Nurse Practitioners In Community And Occupational Health Settings was developed.

During this brief time I have attempted to describe to you the scope of nursing practice in a Comprehensive Cancer Center. I would like to add that along with the technical expertise inherent in each of these roles is a commitment to nurture and comfort those who entrust themselves to our care.

CONGRESS SYMPOSIA

HOSPICE: CONCEPT AND ROLE Mount, B., Canada,
Chairman; Kirchner-Katterhagen, A., USA,
Co-Chairman; Flag Pavilion A

Hospice Care: 'What We Can Do When Nothing More
Can Be Done.' *Mount, B. M., Montreal, Quebec,
Canada. (By Title Only)

Symptom Management in Advanced Disease.
*Scott, J. F., Toronto, Ontario, Canada.
(By Title Only)

Bereavement Programmes and Interventions in
Palliative Care. *Vachon, M. L. S., Toronto,
Ontario, Canada.

Physical-Emotional-Intellectual-Spiritual
Support Systems of the Whole Person/Family with
Cancer in a Hospital Setting. *Bigler, L. R.,
Buffalo, NY USA. (By Title Only)

The Critical Role of a Home Care Component in a
Complete Hospice Program. *Katterhagen, J. G.,
Tacoma, WA USA. (By title only)

Please note: Papers that are listed as "By Title
Only" were presented at the 13th International
Cancer Congress, but are not included in these
volumes.

13th International Cancer Congress, Part E
Cancer Management, pages 451–461
© 1983 Alan R. Liss, Inc., 150 Fifth Avenue, New York, NY 10011

BEREAVEMENT PROGRAMMES AND INTERVENTIONS IN PALLIATIVE CARE

Mary L.S. Vachon, R.N., Ph.D.

Research Scientist, Clarke Institute
of Psychiatry, 250 College Street,
Toronto, Canada M5T 1R8

One of the integral components of an effective system of Palliative Care is the provision of programmes of intervention for the bereaved relatives or significant others. While most Palliative Care programmes attempt to develop bereavement services, their staff resources are often limited. In addition, the personalities of staff members best suited for the care of the dying may or may not be most appropriate in dealing with bereaved survivors. All too often the bereaved are left to fend for themselves, perhaps having received a card from the staff which says "call if you need us".

For most, but not all people, the experience of bereavement is a painful process. It may involve significant role changes; the loss of one's best friend, sexual partner, financial security; and changes in one's identity and sense of self. When someone dies, very often the meaning seems to go out of the lives of those with whom the deceased person was most intimately involved (Morris 1974).

This loss of the familiar can often be most acute following a lingering illness. For so long so much of the family's life space has centred around the care needed by the dying person. Daily routines come to revolve around visiting the hospital or caring for the person at home - always being on call, lest "something happen". Often in the midst of all this awareness of dying, relatives (and caregivers as well) cease to believe that death will actually occur. Time seems to stand still and relatives often expect at some levels that this dying will go on forever, while at the same time they may openly talk about impending death.

In this type of situation death then means not only the loss of the person, but as well the loss of routine and the loss of the caregivers and hospital system with which one has been so intimately connected.

Clearly for most people the losses already mentioned and the accompanying grief are normal, albeit painful, processes from which they will recover. However for some people bereavement has been shown to lead to physical, psychological and social problems (See Vachon 1976 for a review of this literature). The challenge and therapeutic task facing Palliative Care staff becomes one of identifying those most at risk of a poor bereavement outcome and of providing them with intervention to decrease their risk. Parkes (1980) and Raphael (1977) have already made significant contributions to this field. Parkes defined risk through assessments made by nursing staff at St. Christopher's Hospice at the time of the patient's death. "Risk factors included clinging to the patient before death, angry or self-reproachful behaviour, lack of supportive family, low socio-economic status, young age and an intuitive guess by nursing staff that the bereaved relative was likely to cope badly" (Parkes 1980, p.5). In that study after exclusion of an "imperative need" group for whom it would have been unethical to withhold support, the rest of the high-risk relatives were randomly assigned to an experimental (N=32) or control (N=35) group and the experimental group were offered the help of volunteers. Over a four year period the supported group did better in two out of three measures of change in health - a checklist of new or worse autonomic symptoms and a measure of increased consumption of drugs, alcohol and tobacco.

In Raphael's study the principal elements relevant to predicting widows at high risk of bad health outcome following bereavement were the bereaved's perception of non-support for grief and mourning and a high level of ambivalence in the previous relationship (Raphael 1977). Raphael's subjects were randomly assigned to experimental (N=27) or control groups (N=29) and experimental subjects received short-term grief therapy of three months duration from Dr. Raphael. Her study showed that thirteen months after the death the experimental group had a significant lowering of morbidity which was most marked in those who perceived their social network as non-supportive (Raphael 1977).

This paper will present an overview of a study conducted by the author and her colleagues at the Clarke Institute of Psychiatry. The study provides further evidence on the prediction of risk and development of programmes of intervention for the newly bereaved.

PROCEDURE

The two year longitudinal study was conducted with 162 Toronto widows of men aged 67 and under who died in one of seven Toronto hospitals. The women were interviewed in their homes approximately one month after bereavement. Subsequent interviews took place at 6, 12 and 24 months after the husband's death.

Description of the Sample

The median age of the 162 participants was 52 with a range from 22 to 69 years. The sample was predominantly middle class on the Hollingshead two factor SES index. (See Vachon, Lyall et al 1980 for further description of the sample). Forty-five percent of the husbands died of cancer, and 38% of chronic cardiovascular disease. The median length of the final illness was about 6 months. Only 19% of the husbands had a final illness of two weeks or less.

A high attrition rate is the general rule in studies of bereavement, due both to refusals and

to losses in follow-up because of the increased
mobility of the newly bereaved. The refusal rate
in this study was exceptionally low (12% initially,
2% at 12 months and 1% at 24 months). With regard
to subjects being lost to follow-up, however, the
usual difficulties were experienced. The overall
attrition rate was 33% at 6 months, and 39% by 24
months. Follow-up interviews were conducted with
108 women at 6 months, and 99 at 24 months.

Available data suggest that those lost to
follow-up were a more highly stressed group so this
study may under-represent the problems of bereavement.

Measures

Structured interviews and self-administered
questionnaires were used to gather data on sociodemographic variables; pre-bereavement situational
variables (quality of marriage, years married, previous health, etc.); the circumstances surrounding
the husband's death and funeral; and various correlates of distressful response (use of medication,
changes in health, socialization patterns, etc).

The principal outcome measure of the study
was the score on the 30-item Goldberg General
Health Questionnaire (GHQ) (Goldberg 1972). This is
a self-administered screening test originally developed to detect non-psychotic psychiatric disorders in a general medical practice setting. Items
of the scale focus on ability to carry out one's
normal functioning, role satisfaction and outward-
ly observable behaviour (Goldberg 1978). On the
30-item GHQ a score of 5 or more was found to indicate a level of distress sufficient to warrant
further psychiatric assessment.

In our own study, at each interview time,
statistically significant correlations were obser-

ved between various questionnaire items indicative
of poor adaptation to bereavement and GHQ scores of
5 or more (Chi Square analyses; p values from .0001
to .02). These included consistent self-ratings of
health as less than good; use of tranquillizers,
sedatives or antidepressants; the identification of
widowhood as "very stressful" or "the worst possible
disaster" with the expectation of poor adjustment;
and feeling the need to keep up a front instead of
expressing feelings. The consistent correlations
between high GHQ scores and items of this type
support the validity of using the GHQ to define
distress in this population.

RESULTS

Factors Specific to Death from Cancer

        Elsewhere we have reported the specific prob-
lems reported by women whose husbands died of
cancer so these will be only briefly reported here.
Forty-nine percent of the men with cancer had a
final illness of more than 6 months. The final illness period was rated as being extremely or very
stressful by 81% of the widows. As a group the
women tended to deny their husbands' impending
death and most couples had not discussed the possibility of death. In two year follow-up studies
there is no evidence that talking or not talking
made any difference in long-term outcome. Other
problems reported by women whose husbands died of
cancer included quality of nursing care, accessi-
bility of physicians and accuracy of information
(Vachon et al 1977).

Psychosocial Factors Associated with High Distress
One Month after Bereavement

        At the time of the one-month interview, the
median GHQ score for the widows was 10.4. Seventy
percent (N=114) had a score of 5 or more; 31% (N=
50), a score of 15 or more. By comparison, in an
Australian community sample, Finlay-Jones and Burvill (1977) found that only 16% of women of the

same age range as our subjects had scores of 5 or
more.

Social support variables were the most important in explaining the level of distress one month
after bereavement (Vachon, Rogers et al in press).
Among these, the most relevant accounting for 19%
of the variance was the woman's perception that she
was seeing old friends less than before the death
of her husband.

The significant sociodemographic variables
associated with high distress included ethnic background, defined as not having English as a primary
language and/or Jewish subjects, and younger age.
The pre-bereavement variables of relevance were
the sudden death or short (under 2 months) final
illness of the husband, poor health pre-bereavement
in the wife, previous psychiatric help, a stressful
last illness and a good marriage. Significant
variables included rating religion as not being
very helpful and having problems in addition to
bereavement (Vachon, Rogers et al. in press).

Psychosocial Factors Predictive of Distress Two
Years After Bereavement

Two years following bereavement, 58% of the
1-month high distress group (GHQ $\geq$ 5) and 67% of
the 1-month low distress group (GHQ $<$ 5) remained
in the study. In the high distress group, 25 of
the 66 women (38%) still had a GHQ score of 5 or
more at 2-years post-bereavement. In the low distress group, 30 of the 33 women (91%) had low distress at 2-years. Low distress on the 1-month GHQ
was, therefore, a good predictor of low distress
2 years later.

Analysing the 2 year data for the 99 women
who remained in the study, three distinct distress
patterns emerge: those who never experienced high
distress (30%); those who initially experienced
high distress but gradually returned to normal levels (41%); and those who continued to have marked
distress levels even at the end of two years (25%).

Only 3 subjects had low 1-month distress levels and high distress at one or more follow-up times (Vachon Rogers et al. in press).

Using data available one month after bereavement a regression analysis was performed. A combination of 10 variables explained 43% of the variance and correct classification of 85% in predicting good (low GHQ) or poor (high GHQ) outcome at two years. Some of the factors predictive of high distress two years after bereavement included high initial distress as measured by the GHQ, short final illness, low satisfaction with help, lower social class, poor health pre-bereavement, finding religion not helpful and having a sense of huband's presence at one month (Vachon, Rogers et al. in press).

Psychosocial Factors Correlated With High Distress Two Years After Bereavement

A combination of three out of four variables was found to be correlated with high distress two years after bereavement. Widows who had high initial levels of distress and a lack of social support and either health or financial problems were at great risk of having high levels of distress two years after bereavement (Vachon, Sheldon et al. in press).

Intervention Following Bereavement

Is it possible to decrease the distress associated with bereavement? In our study we found that a self-help widow-to-widow programme was able to accelerate the pathway of adaptation to bereavement through improved interpersonal adaptation at 6 months after bereavement and improved interpersonal adaptation at 12 months. Twenty-four months after bereavement the widows with high initial distress who had participated in the widow-to-widow programme were significantly less likely to still be under high distress compared with the control group of previously high distress widows

(Vachon, Lyall et al. 1980).

IMPLICATIONS FOR PALLIATIVE CARE

What are the implications for the Palliative Care system of these findings? First, a certain percentage of bereaved persons do not experience measurable distress at any point during bereavement. In the author's study almost all women who had low distress initially continued to have low distress over the first two years of bereavement. This group of women (perhaps men as well but that has not been researched) manage to cope quite well during bereavement with the help of their family and friends and a reasonably caring attitude of the professionals. They might join a voluntary or self-help group or return to the Palliative Care system for monthly bereavement meetings but these would generally be incidental to their adjustment. This group might want to return to the system as volunteers and can often function well in that role providing that they are tolerant of others who are more overtly upset.

The largest percentage of the bereaved (41% in our study) have high initial distress which gradually decreases. This group can benefit from ongoing contact with staff members of the Palliative Care system who do bereavement follow-up or they might be seen individually by bereaved volunteers or join a self-help programme associated with the Palliative Care system or operating within the community. Those in this group with low social support can particularly benefit from this follow-up.

The third group of bereaved (25% in this study) continue to have high distress in response to bereavement. This group may well have the combination of high initial distress, low social support and health or financial problems. This group should be followed. They may profit from a volunteer or self-help programme but may well also need to be involved with a mental health professional especially if they are having suicidal fantasies, abusing drugs and/or alcohol or showing major personality

changes. This mental health professional may be a
part of the Palliative Care team or may be an out-
sider.

Palliative Care systems must address three
major issues regarding bereavement care. The first
is whether such care should be provided - my answer
to this is that some provision must be made at
least for the high risk bereaved. Secondly, the
issue must be addressed whether such care will be
done by professionals or volunteers. Here I am
inclined from experience to feel that much of the
work can be done by volunteers but that professionals must be available and probably must be involved
with the highest risk group at least until volunteers are quite skilled. For some Palliative Care
staff the opportunity to do bereavement follow-up
work is a very rewarding experience. Seeing the
bereaved gradually come to terms with their loss
and begin a new life can make it easier to work
with those currently going through the crisis of
death.

Thirdly, Palliative Care systems must decide,
if they are going to use volunteers, whether these
will be non-bereaved volunteers or, following the
self-help model, whether they will use those who
have resolved their bereavement experience to help
others now undergoing such an experience. This decision has to be made according to the resources
available to a particular Palliative Care system.
Parkes (1980) and Hampson (1980)have had considerable success using non-bereaved volunteers who have
had an extensive training programme. In our experience we have found a widowed-to-widowed self-help
programme to be particularly effective. Community
Contacts for the Widowed incorporated in 1976 has
served over 2000 widows and a small number of
widowers. Between 600-700 persons are served
annually. The service is run by ten widow contacts
who are paid a small salary for working 6-12 hours
a week. They are assisted by about 100 volunteers.
Self-help programmes can provide the bereaved with
understanding; social support to deal with the
loneliness and isolation of bereavement; advice
and practical help in dealing with grief and coping

with families, social, vocational and financial matters and education regarding the stages and phases of grief so that the bereaved have a cognitive framework within which to view their experience which will allow for enhanced coping skills. (Rogers, Vachon et al. 1980).

CONCLUSIONS

Bereavement services are essential for the high risk bereaved. This group can be identified through initial high distress, low social support, health and/or financial problems. Programmes of intervention can be run by professionals but the cost-effectiveness and good results obtained by volunteers suggests that they have an important role to play in bereavement care.

Research on the study "A Preventive Intervention For The Newly Bereaved" was funded by the Ontario Ministry of Health (DM 158). Co-investigators are: J. Rogers, W.A.L. Lyall, K. Freedman, S.J.J.Freeman.

References

Andrews G, Tennant C, Hewson DM & Vaillant GE (1978) Life event stress, social support, coping style and risk of psychological impairment. J of Ner & Ment Dis 166: 307-16.
Finlay-Jones RA, Burvill PW (1977) The prevalence of minor psychiatric morbidity in the community. Psychol Med 7: 475-89.
Goldberg D (1972) The detection of psychiatric illness by questionnaire. A technique for the identification of non-psychotic psychiatric illness. "Institute of Psychiatry, Maudsley Monographs #21", London: Oxford University Press.
Goldberg D (1978) "Manual of the general health questionnaire". Windsor, England: NFER Publishing Co.
Hampson A (1980) Palliative care service bereavement program. In Ajemian I & Mount B (eds.)

"The RVH manual on palliative/hospice care".
New York: ARNO Press.

Morris P (1974) "Loss and Change", New York:
Panthean Books.

Parkes CM (1980) Bereavement counselling: does
it work? Br Med J 5 July.

Raphael B (1977) Preventive intervention with the
recently bereaved. Arch Gen Psych 34: 1450-54.

Rogers J, Vachon MLS, Lyall WAL, Sheldon A & Freeman SJJ (1980) An urban widow-to-widow programme: from demonstration model grant to
independent community service. Hosp and Comm
Psych 31: 844-7.

Vachon MLS (1976) Grief and bereavement following
the death of a spouse. Can Psych Assoc J 21:
35-43.

Vachon MLS, Freedman K, Formo A, Rogers J, Lyall
WAL & Freeman SJJ (1977) The final illness
in cancer: the widow's perspective. Can Med
Assoc J 117: 1151-4.

Vachon MLS, Lyall WAL, Rogers J, Freedman-Letof-
sky K, Freeman SJJ (1980) A controlled study
of self-help intervention for widows. Am J
Psychiatry 137: 1380-4.

Vachon MLS, Rogers J, Lyall WAL, Lancee WJ, Sheldon AR & Freeman SJJ (in press) Predictors
and correlates of high distress in adaptation
to conjugal bereavement. Am J Psychiatry
expected publication August or September 1982.

Vachon MLS, Sheldon AR, Lancee WJ, Lyall WAL,
Rogers J & Freeman SJJ (in press) Correlates
of enduring distress patterns following
bereavement: social network, life situation
& personality. Psychol Med expected publication Fall 1982.

CONGRESS SYMPOSIA

SCREENING FOR CANCER Ebeling, K., GDR, Chairman; Berlin, N., USA, Co-Chairman; Opera House

Screening for Early Breast Cancer Detection. *Strax, P., New York City, NY USA.

Status of Screening for Large Bowel Cancers. *Gilbertsen, V. A., Minneapolis, MN USA. (By Title Only)

Research on High Risk Groups of Primary Hepatocellular Carcinoma (PHC). *Yu, L-y., Changhai, China.

The Current Status of Screening for Uterine Cancer. Boyes, D. A., Vancouver, British Columbia, Canada.

Screening for Carcinoma of the Stomach and Esophagus. *Ichikawa, H. and Iizuka, T., Tokyo, Japan.

Please note: Papers that are listed as "By Title Only" were presented at the 13th International Cancer Congress, but are not included in these volumes.

13th International Cancer Congress, Part E
Cancer Management, pages 465–473
© **1983 Alan R. Liss, Inc., 150 Fifth Avenue, New York, NY 10011**

SCREENING FOR EARLY BREAST CANCER DETECTION

Philip Strax, M.D.

Medical Director
Guttman Institute
New York City, New York   10001

The definitive diagnosis of breast cancer is made by the pathologist. The step before that involves the clinician, be he internist, gynecologist or surgeon, who is faced with a more or less frightened woman who comes in with a lump, a localized pain or a nipple discharge. A differential diagnosis is called for with the subsequent and sometimes difficult decision to explore the breast or do watchful waiting. The clinician uses all the resources available in the community in addition to palpation and inspection. An opinion from a colleague perhaps more expert in palpation is obtained. The woman is referred for evaluation by breast imaging modalities, such as mammography, thermography, ultrasound, transillumination or aspiration. All of these procedures are vital and most important to get as much information as possible to help the clinician make the decision to have the patient explored or not and to avoid delay in doing so.

However, there is a step before the clinical one and that is detection of an abnormality that will propel the woman into the stream of medical care to lead, hopefully, to the differential diagnosis. That initial step may be a suspicion on the part of the woman herself that a problem may be present, as found by her on periodic or accidental breast self-examination or by accidental detection of pathology by a physician in the course of an examination for a non-breast condition. Unfortunately, however, waiting for a woman to find her own abnormality or hoping that a physician will even bother to examine the breast when the patient's symptoms point elsewhere is what we've been doing for the most part up to now - and our results in terms of saving lives of women from breast cancer have not been as good as they might be. More than half the time the breast cancer is detected in too late a stage for a cure. Overall, probably not more than 30% of women are alive and free of disease 10 years after diagnosis. We need a better way.

Breast cancer is vulnerable on 3 fronts. Our ultamate goal in control of the disease is primary prevention. Much effort is properly being expanded in finding the cause or causes to lead, hopefully, to preventing the disease. Unfortunately, we are still not close to the goal. Another method of attack in breast cancer is through treatment. A cure of the disease at any stage would be a real breakthrough. Success in this area still eludes us. All we have is lots of evidence that detection of breast cancer at an early stage, when it is presumably localized, leads to considerable increase in survival after treatment. This indicates the third possible approach - secondary prevention or detection of the disease at an earlier stage than is usually the case in general medical practice.

There has been an increasing awareness in recent years that breast cancer may be a systemic disease early in its onset. It is also becoming apparent that most breast cancer when it is brought to the physician by the patient is already in a late stage. The obvious lesion may be removed, but micrometastases are in sufficiently advanced stage of development or the body resistance to them has sufficiently deteriorated so that the patient is not cured. That is the basis for the concept of adjuvant chemo or hormone therapy. However, it should be emphasized that new information, particularly from the Health Insurance Plan and other screening studies, now teaches us that in breast cancer the disease can be detected at a stage far earlier than is the usual case in general medical practice. At this optimal stage, the lesion is small and detectable when the body's immune mechanism is sufficiently intact to remove micrometastases. We may then be in a position to treat breast cancer when it is potentially curable.

It is well known that breast cancer found in a localized state has an 85% five-year survival compared to 53% when glands are involved. Since most breast cancer today is not localized when first seen by the clinician, a means must be found to have women present themselves for examination with their disease at an earlier stage than is commonly the case. This means, in a practical way, detection of pre-clinical cancer in apparently "well" women, when the disease is unsuspected by patient or physician - as is the case in mass screening.

Screening as defined by the World Health Organization is "the presumptive identification of unrecognized disease or defect by the application of tests, examinations or other procedures which can be applied rapidly. Screening tests sort out apparently well persons who probably have a disease from those who probably do not." The disease in-volved should in a practical way stand a reasonable chance of being cured if detected early, whereas if not diagnosed until the patient comes to the physician with clear cut symptoms, it may be incurable.

What was needed for widespread efforts in mass screen-ing was statistical proof that such screening for breast cancer would result not only in prolonged survival, but in actual reduced mortality. That was the concept in back of the mass screening study of the Health Insurance Plan of New York conducted under contract with the National Cancer Institute and begun in 1963. The project was initiated against a background of a stationary death rate from breast cancer and a revised interest in mammography as an effective means for detecting the disease in a non-palpable and per-haps more curable stage (Gershon-Cohen, Hermel, Berger 1961; Egan 1962). The two questions to be answered, therefore, were: 1. Could such a mass screening result in reduction of mortality from breast cancer and 2. What would be the con-tribution of mammography in such a program?

In this study 62,000 women aged 40 to 64 chosen as 31,000 carefully matched pairs were picked at random from lists at H.I.P. headquarters. One pair was the "study group" and the other the "control group". The study women received palpation and mammography initially and then annually for 3 years. These were done in completely inde-pendent fashion. Two-thirds of the invited women in the study group came at least once. One-third never came in spite of strenuous attempts, but have been continued as part of the study group in statistics in comparison with the con-trol group. The control group women received their usual medical care. Data have been and still are being collected.

One-third of the cancers in the study group were found on mammography alone and were not palpable by the expert surgeons of the group. Two-fifths were found on clinical examination, and not seen on the x-ray. It was concluded that in screening, both modalities were essential for proper yield.

Table 1

Modality*	Breast Cancers Number	Percent
Total	127	100.0
Mammography only	42	33.1
Clinical only	56	44.1
Both	29	22.8

*Initial evidence resulting in biopsy recommendation.

It was also found that 79% of those found only on the x-ray had no nodal involvement. 75% of those found on palpation alone were localized. Obviously, the mammogram was finding non-palpable cancers in a localized, more curable stage. Of 44 cancers found on mammography alone only 3 women have died in an 8 year period of follow-up. Six of these were under 50 and only one of these has died. In the control group more than one-half of the cancers had nodal involvement (Strax, Venet, Shapiro 1973; Shapiro, Venet, Strax, Venet, Roeser 1982).

After 7 years of follow-up there was a one-third reduction in mortality from breast cancer in the study group compared to the control (70 vs. 108). In other words, the screening procedure had resulted in a substantial saving of lives from the disease.

After 9 years of follow-up a similar death rate reduction was present (91 vs. 128).

The mortality reduction of 30% has persisted after 13 years. Over a 13 year follow-up the number of deaths from breast cancer within 5 years of onset of the study in both study and control groups was essentially the same in women aged 40 to 50. The entire reduction in mortality appeared to be concentrated in women over 50. This is true if we compare number of deaths at age of death (15 vs. 17) or age at diagnosis (36 vs. 36).

However, it is interesting to note that if we take the age of a woman at entry into the study and not the age at death or age at diagnosis there is increasing evidence of mortality benefit in women under 50, although not statistically significant, according to Shapiro, the study's statistician.

Other statisticians, like Dubin from New York University Medical Center and Seidman from the American Cancer Society on review of the H.I.P. data, however, insist that a definite mortality benefit was demonstrated in women under 50, though not as significant as in women over 50 (Dubin, 1979; Seidman, 1979). The number of cancers in the under 50 age group was perhaps too small for statistical purposes. However, the statistical mortality benefit has been increasing in 5 to 14 years of follow-up.

Table 2
Breast Cancer Deaths By Age At Entry
5 and 13 Years From Entry

| | 5 Years | | 13 Years | |
	Study	Control	Study	Control
Total	39	63	116	148
Age at Entry				
40-49	19	20	45	59
50-59	15	33	52	66
60 and Older	5	10	19	23

These considerations led to the development in 1968 of the Guttman Breast Diagnostic Institute in New York City with the basic objective of developing a mass screening approach that would be feasible and could reach the general population of women (Strax, 1971). Cooperation with the New York City Division of the American Cancer Society has been a key to stimulating women to come in. Up to 50,000 examinations per year have been made with such cooperation. Hundreds of cancers have been found in the past 14 years with a large proportion in the localized stages. Film-screen techniques have been developed which use minute amounts of radiation, down to .2R to .3R to the skin per exposure and to less than .05 rad to the mid breast for the two views used. Such a radiation dose has been considered negligible by most authorities even on a repetitive screening basis and the hazard probably not measurable. Fortunately, too, the newer techniques lead not only to much reduced radiation compared to that used in the H.I.P. study, but to films of much enhanced quality which lend themselves to greater accuracy and ease in interpretation.

The success of the H.I.P. study and that of the Guttman Institute stimulated the large-scale national breast screening program supported by the American Cancer Society and the National Cancer Institute, involving some 280,000 women, using the Guttman Institute as a prototype (the Breast Cancer Detection Demonstration Project. Mammography, with techniques improved over those used in the H.I.P. study, was particularly effective in detecting early and very small cancers with a substantial degree of no nodal involvement. Similar programs are under way in England, Sweden, Italy, Greece, Germany, France and Brazil.

It is interesting to compare findings in the H.I.P. study with those in the screening centers - where the much improved mammography technique has been used. Under age 50 - which is a particularly important group - 44% of the cancers were found in the centers' groups on mammography alone compared to 19% in H.I.P., 91% of all cancers under age 50 were found on mammography vs. 40% in H.I.P., and 13.8% of the cancers were under 1 cm. in size vs. 3.5% in the H.I.P. study (Baker, 1982). Apparently, the improved mammographic techniques used in the new studies resulted in a substantial increase in cancers found on mammography alone, especially in women under 50 and especially in cancers under 1 cm. in size. The intriguing thought persists that if the H.I.P. study were repeated today using the improved mammographic techniques significantly improved statistical results might result in the under 50 age group.

Table 3

Findings	HIP data (132 cancers)	BCDDP data (2379 cancers)
CA-Mammo. alone	33%	48%
negative nodes	79%	77%
CA-Mammo. alone (under 50)	19%	45%
negative nodes	68%	73%
Minimal CA	3.5%	13.8% (58.6% of these found on Mammo. alone)

Such a study has indeed begun in Canada by Anthony Miller, but definitive results will probably not be available for at least 5 years (Miller, Howe, Wall in Press).

There are 2 problems, however, that need further attention: The first is the so-called "interval" cancer. About 10-15% of cancers in screening become apparent after a negative examination and before the next scheduled annual study. These "interval" cancers need to be detected by the women themselves. In the H.I.P. study women were not taught or made aware of the possibility of an "interval" cancer. The degree of nodal involvement in these cases was almost the same as in control women. At the Guttman Institute women are indoctrinated into B.S.E. and strongly urged to follow through on a regular monthly basis. Interval cancers are being detected with reasonably reduced nodal involvement. It is suspected that many, if not most, of the interval cancers are of a more rapidly growing type.

Another problem with the mass screening concept is that the vast majority of women do not have such a program available to them or do not have the motivation to become involved. Thus, for women in general, breast self-examination on a regular periodic basis becomes our only means for early detection. However, B.S.E. does have some important limitations (Strax, Greenwald 1979).

The female breast varies greatly in size, texture and nodularity. The small, firm breast in the nulliparous woman differs remarkably from the large pendulous breast of most postmenopausal, multiparous women. The young woman finds little difficulty in following the B.S.E. instructions, but the older woman may become frustrated when she attempts to examine her breasts. Palpation of the large, pendulous breast is difficult even for the experienced physician; it is almost an impossible task for the average postmenopausal woman.

The importance of routine periodic breast examination by medical personnel must be emphasized and its relationship to B.S.E. clarified. If at all possible, B.S.E. instruction should be given at the time of a clinical examination to be reasonably sure that a cancer is not, in fact, present at the time of indoctrination.

There is need for a comprehensive study evaluating B.S.E. in women of different ages, ethnic groups, and under different techniques of instruction. We need more evidence that the effort, expense, and difficulties involved in B.S.E. instruction are truly worthwhile, but most authorities agree that B.S.E. instruction and indoctrination should be continued and expanded even while attempts to validate the procedure continue to be made.

What is really needed to improve the status of breast self-examination is an objective method that is simple, easy to follow, safe and inexpensive so that a woman does not have to rely on subjective palpation. She must also be assured that the method has not been devised to detect cancer, but only to let her know that a difference exists between the two breasts which requires evaluation by her physician. The device should be available for regular, periodic examination at home.

Finally, what we now need to further our objectives is as follows:
1. We need a preventive - a vaccine that will protect our girl babies against the disease. We are not near this goal.
2. We need a method of curing breast cancer at any stage. All we have now are good techniques to cure the disease only when it is localized. This requires mass screening to bring women in at the right time.
3. We need improved techniques in screening, such as involvement of trained paramedical personnel in breast palpation and in interpretation of mammograms. We also need to evaluate factors leading to improved knowledge of frequency of examination in screening.
4. We have a pressing need to find true high risk markers which will tell us which women need to be examined more frequently and which can afford to wait several years between examination. After all, only 1 woman in 11 develops breast cancer. We would like to know which is that woman.

Efforts are being made to find the magic marker in the blood or sputum that can signal the woman who is truly at high risk. A project is being mounted in this direction under the auspices of New York University School of Medicine and involving the Guttman Institute of New York, the Imperial Cancer Research Fund in London and the Netherlands Cancer Institute. If it succeeds, we may be closer to our objective of making it possible to save 3 out of 4 women with breast cancer instead of perhaps 1 out of 4 as at present.

Acknowledgement - The H.I.P. study was initiated by Philip Strax, but it is the result of a collaborative effort between himself and Sam Shapiro, Louis Venet and Ruth Roeser.

References

Baker LH (1982). Breast cancer demonstration project: five year summary report. CA 32:194.

Dubin N (1979). Analysis of the benefits of mammographic screening for breast cancer to women under 50 years of age. In proceedings of Third Annual Conference of the American Society of Preventive Oncology. New York City, March.

Egan RL (1962). Mammography, an aid to diagnosis of breast carcinoma. JAMA 182:938.

Gershon-Cohen J, Hermel MB, Berger SM (1961). Detection of breast cancer by periodic x-ray examination. JAMA 176: 1114.

Miller AB, Howe GR, Wall C (1982). The national study of breast cancer screening. Clin. and Invest. Med. in Press.

Seidman H (1979). Lessons from the BCDDP - Possible gains in life expentancy from screening women under 50 for breast cancer. In Control of Breast Cancer Through Mass Screening. p 37 Ed. Philip Strax, PSG Publishing Co., Littleton, Mass.

Shapiro S, Venet W, Strax P, Venet L, Roeser R (1982). Ten to fourteen year effects of breast cancer screening on mortality. Jour. Nat. Cancer Inst. in Press.

Strax P (1971). New techniques in mass screening for breast cancer. Cancer 28:1563.

Strax P, Venet L, Shapiro S (1973). Value of mammography in reduction of mortality from breast cancer in mass screening. Amer. Jour. Roentgenology 117:686.

Strax P, Greenwald P (1979). Potential and limitations of breast self-examination. The Cancer Bulletin 31:142.

13th International Cancer Congress, Part E
Cancer Management, pages 475–482
© 1983 Alan R. Liss, Inc., 150 Fifth Avenue, New York, NY 10011

RESEARCH ON HIGH RISK GROUPS OF PRIMARY HEPATOCELLULAR
CARCINOMA (PHC)

Lu-yi Yu, M.D.

Cancer Hospital
Shanghai First Medical College
Shanghai, China

PHC is the third frequently occurring malignancy in
China, considerable efforts have been concentrated on
population screening for PHC by alpha fetoprotein (AFP)
assay since 1971 (Coordinating group for the research on
liver cancer 1974). The positivity of AFP assay was
improved from 67.9 % by using agar gel diffusion (AGD) in
1971 to 96.3 % by applying reverse passive hemagglutina-
tion (RPHA) and radiorocket electrophoresis autography
(RREA) in 1974 (Zhu 1981). In addition to the conventional quantitative assay, e.g. radioimmunoassay (RIA),
other sensitive, simple and reliable technic, i.e.
enzyme-linked immunosobent assay (ELISA), is being
investigated (Tian, Wu, Zeng, Yong 1982).

Study on population screening for PHC showed that
AFP assay had not only improved the diagnostic rate of
stage I PHC from 4.7 % to 60 % (Coordinating group for
the research on liver cancer 1979), but also discovered
individuals with persistent low-level AFP, among whom the
incidence of developing PHC was fairly high. These
individuals could be considered high risk groups for PHC
(Yu 1981), investigation of these high risk groups has
given new insights into early diagnosis and treatment as
well as prevention. This overview deals mainly with its
present status and prospects.

The criteria (Coordinating group for the research on
liver cancer 1978) for the individual with persistent
low-level AFP are defined as follows: (1) the concentra-

tion of the AFP is 50-300 ng/ml, and clinical diagnosis of PHC cannot be ascertained; (2) the AFP level persists at 50-300 ng/ml during the subsequent 2-month follow-up, as established by a 2-week serial determination of the AFP level; (3) the possibility of serum glutamic pyruvic transaminase (SGPT) related to AFP or the presence of other malignancy has been ruled out.

According to a survey in Shanghai concerning a group of 525 individuals with persistent low-level AFP, the incidence of PHC within one, two and three years was 3.4 %, 4.6 % and 5.0 % respectively (Li, Zhang, Zhang, Zhou, Chen, Yu, Zheng, Tang, Shen, Zhu 1979). In another study, 282 individuals with persistent low-level AFP were found through 115,000 urban population screened for PHC. Of this group, 270 individuals were followed for two years, 9 cases of PHC developed with an incidence of 3.3 %, 233 with AFP turned negative and 38 remained unchanged during this period (Xu, Li, Guan, Yu, Song, Shen, 1980).

In Qidong county of Kiangsu province, a survey on 287 individuals with persistent low-level AFP revealed that 35 cases of PHC developed within one year denoting an incidence of 12.2 % (35/287) (Lu, Huang, Zhang 1981). Of these 35 cases with PHC, diagnosis of PHC in 24 cases was established at 6 months duration since the discovery of initial low-level AFP. This higher incidence was also demonstrated in Qidong county to the extent that the occurrence of PHC in the individuals with persistent low-level AFP was a hundred-fold greater than that in the general population (Table 1) (Ji, Sun, Wang, Ding, Chu, Li 1979).

Table 1. Incidence of PHC between high risk group and general population

	PHC developed within 2-yr	Annual incidence of PHC
Individuals with persistent low-level AFP	4/25	8×10^{-2}
General population	12/33,000	2×10^{-4}

Furthermore, close follow-up of individuals with persistent low-level AFP not only resulted in detecting more cases of stage I or subclinical PHC (Table 2) (Zhu

1981), but also uncovered some small liver cancer (SLC). The latter was documented in a series of 46 cases with SLC (Tang, Yu, Lin, Yang, Lu, Zhou, Tang, Zhou 1981), among which 15 cases, being individuals with persistent low-level AFP, were proved to be through serial determinations for AFP, with a median duration of follow-up of 8.7 months and the longest being 14 months. Intensive study on the SLC would enable a better scrutiny into the "detectable preclinical phase (DPCP)" of PHC, which might be essential in studying the biological behavior of PHC, as the prevalence of the DPCP is effectively increased by the use of a test which can detect earlier lesions (Cole, Morrison 1978). This is of practical significance in implementing effective therapy as well as improving survival.

Table 2. Comparison of stage I PHC between the general population and high risk group (1974-1976)

	No. screened or followed	No. of cases with PHC	Stage I PHC No.	%
General population	208,542	167	58	34.7
Individuals with persistent low-level AFP	233	45	25	55.6

Since several factors might be implicated in the development of persistent low-level AFP, investigation in these high risk groups with various parameters has been conducted so as to ensure a better differential diagnosis for PHC. The prevalence rate of hepatits B surface antigen (HBsAg) in 104 individuals with persistent low-level AFP was studied during a 2-yr follow-up, 39/104 (37.5 %) were HBsAg (+) , among whom PHC developed in 8 cases, whereas no PHC occurred among the 53 cases with both HBsAg and antibody to hepatitis B surface antigen (anti-HBs) negative, and 12 cases with anti-HBs (-) (Yu, Wang, Xu 1980). In a $1\frac{1}{2}$ to $2\frac{1}{2}$-yr follow-up of 75 individuals with persistent low-level AFP, the prevalence rate of HBsAg was 19/25 (76.0 %) in 25 cases with PHC developed, 13/15 (86.7 %) in 15 cases with persistent low-level AFP, and 16/35 (45.7 %) in 35 with **AFP turned** negative. It appears that the prevalence of HBsAg might influence or hinder the AFP from turning negative and possibly increase the risk of PHC (Sun, Gu, Lu, Gu 1979).

It was noteworthy to mention that liver function tests were performed concurrently with the monitoring for AFP in the 3-yr follow-up of 525 individuals with persistent low-level AFP as already stated, fewer cases with abnormal liver function tests, particularly those indicating chronic hepatic damage, became AFP negative and showed high incidence of PHC (Li, Zhang, Zhang, Zhou, Chen, Yu, Zheng, Tang, Shen, Zhu 1979).

An analysis of γ-glutamyl transpeptidase (γ-GT) isoenzyme pattern in 330 cases with persistent low-level AFP showed that PHC developed in 8 (6.4 %) out of the 125 cases with positive -GT isoenzyme during one-year follow-up, as compared with only one PHC among 205 cases with negative γ-GT isoenzyme (Guan, Xu, Li, Chen 1982). 5'-nucleotide phosphodiesterase isoenzyme-V (5'-NPDase) was determined in 10 cases with persistent low-level AFP revealing a positive rate of 8/10 (80 %) (Table 3) (Lu, Chen, Liu, Yang, Hu, Jiang, Ding, Xu 1981). Determination of alpha$_1$ antitrypsin (A_1AT) showed that 12 out of 18 PHC cases (66.67 %) with negative or low-level AFP had high level of A_1AT (Xu, Guan, Wang, Chen, Yu, Xu 1981). All these assays may be used concurrently with AFP as complementary means. Other studies such as chromosome studies on peripheral blood lymphocytes were investigated as well (Xu, Li 1982).

Table 3. Correlation between positive rate of 5'-NPDase-V and AFP concentration

AFP (ng/ml)	Total no.	5'-NPDase-V (+) No.	%
0–31	24	19	79.2
32–500	10	8	80.0
500	66	56	84.8

It is suggested that several paramaters cited above might be employed in combination with monitoring for AFP during the survey on these high risk groups so as to identify PHC as early as possible. Furthermore, tumor-localizing procecure, e.g. selective hepatic arteriography, is also essential in order to make the assessment of the earlier lesion as precisely as possible (Wang, Chen, Wang 1982).

Clinical trial with traditional Chinese Medicine was conducted on 270 individuals with persistent low-level AFP, and resulted in 82.6 % (223/270) cases with AFP turned negative and 3.3 % (9/270) cases with PHC developed during a 2-yr follow-up (Table 4). Another group of 116 individuals with persistent low-level AFP without treatment was selected for comparison, and a marked difference in the incidence of PHC was shown (Table 5). 7 out of 270 (2.6 %) treated cases developed PHC within one year, whereas 12 out of untreated 116 cases developed PHC in the same period (Xu, Li, Guan, Yu, Song, Shen 1980).

Table 4. Follow-up of 270 individuals with persistent low-level AFP treated with traditional Chinese medicine

	AFP turned negative		PHC developed	
	1-yr	2-yr	1-yr	2-yr
No.	187	223	7	9
%	69.2	82.6	2.6	3.3

Table 5. Comparison of PHC incidence within 1-yr follow-up between the treated and untreated groups

	No. of individuals	PHC developed	
		No.	%
Treated group	270	7	2.6*
Untreated group	116	12	10.3

*$P<0.01$

Cytoplasmic RNA prepared from animal liver was given to 116 cases with persistent low-level AFP for three or four months, the percentages of AFP turned negative for treated group and control were 25/38 (65 %) and 46/97 (47 %) respectively for 1-yr follow-up. The incidence of PHC for the treated group and control were 3/38 (7.6 %) and 36/97 (37 %) respectively for 1-yr follow-up (Huang, Chen, Zhou, Hu, Cao 1981). Further trials appear necessary in evaluating the possible beneficial effects as well as in exploring some clues for preventive measures.

In conclusion, individuals with persistent low-level AFP were found through population screening for PHC among whom the incidence of developing PHC was fairly high, and they could be considered as group at high risk. From the cost-effectiveness viewpoint of screening for PHC, it is essential to focus screening and preventive program on these high risk groups. It is evident that the simultaneous use of several parameters in combination with the monitoring for AFP is often necessary in enhancing the predictability for subclinical PHC or SLC which is of vital improtance in improving the survival. Furthermore, the preliminary observations in clinical trials seem promising. It is hoped that further study on high risk groups for PHC might represent a rewarding research area in the foreseeable future.

Cole P, Morrison AS (1978). Basic issues in cancer screening. In Miller AB (eds):"Screening in Cancer," Geneva: U I C C, p 7.
Coordinating group for   research on liver cancer (1974). Application of serum alph feto-protein assay in mass survey'of primary carcinoma of liver. In Maltoni C (eds):"Proceedings of the 2nd International Symposium on Cancer Detection and Prevention," Amsterdam: Excerpta Medica, p 55.
Coordinating group for research on liver cancer (1978). Further investigation on α-fetoprotein in mass survey and follow-up studies of primary hepatocellular carcinoma. Res Cancer control 6:6
Coordinating group for research on liver cancer (1979). Further investigation on α-fetoprotein in mass survey and follow-up studies of primary hepatocellular carcinoma. In Canonico O, Estevez R, Chacon R. Barg S (eds):"Proceedings of 12th International Cancer Congress", Oxford: Pergamon Press, p 721.

Guan SF, Xu SK, Li ML and Chen FH (1982). Clinical studies on γ-glutamyl transpeptidase (γ-GT) isoenzyme. Tumor 2(1):13.

Huang JK, Chen ZJ, Zhou XM, Hu LF, Cao CM (1980): The analysis of therapeutic effect of animal liver RNA in treating patients with persistent low-level alpha fetoprotein. Jiangsu Med J 6(7):12.

Ji Z, Sun ZT, Wang LQ, Ding GS, Chu PP, Li FM (1979). Characteristics of AFP serology in early primary hepatocellular carcinoma and the high-risk group. Chin J Oncol 1:96.

Li ML, Zhang PL, Zhang MX, Zhou J, Chen FH, Yu EX, Zheng P, Tang JX, Shen FX, Zhu FC (1979). The follow-up and clinical significance of individuals with low-level alpha-fetoprotein. Res Cancer Control 7:9.

Lu HM, Chen Q, Liu CY, Yang BH, Hu HK, Jiang KL, Ding CR, Xu WJ (1981). A comparison of 5'-nucleotide phospho-diesterase isoenzyme and other enzymes in primary hepatic carcinoma. Ch J of Digestion, 1:82.

Lu PX, Huang JK, Zhang JX (1981). Clinical study on serum low-level AFP. Qidong Liver Cancer Res p 47.

Sun C, Gu BC, Lu JH, Gu XH (1979). Relationship between hepatitis B surface antigen carriers and incidence of primary liver cancer. Shanghai Med J 2:1.

Tang ZY, Yu YQ, Lin ZY, Yang BH, Lu JZ, Zhou XD, Tang Cl, Zhou NQ (1981). Discussion on some problems concerning small hepatocellular carcinoma. Tumor 1(1): 14.

Tian AD, Wu GD, Zeng QY, Yong JM (1982). Enzyme-linked immunosobent assay of AFP-quantitative determination of serum AFP in different groups of subjects. Tumor 2(1):10.

Wang SZ, Chen XR, Wang GX (1982). Selective angiography in 50 cases of primary hepatocellular carcinoma. Ch Med J 95(3):170.

Xu KL, Li ML, Guan SF, Yu EX, Song MZ, Shen FX (1980). Clinical analysis of low AFP level cases and their prognosis. Chin J Oncol 2:45.

Xu SK, Guan SF, Wang BL, Chen FH, Yu EX, Xu WQ (1981). Assay of -antitrypsin activity in the diagnosis of hepatocellular carcinoma. Tumor 1:5.

Xu LZ, Li ML (1982). Chromosome studies on peripheral blood lymphocytes on low AFP level cases. Tumor 2(4): 15.

Yu EX, Wang BL, Xu SK (1980). Further study on the relation between the primary hepatocellular carcinoma, the individuals with persistent low-level alpha-fetoprotein, and hepatitis B surface antigen and antibody to hepatitis B surface antigen. Res Cancer Control 8(5):3.

Yu LY (1981). Detection of primary hepatocellular carcinoma (PHC): Study of individuals with persistent low-level α-fetoprotein (AFP). In Friedman M, Ogawa M, Kisner D (eds):"Diagnosis and treatment of upper gastrointestinal tumors," Amsterdam: Excerpta Medica, p 102.

Zhu YR (1981). AFP sero-survey and early diagnosis of liver cell cancer in the Qidong field. Chin J Oncol 3:35.

13th International Cancer Congress, Part E
Cancer Management, pages 483–493
© **1983 Alan R. Liss, Inc., 150 Fifth Avenue, New York, NY 10011**

THE CURRENT STATUS OF SCREENING FOR UTERINE CANCER

David A. Boyes, M.D.

Director, Cancer Control Agency of B.C.
Clinical Professor, Dept. of Obs. & Gynec.,U.B.C.
#700-686 West Broadway, Vancouver, B.C.V5Z 1G1

Since 1949 a screening program for carcinoma of the cervix has been in operation in the Province of British Columbia. We have reached approximately 85% of our population and are at the present processing 2200 specimens per day in our one central laboratory.

For the first 25 years of operation the main objective was to prove the worth of the pap smear program as a service that could reduce the incidence and mortality of carcinoma of the uterine cervix. We used as endpoints the incidence and mortality of clinical squamous carcinoma and Table 1. shows the incidence of clinical squamous carcinoma in women over 20, and Table 2. the mortality in this same group of women.

INCIDENCE OF CLINICAL INVASIVE SQUAMOUS CARCINOMA
OF THE CERVIX UTERI IN WOMEN OVER 20 YEARS OF AGE
IN BRITISH COLUMBIA

Year	Population in Thousands	Total Cases	Incidence per 100,000
1955	422.9	120	28.4
1959	478.7	108	22.6
1963	513.0	98	19.1
1967	592.4	85	14.3
1971	687.2	73	10.6
1975	805.5	70	8.7
1979	892.2	74	8.3

Table 1.

CRUDE AND REFINED MORTALITY RATES FOR SQUAMOUS CARCINOMA OF THE CERVIX
IN WOMEN OVER 20 YEARS OF AGE IN BRITISH COLUMBIA

YEARS	POPULATION in thousands	CRUDE*		REFINED	
		No. of Deaths	Rate 1/100,000	No. of Deaths	Rate 1/100,000
1959	478.7	65	13.6	51	10.6
1963	513.0	60	11.7	57	11.0
1967	592.4	52	8.8	38	6.4
1971	687.2	69	10.0	55	8.0
1975	805.5	68	7.2	42	5.2
1979	892.2	47	5.3	35	3.5

* Includes adenocarcinoma

Table 2.

It can be seen that the incidence of clinical squamous carcinoma has dropped by about 75% and the mortality about two thirds.

Table 3. shows the patients screened up to the end of 1979, the in situ carcinomas treated and also the preclinical invasive lesions, microscopic foci of invasion (FIGO stage Ia) and occult invasive carcinoma (FIGO stage Ib1).

CASES OF IN SITU AND PRECLINICAL INVASIVE SQUAMOUS CARCINOMA
1949 - 1979

YEARS	WOMEN SCREENED	IN SITU CARCINOMA	IN SITU WITH MICRO-INVASION	OCCULT INVASIVE CARCINOMA
1949-51	3,101	20	1	2
1952-53	9,644	54	1	6
1954-55	20,555	89	8	3
1956-57	33,825	171	11	6
1958-59	68,718	283	18	13
1960-61	136,458	446	35	31
1962-63	225,468	638	51	.43
1964-65	300,256	961	47	56
1966-67	391,800	1290	47	58
1968-69	502,270	1364	69	77
1970-71	619,843	1490	37	70
1972-73	713,748	1582	42	48
1974-75	805,794	2093	41	51
1976-77	822,132	2782	37	47
1978-79	847,465	3489	42	38
TOTAL:	5,501,077	16752	487	549

Table 3.

By 1974 it was felt that the data that had been accumulated supported the worth of the service. The emphasis was then switched from that of a research project, attempting to evaluate the technique, to a service that would be as convenient and safe for the patient as possible.

An aspect of the program in the province that is of interest to us is that we appear to have reached a stable state in patient accrual and our incidence rates for invasive carcinoma have levelled off. In terms of patient accrual, we feel it is not possible in a voluntary program to reach more than 85% of the population in any one year, because by the end of the year, many of the patients screened 20 to 30 years ago will have died or moved away and many younger women will have moved into the population or grown into the study years. A simple sum can be carried out to estimate the maximum gain from a voluntary program of this type, but first the material shown in Table 4. is necessary. This is a table showing disease in the screened population and the unscreened population.

REVISED INCIDENCE OF SQUAMOUS CARCINOMA OF THE CERVIX IN WOMEN OVER 20 YEARS OF AGE
IN BRITISH COLUMBIA IN SCREENED AND UNSCREENED SEGMENTS OF THE POPULATION

YEARS	S C R E E N E D			U N S C R E E N E D		
	Estimated women screened to previous year (in thousands)	Clinical invasive carcinoma cases	Rate per hundred thousand	Estimated women unscreened to previous year (in thousands)	Clinical invasive carcinoma cases	Rate per hundred thousand
1961	120.9	5	4.14	375.1	110	29.33
1962	164.2	7	4.26	338.8	71	20.96
1963	214.9	10	4.65	298.4	88	29.52
1964	260.0	12	4.6	266.8	74	27.8
1965	300.7	13	4.3	242.5	67	27.7
1966	342.7	17	4.9	223.8	60	26.8
1967	383.8	22	5.7	208.6	63	30.2
1968	423.0	17	4.7	192.4	60	31.2
1969	463.0	17	3.7	175.2	72	41.1
1970	507.8	27	5.3	156.6	55	35.1
1971	553.3	28	5.1	133.9	45	33.6
1972	593.4	27	4.5	119.7	39	32.6
1973	632.4	22	3.5	109.0	49	44.9

Table 4.

Table 5. shows the use that can be made of this sum and it can be seen that the best we should expect from this type of program is to reduce the incidence and mortality from this disease by about 72%. We appear to have reached this point and should not expect much more in the way of improvement in either the incidence or the mortality.

CALCULATED EXPECTED MAXIMUM DROP IN INCIDENCE*

Incidence of invasive squamous ca of cervix

in unscreened women	28.5
in screened women	4.5

Percentage of women screened after 30 years -   85 %

Calculation of the effect in incidence of the program

28.5	-	4.5	=	24
85%	of	24	=	20.4
28.5	-	20.4	=	8.1 (maximum)

*The B.C. screening program for cervical cancer - rates per 100,000 female population over the age of 20

Table 5.

In the early 1970's it became apparent to us that there was a real increase in preclinical disease in young women, many of whom have not had their children. Graph.1. shows the change in cases found by age of in situ carcinoma from our population and it became apparent that many young women were developing this disease. For this reason and because we felt that the main thrust of the project was now patient convenience and safety, rather than research, a colposcopy program was designed. We now have 18 clinics in the province to which patients are referred with suspicious or positive smears. These are manned by gynecologists with a least one month's training in colposcopy, and as they see a high volume of suspicious and positive cases regularly, they are able to maintain their expertise. This program has produced a significant change in our data and we suspect in other communities' data as well. There are several reasons for this. The most important one stems from an observation from our results in the early 1970's as is shown in Table 6. It can be seen that two thirds of moderate to severe dysplasias either persist or advance within a 5 year period. With this knowledge and with the ability to treat many of these early lesions with

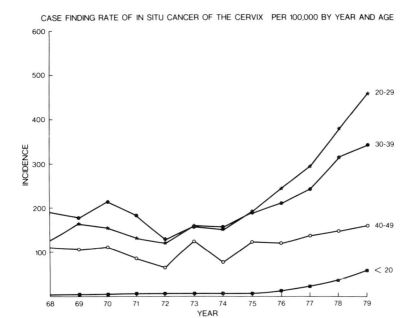

Graph. 1.

SIGNIFICANCE OF CYTOLOGIC DYSKARYOSIS

Age Group	Total No. of Cases	No.of Cases Progressing or Persisting	No.of Cases Regressing
		COHORT II*	
25 - 29	126	82 (65%)	44 (35%)
30 - 34	632	434 (69%)	198 (31%)
		COHORT I**	
40 - 44	193	122 (63%)	71 (37%)
45 - 49	402	257 (64%)	145 (36%)

* -Born 1929-33
** -Born 1914-18
   Followed until the end of 1969

Table 6.

cautery, cryotherapy or laser therapy in the colposcopy
clinics, we changed our policies in this regard. For the
first 25 years cases with cytologic dyskaryosis were followed
until the atypia suggested the presence of in situ carcinoma
and then a cone biopsy was used for diagnosis. Since 1974
the investigation has been changed in that patients are referred to the colposcopy clinics with moderate and marked
dyskaryosis for biopsy and treatment. Another change took
place about 1974 for the reasons given above. Prior to this
time all of the material arising from the investigation of
suspicious and positive smears was reviewed by a core group
and management recommended by this group. With the advent
of colposcopy the decision-making was decentralized to the
colposcopist and his supporting pathologist, so uniformity
of diagnosis was no longer a feature of this program. As
well, a colposcopy biopsy is normally rather small, often
with little supporting stroma. A pathologist who would be
very comfortable calling a lesion dysplasia from a cone biopsy
would occasionally, in order to protect the patient, call a
small bite biopsy a bit higher, suspecting there might be
worse disease in adjacent areas. Similarly, with in situ
carcinoma in a small biopsy, pathologists are reluctant to
make a firm diagnosis of in situ cancer without adequate
supporting stroma in which to search for invasion, so frequently the diagnosis becomes 'squamous carcinoma in the
tissue received'. As these results are sent to the cancer
registry to form the basis of our registration procedures,
we are able to show that they produce a marked change in
our data, as seen in Table 7.

REGISTRY REPORTING VERSUS PATHOLOGY REVIEW
OF INCIDENCE OF INVASIVE SQUAMOUS CERVICAL CANCER

1975

REGISTRY REPORT		161 cases
Review of Registry Cases:		
Negative	3	
Dysplasia	2	
In situ ca	51	
Preclinical inv.ca	35	
Wrong year	8	
	99	− 99 cases
		= 62 cases
NOT recorded by Registry		+ 8 cases
CANCER CONTROL AGENCY REPORT		70 cases

Table 7.

Here we see that the cancer registry reported 161 cases of invasive squamous carcinoma when there actually were 70. Fifty of those cases were in situ carcinoma on review. We have now taken over the cancer registry into our organization so this should no longer be happening, but epidemiologists should be aware that data concerning squamous cell carcinoma of the cervix coming out of cancer registries in other areas may contain this same type of error.

Throughout the years of this project we have classified several types of preclinical invasive carcinoma as mentioned previously as in situ carcinoma with microscopic foci of invasion and occult invasive carcinoma. We have recently been able to report on the results of treatment of these groups of patients and it is apparent that cases with micro-scopic foci (FIGO Ia) can be treated safely with a simple total hysterectomy as is shown in Tables 8. and 9. There has been only one death in this series up to date.

TREATMENT METHODS OF IN SITU SQUAMOUS CARCINOMA WITH MICROSCOPIC FOCI OF INVASION

Treatment Methods	Number of Cases
Stumpectomy	6
Cone Biopsy	14
Hysterectomy	283
Radical Hysterectomy	7
Radiotherapy	40
Other	3
Total	353

Table 8.

FOLLOW-UP OF IN SITU CARCINOMA WITH MICROSCOPIC FOCI OF INVASION

Follow-up (years)	Number of cases	Alive	Dead of disease	Dead of other disease	Contact lost
5	353	316	1	17	19
10	249	192	1	24	32
15	120	80	-	19	21

Table 9.

Cases with stage Ib1, or occult carcinoma, have been
treated more radically and their results are shown in
Tables 10. and 11.   There is a significant mortality in this
group even with radical treatment.   The validity of the
FIGO staging is, I think, supported by this data.

TREATMENT METHODS OF OCCULT INVASIVE SQUAMOUS CARCINOMA OF THE CERVIX

Treatment Method	Number of Cases
Cone Biopsy	3
Hysterectomy	58
Hysterectomy and Radiotherapy	45
Radiotherapy	262
Radical Hysterectomy	19
Other	4
Total	391

Table 10.

FOLLOW-UP OF OCCULT INVASIVE SQUAMOUS CARCINOMA OF THE CERVIX

Follow-up (years)	Number of cases	Alive	Dead of disease	Dead of other disease	Contact lost
5	391	335 (85.7)	24 (6.1)	18 (4.6)	14 (3.6)
10	252	184 (73.0)	17 (6.7)	35 (13.9)	16 (6.4)
15	102	65 (63.7)	9 (8.8)	22 (21.6)	6 (5.9)

Percentages shown in paratheses

Table 11.

An additional graph (Graph 2.) shows another observation
that we were able to make from the occult cases.   It can be
seen that patients where lymphatic permeation is observed in
a biopsy specimen, have a worse prognosis than those where
no such feature is observed.   We have changed our treatment
policy now and patients showing lymphatic permeation are
treated with radiotherapy rather than radical surgery.

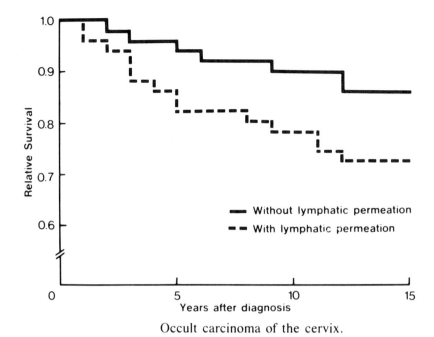

Occult carcinoma of the cervix.

Graph 2.

Our program has been basically designed to detect cervical in situ carcinoma. An Ayre's spatula scrape has been the most common way of collecting specimens. It is of no surprise to us that our detection rates for endometrial carcinoma are in the vicinity of 50%. We still state strongly to our physicians that peri- or postmenopausal women with bleeding must have a curettage regardless of pap smear results.

Throughout the years we have tried many methods of improving the detection rate of endometrial carcinoma. Many of these worked well in the hands of gynecologists in hospital outpatients or in their private offices, but thus far we have not found a technique that we could use in a program such as ours where we have more than 3,000 general practitioners obtaining specimens for us throughout the province. Our incidence rate for endometrial cancer and the mortality from it in our province is shown in Graph 3.

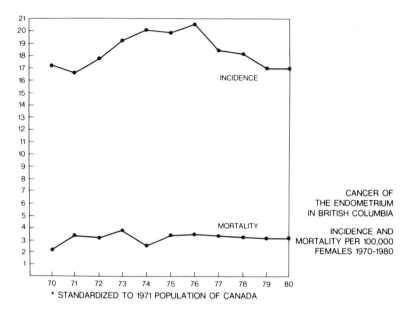

CANCER OF
THE ENDOMETRIUM
IN BRITISH COLUMBIA

INCIDENCE AND
MORTALITY PER 100,000
FEMALES 1970-1980

* STANDARDIZED TO 1971 POPULATION OF CANADA

Graph 3.

Unlike other reported series, we have not seen a major increase in this disease in our province and our mortality is similarly stable. Coupled with the above, the survival rate for stage Ia endometrial carcinoma, which make up about 70% of our cases, is just over 90% when a relative survival rate is used. From our previous experience with screening it is our feeling that patients who would come for screening for endometrial cancer would be those with fairly early disease, as this has been the case with cervix. The same patient who gets screened is the same patient patient who reports early symptoms. We are in doubt that we could improve the results of treatment of stage Ia by earlier detection as it could well be similar to occult cervix cancer where we have about a 92% - 5 year survival rate. We also feel that patients who come in with more advanced disease are likely those who would not respond to a screening program, as we have seen in cervical cancer screening. We therefore do not plan to undertake a program for screening for endometrial cancer unless a perfectly safe method could be developed for wide application.

Summary

The screening program for cervix cancer in the Province of British Columbia appears to have reached a stable state. It has achieved a reduction in incidence of clinical squamous carcinoma in women over 20 of about 75% and reduction in mortality of about two thirds. Data has been presented to suggest that no further improvement in these rates should be forthcoming in a voluntary program such as ours.

There has been a real increase in the numbers of in situ carcinomas found in our population but despite this increase clinical invasive carcinoma has not risen and we attribute this to the success of the program in intercepting disease before it becomes invasive.

Endometrial carcinoma has not increased in our population and we do not feel that the current methods for early detection of this disease are applicable to a province-wide study. We intend to continue to emphasize the earliest possible investigation of abnormal peri- and postmenopausal bleeding by fractional curettage, as our mainstay of detection.

13th International Cancer Congress, Part E
Cancer Management, pages 495–499

SCREENING FOR CARCINOMA OF THE STOMACH AND ESOPHAGUS

Heizaburo Ichikawa, M.D.
Toshifumi Iizuka, M.D.
National Cancer Center Hospital
Tokyo, Japan

INTRODUCTION

Since double contrast radiography for the stomach was developed firstly in Japan around 1955, this technique has been not only refined year by year but also distributed almost all institutions, hospitals and even small dispensaries in Japan during the last 25 years. As the result of it, number of early gastric cancer cases detected and treated in these organizations has been markedly increased.

However, the authors feel that there are some misunderstanding still remained saying that a large number of early gastric cancer has been detected in Japan "because mass-screening programs for asymptomatic population are conducted in Japan." It must be said that "because mass-screening with double contrast radiography has been well conducted." As the matter of fact, during the early stage of history of mass-screening, detection rate of early gastric cancer out of all detected gastric cancer was less than 10%. However, after application of double contrast technique in the field of mass-screening since the last 15 years, detection rate of early gastric cancer has been increased year by year and now become more or less 40% in average.

The authors presented the recent results of mass-screening for stomach in Japan, and some approaches of screening to the early detection of esophageal cancer.

STOMACH

The author presented 6 cases of early gastric cancer clearly demonstrated with double contrast radiography. One of the lesions was not defined macroscopically after resection even by pathologist, though the lesion was clearly demonstrated by this method preoperatively.

5,475 cases collected from 103 leading hospitals in Japan indicate that the 5 year survival rate shows beautiful correlation with the degree of depth invasion.

1,210 early gastric cancer cases have been detected and treated in the National Cancer Center Hospital, Tokyo, during the past 20 years since the opening of the hospital in 1962. 5, 10, 15 and 20 years survival rates of 1,000 cases of early gastric cancer cases were calculated recently, and showed 99.1% of 20 year survival rate for mucosal cancer, 90.2% of 20 year survival rate for submucosal cancer, and 95.0% for total 1,000 cases of early gastric cancer cases (Fig. 1).

Fig. 1

Survival Rate after Surgery for Early Gastric Cancer

National Cancer Center Hospital (1962~80)

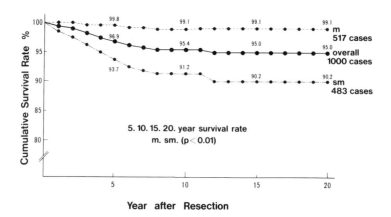

According to the analysis made by Dr. Hirota, pathologist, out of 1,084 lesions of early gastric cancer resected
in the National Cancer Center Hospital, lesions smaller than
2 cm in diameter was 14% in 1962-3, but 40% in 1979.

Annual report of the Japanese Society of Gastric Mass
Survey reveals that the total number of examinees exceeded
3 million every year after 1973. In 1980, out of 3,079,236
examinees, 2,992 (0.10%) cases of gastric cancer were
detected which include 1,116 (0.04%) cases of early gastric
cancer.

As to the effectiveness of mass-screening for stomach
cancer in the communities, Dr. Tominaga has made a new
comparison study, and revealed that age-adjusted death rate
in 14 model areas has changed 25% down within 5 years, but
it has not changed in the 28 control areas (Table 1).

Table 1

Comparison of Age-adjusted Death Rates

for Stomach Cancer

between the Model Areas & the Confrol Area

Area	No. of Municipalities	Coverage Rate of Screening (1969-78)	Age-adjusted Death Rate per 100,000		Change in the Death Rate
			(1969-72)	(1973-77)	
Model	14	17.7%	97.5	73.0	**−25.2**
Control	28	7.2%	83.6	83.7	**+ 0.2**

by. Dr. S. Tominaga, 1982

Cost-benefit analysis of gastric mass-screening has
been studied for a company with 10,000 employees by Dr.
Yoshikawa, showing that cost-benefit ratio was 1:3.7.

ESOPHAGUS

Double contrast radiography is playing a great role
also in detecting early esophageal cancer. 4 early cases,

mucosal and submucosal cancer, beautifully demonstrated by this technique were presented.

However, the incidence of esophageal cancer in Japan is quite low, showing approximately 10% of the incidence of gastric cancer. So that, Dr. Iizuka and his group have been trying a new balloon method (Esoballoon Method). Specially designed balloon is inserted through gastric fiberscope, and after gastroscopic examination the balloon is blown up and pulled out, taking cytological materials. This method was tried for 267 cases including 13 carcinomas of the esophagus. 11 cases showed positive cytology by this method.

From the experience of 451 cases of esophageal carcinoma in our National Cancer Center Hospital, 16 early cases, mucosal and submucosal cancer, showed 67% of 10 year survival rate (Fig. 2).

Fig. 2

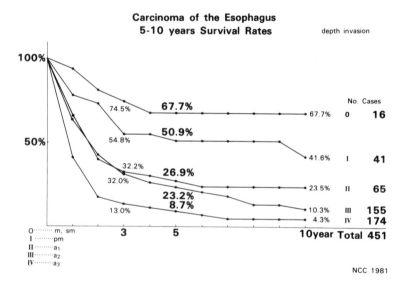

5 and 10 year survival rates of all 451 cases treated in the National Cancer Center Hospital is shown in Fig. 3, indicating 24% of 5 year survival rate and 18% of 10 year survival rate respectively.

Fig. 3

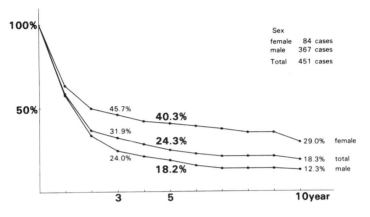

Carcinoma of the Esophagus
5-10 years Survival Rates

CONCLUSION

As the conclusion of this paper, the importance of early diagnosis for stomach and esophageal cancer is strongly emphasized. And for this purpose, effective application of double contrast radiography is positively recommended.

Index

PROGRESS IN CLINICAL AND BIOLOGICAL RESEARCH

Series Editors

Nathan Back
George J. Brewer
Vincent P. Eijsvoogel
Robert Grover

Kurt Hirschhorn
Seymour S. Kety
Sidney Udenfriend
Jonathan W. Uhr